CLINICAL NEUROSURGERY

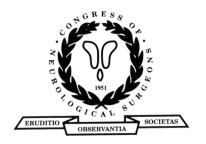

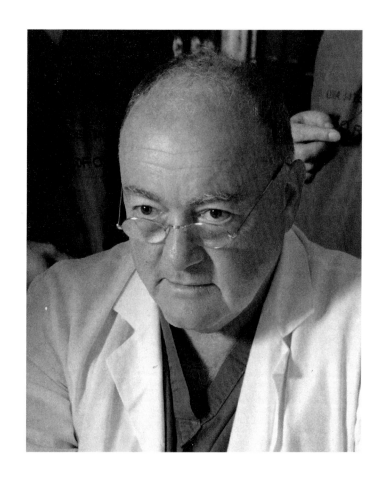

JOHN A. JANE, M.D., PH.D.

CLINICAL NEUROSURGERY

Proceedings

OF THE
CONGRESS OF NEUROLOGICAL SURGEONS

San Francisco, California
1995

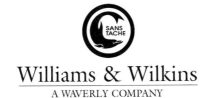

Williams & Wilkins
A WAVERLY COMPANY

BALTIMORE • PHILADELPHIA • LONDON • PARIS • BANGKOK
BUENOS AIRES • HONG KONG • MUNICH • SYDNEY • TOKYO • WROCLAW

Copyright © 1996
THE CONGRESS OF NEUROLOGICAL SURGEONS

Accurate indications, adverse reactions, and dosage schedules for drugs are provided in this book, but it is possible that they may change. The reader is urged to review the package information data of the manufacturers of the medications mentioned.

Printed in the United States of America   96 97 98 99
(ISBN 0-683-18300-1)   1 2 3 4 5 6 7 8 9 10

Reprints of Chapters may be purchased from Williams & Wilkins in quantities of 100 or more. Contact Trudy Rutherford, telephone (800) 882-0483 or 410-361-8036.

Preface

The 45th annual meeting of the Congress of Neurological Surgeons, with a program theme of "Innovations in Neurosurgery," was held at the Moscone Center in San Francisco, California, from October 14–19, 1995. The success of the meeting was due in large part to the efforts of the Scientific and Annual Meeting Committees, led by Annual Meeting Chairman Marc R. Mayberg and Scientific Program Chairman Stephen M. Papadopoulos. This year's Honored Guest of the Congress was John A. Jane, M.D., Ph.D., a distinguished neurosurgical educator, editor of the *Journal of Neurosurgery,* and Professor and Chairman of Neurosurgery at The University of Virginia. This book, then, the 43rd edition of *Clinical Neurosurgery*, catalogs and presents the invited scientific manuscripts from the plenary sessions, the biographic and bibliographic information of the honored guest, and the presidential address. Dr. Jane in particular has contributed four outstanding manuscripts to this volume.

Ralph Dacey, the president of the Congress of Neurological Surgeons for 1994–1995, delivered the extraordinarily witty and clever allegorical Presidential Address, reproduced as Chapter 1. The remainder of the book, as is our custom, is organized according to the underlying principles of the daily scientific sessions. These four sessions were, sequentially "Innovations in Cranial Approaches and Exposures," "Innovations in the Treatment of Craniofacial Disorders and Spinal Dysraphisms," "Lumbar Disk Disease: Current Trends in Management," and "Innovations in Minimalism." As we did in Volume 42, the tabulated IRIS audience response data is presented as a final chapter edited by Mark Hadley. I once again express my gratitude to Dr. Hadley for taking on this task at the last moment. Unfortunately, the number of respondents in the IRIS sessions was not enough to give particularly great significance to the information, and it is unclear whether or not this form of data will be available in future volumes.

With the publication of Volume 43, my 3-year term as editor-in-chief of *Clinical Neurosurgery* is complete. The editorship of this publication has been a rewarding experience, and I am grateful to the Congress of Neurological Surgeons, and in particular Dr. Arthur Day, for affording me this opportunity. I would like to express my gratitude to the members of the editorial board, who have served continuously for the 3-year period with great distinction to themselves and to the Congress. My secretary at The University of Iowa, Kathy Escher, who recently moved on to other pursuits, worked diligently in the preparation of all three volumes, and she has my gratitude. The publication staff at Williams & Wilkins who are responsible for *Clinical Neurosurgery*, including Timothy Grayson, Carole Pippin, and Trudy Rutherford, have been unfailing in their willingness to assist and speed up publication, particularly in those instances where deadlines were overextended and delinquent authors were being rounded up.

Dr. M. Sean Grady from the University of Washington has been appointed to succeed me as the editor-in-chief for *Clinical Neurosurgery,* Volume 44. He has served well as a member of the editorial board, and I have no doubt that he will distinguish himself as editor-in-chief. He has my congratulations and best wishes for completion of three more successful volumes of *Clinical Neurosurgery.*

Christopher M. Loftus MD, FACS
Editor-In-Chief

Editorial Board

ISSAM A. AWAD
KEITH L. BLACK
ROBERT J. DEMPSEY
JAMES T. GOODRICH
M. SEAN GRADY
MARY LOUISE HLAVIN
FREDRIC B. MEYER
JEFFREY J. OLSON
VINCENT C. TRAYNELIS

Editors-in-Chief
Clinical Neurosurgery

Volume	Date	Editor-in-Chief
1	1953	Raymond K. Thompson, M.D.
2	1954	Raymond K. Thompson, M.D. & Ira J. Jackson, M.D.
3	1955	Raymond K. Thompson, M.D. & Ira J. Jackson, M.D.
4	1956	Ira J. Jackson, M.D.
5	1957	Robert G. Fisher, M.D.
6	1958	Robert G. Fisher, M.D.
7	1959	Robert G. Fisher, M.D.
8	1960	William H. Mosberg, Jr., M.D.
9	1961	William H. Mosberg, Jr., M.D.
10	1962	William H. Mosberg, Jr., M.D.
11	1963	John Shillito, Jr., M.D. & William H. Mosberg, Jr., M.D.
12	1964	John Shillito, Jr., M.D.
13	1965	John Shillito, Jr., M.D.
14	1966	Robert G. Ojemann, M.D. & John Shillito, Jr., M.D.
15	1967	Robert G. Ojemann, M.D.
16	1968	Robert G. Ojemann, M.D.
17	1969	Robert G. Ojemann, M.D.
18	1970	George T. Tindall, M.D.
19	1971	George T. Tindall, M.D.
20	1972	Robert H. Wilkins, M.D.
21	1973	Robert H. Wilkins, M.D.
22	1974	Robert H. Wilkins, M.D.
23	1975	Ellis B. Keener, M.D.
24	1976	Ellis B. Keener, M.D.
25	1977	Ellis B. Keener, M.D.
26	1978	Peter W. Carmel, M.D.
27	1979	Peter W. Carmel, M.D.
28	1980	Peter W. Carmel, M.D.
29	1981	Martin H. Weiss, M.D.
30	1982	Martin H. Weiss, M.D.
31	1983	Martin H. Weiss, M.D.
32	1984	John R. Little, M.D.
33	1985	John R. Little, M.D.
34	1986	John R. Little, M.D.
35	1987	Peter McL. Black, M.D., Ph.D.
36	1988	Peter McL. Black, M.D., Ph.D.
37	1989	Peter McL. Black, M.D., Ph.D.
38	1990	Warren R. Selman, M.D.
39	1991	Warren R. Selman, M.D.
40	1992	Warren R. Selman, M.D.
41	1993	Christopher M. Loftus, M.D.
42	1994	Christopher M. Loftus, M.D.
43	1995	Christopher M. Loftus, M.D.

Officers of the Congress
of
Neurological Surgeons
1995

RALPH G. DACEY, JR., M.D.
President

STEPHEN J. HAINES, M.D.
President-Elect

MARC R. MAYBERG, M.D.   DANIEL L. BARROW, M.D.
Vice-President   *Secretary*

WILLIAM A. FRIEDMAN, M.D.
Treasurer

Honored Guests

1952—Professor Herbert Olivecrona, Stockhom, Sweden
1953—Sir Geoffrey Jefferson, Manchester, England
1954—Dr. Kenneth G. McKenzie, Toronto, Canada
1955—Dr. Carl W. Rand, Los Angeles, California
1956—Dr. Wilder G. Penfield, Montreal, Canada
1957—Dr. Francis C. Grant, Philadelphia, Pennsylvania
1958—Dr. A. Earl Walker, Baltimore, Maryland
1959—Dr. William J. German, New Haven, Connecticut
1960—Dr. Paul C. Bucy, Chicago, Illinois
1961—Professor Eduard A. V. Busch, Copenhagen, Denmark
1962—Dr. Bronson S. Ray, New York, New York
1963—Dr. James L. Poppen, Boston, Massachusetts
1964—Dr. Edgar A. Kahn, Ann Arbor, Michigan
1965—Dr. James C. White, Boston, Massachusetts
1966—Dr. Hugo A. Krayenbühl, Zurich, Switzerland
1967—Dr. W. James Gardner, Cleveland, Ohio
1968—Professor Norman M. Dott, Edinburgh, Scotland
1969—Dr. Wallace B. Hamby, Cleveland, Ohio
1970—Dr. Barnes Woodhall, Durham, North Carolina
1971—Dr. Elisha S. Gurdjian, Detroit, Michigan
1972—Dr. Francis Murphey, Memphis, Tennessee
1973—Dr. Henry G. Schwartz, St. Louis, Missouri
1974—Dr. Guy L. Odom, Durham, North Carolina
1975—Dr. William A. Sweet, Boston, Massachusetts
1976—Dr. Lyle A. French, Minneapolis, Minnesota
1977—Dr. Richard C. Schneider, Ann Arbor, Michigan
1978—Dr. Charles G. Drake, London, Ontario, Canada
1979—Dr. Frank H. Mayfield, Cincinnati, Ohio
1980—Dr. Eben Alexander, Jr., Winston-Salem, North Carolina
1981—Dr. J. Garber Galbraith, Birmingham, Alabama
1982—Dr. Keiji Sano, Tokyo, Japan
1983—Dr. C. Miller Fisher, Boston, Massachusetts
1984—Dr. Hugo V. Rizzoli, Washington, D.C.
      Dr. Walter E. Dandy (posthumously), Baltimore, Maryland
1985—Dr. Sidney Goldring, St. Louis, Missouri
1986—Dr. M. Gazi Yasargil, Zurich, Switzerland

1987—Dr. Thomas W. Langfitt, Philadelphia, Pennsylvania
1988—Professor Lindsay Symon, London, England
1989—Dr. Thoralf M. Sundt, Jr., Rochester, Minnesota
1990—Dr. Charles Byron Wilson, San Francisco, California
1991—Dr. Bennett M. Stein, New York, New York
1992—Dr. Robert G. Ojemann, Boston, Massachusetts
1993—Dr. Albert L. Rhoton, Jr., Gainesville, Florida
1994—Dr. Robert F. Spetzler, Phoenix, Arizona
1995—Dr. John A. Jane, Charlottesville, Virginia

Contributors

EBEN ALEXANDER, III, M.D., Associate Professor of Surgery (Neurosurgery), Harvard Medical School, Boston (Chapter 24)

PAUL J. APOSTOLIDES, M.D., Division of Neurological Surgery, Barrow Neurological Institute, St. Joseph's Hospital and Medical Center, Phoenix (Chapter 16)

ISSAM A. AWAD, M.D., Msc, FACS, MA (Hon.), Professor of Surgery (Neurosurgery), Yale University School of Medicine, New Haven (Chapter 21)

MITCHEL S. BERGER, M.D., University of Washington Department of Neurological Surgery, Seattle (Chapter 23)

CHARLES L. BRANCH, Jr., M.D., Department of Neurosurgery, The Bowman Gray School of Medicine of Wake Forest University, Winston-Salem (Chapter 18)

JAMES B. CHADDUCK, M.D., Department of Neurosurgery, University of Virginia Health Sciences Center, Charlottesville (Chapter 20)

RALPH G. DACEY, Jr., M.D., Department of Neurological Surgery, Washington University, St. Louis (Chapters 1 and 26)

C. PHILLIP DASPIT, M.D., Division of Neurological Surgery and Neuro-Otology, Barrow Neurological Institute, St. Joseph's Hospital and Medical Center, Phoenix (Chapter 6)

ARTHUR L. DAY, M.D., University of Florida, Gainesville (Chapter 8)

J. DIAZ DAY, M.D., Department of Neurosurgery, Alleghany General Hospital, Pittsburgh (Chapter 5)

CURTIS A. DICKMAN, M.D., Division of Neurological Surgery, Barrow Neurological Institute, St. Joseph's Hospital and Medical Center, Phoenix (Chapter 27)

CHARLES G. DiPIERRO, M.D., Department of Neurosurgery, University of Virginia Health Sciences Center, Charlottesville (Chapter 20)

RICHARD G. FESSLER, M.D., Ph.D., Department of Neurological Surgery, University of Florida, Gainesville (Chapter 19 and 28)

EUGENE S. FLAMM, M.D., Division of Neurosurgery, University of Pennsylvania School of Medicine, Philadelphia (Chapter 15)

TAKANORI FUKUSHIMA, M.D., D.M.Sc., Division of Neurosurgery, Alleghany General Hospital, Pittsburgh (Chapter 5)

STEVEN L. GIANNOTTA, M.D., Professor of Neurosurgery, University of Southern California, Los Angeles (Chapter 5)

P. LANGHAM GLEASON, M.D., Division of Neurosurgery, Alleghany General Hospital and The Medical College of Pennsylvania and Hahnemann University, Philadelphia (Chapter 17)

MARK GILLESPY, M.D., Orthopaedic Clinic of Daytona Beach, Daytona Beach (Chapter 28)

G. T. GILLIES, School of Engineering and Applied Science, University of Virginia, Charlottesville (Chapter 26)

M. S. GRADY, M.D., Department of Neurosurgery, University of Washington, Harborview Medical Center, Seattle (Chapter 26)

DAVID GRUBER, M.D., Department of Neurosurgery, University of Cincinnati College of Medicine, Cincinnati (Chapter 3)

MARK N. HADLEY, M.D., Department of Neurological Surgery, University of Alabama, Birmingham (Chapter 29)

ZACHARY W. HALL, Ph.D., Director, National Institutes of Health, Bethesda (Chapter 14)

GRIFFITH R. HARSH IV, M.D., Associate Professor of Surgery, Harvard Medical School, Neurosurgical Service, Massachusetts General Hospital, Boston (Chapter 2)

GREGORY A. HELM, M.D., Department of Neurosurgery, University of Virginia Health Sciences Center, Charlottesville (Chapter 20)

M. M. HENEGAR, M.D., Department of Neurological Surgery, Washington University, St. Louis (Chapter 26)

M. A. HOWARD III, M.D., Division of Neurological Surgery, University of Iowa Hospitals and Clinics, Iowa City (Chapter 26)

ROBIN P. HUMPHREYS, M.D., FRCSC, FACS, Professor of Surgery, University of Toronto, Senior Surgeon, Division of Neurosurgery, The Hospital for Sick Children, Toronto (Chapter 11)

RONALD JACOBOWITZ, Ph.D., Department of Mathematics, Arizona State University, Tempe (Chapter 16)

JOHN A. JANE, Jr., M.D., Department of Neurosurgery, University of Virginia Health Sciences Center, Charlottesville (Chapter 9, 20)

JOHN A. JANE, Sr., M.D., Ph.D., Department of Neurosurgery, University of Virginia Health Sciences Center, Charlottesville (Chapter 4, 9, 10, 20)

FERENC A. JOLESZ, M.D., Associate Professor of Radiology, Harvard Medical School, Boston (Chapter 24)

MICHAEL P. JOSEPH M.D., Massachusetts Eye & Ear Infirmary, Boston (Chapter 2)

DAVID F. KALLMES, M.D., Department of Radiology, University of Virginia Health Sciences Center, Charlottesville (Chapter 20)

DEAN G. KARAHALIOS, M.D., Division of Neurological Surgery, Barrow Neurological Institute, St. Joseph's Hospital and Medical Center, Phoenix (Chapter 27)

RON KIKINIS, M.D., Departments of Surgery (Neurosurgery) and Radiology, Surgical Planning Laboratory, Brigham and Women's Hospital, Harvard Medical School, Boston (Chapter 24)

MICHAEL T. LAWTON, M.D., Barrow Neurological Institute, St. Joseph's Hospital and Medical Center, Phoenix (Chapter 6)

SHIH SING LIU, M.D., Department of Neurosurgery, University of Cincinnati College of Medicine, Cincinnati (Chapter 3)

JOEL D. MACDONALD, M.D., University of Florida, Gainesville (Chapter 8)

ROBERT MACIUNAS, M.D., FACS, Associate Professor of Neurological Surgery and Biomedical Engineering, Department of Neurological Surgery, Vanderbilt University Medical Center, Nashville (Chapter 25)

MICHAEL MAC MILLAN, M.D., Associate Professor, Department of Orthopaedics, University of Florida, Gainesville (Chapter 28)

ASIM MAHMOOD, M.D., Department of Neurosurgery, Henry Ford Hospital, Detroit (Chapter 3)

JOSEPH C. MAROON, M.D., Division of Neurosurgery, Alleghany General Hospital, The Medical College of Pennsylvania and Hahnemann University, Philadelphia (Chapter 17)

TRACY K. MCINTOSH, Ph.D., Division of Neurosurgery, University of Pennsylvania School of Medicine, Philadelphia (Chapter 15)

DAVID G. MCLONE, M.D., Ph.D., Northwestern University Medical School, Children's Memorial Hospital, Chicago (Chapter 13)

WILLIAM J. MONTGOMERY, M.D., Associate Professor, Department of Radiology, University of Florida, Gainesville (Chapter 28)

THOMAS M. MORIARTY, M.D., Ph.D., Resident in Neurological Surgery, Brigham & Women's Hospital, Boston (Chapter 24)

STEVEN A. NEWMAN M.D., Department of Neuro-Ophthalmology, University of Virginia, Charlottesville (Chapter 4)

W. JERRY OAKES, M.D., University of Alabama, Birmingham (Chapter 12)

ROBERT G. OJEMANN, M.D., Massachusetts General Hospital, Boston (Chapter 2)

LAWRENCE H. PHILLIPS, II, M.D., Department of Neurology, University of Virginia Charlottesville (Chapter 10)

MATTHEW R. QUIGLEY, M.D., Assistant Professor of Surgery (Neurosurgery), Alleghany General Hospital, The Medical College of Pennsylvania and Hahnemann University, Philadelphia (Chapter 17)

R. C. RITTER, Department of Physics, University of Virginia, Charlottesville (Chapter 26)

DONALD A. ROSS, M.D., Section of Neurosurgery, University of Michigan, Ann Arbor (Chapter 22)

CHANDRANATH SEN, M. D., Department of Neurosurgery, The Mount Sinai Medical Center, New York (Chapter 7)

CHRISTOPHER I. SHAFFREY, M.D., Department of Neurosurgery, University of Virginia, Charlottesville (Chapter 20)

GRANT SINSON, M.D., Division of Neurosurgery, University of Pennsylvania School of Medicine, Philadelphia (Chapter 15)

VOLKER K. H. SONNTAG, M.D., Barrow Neurological Institute, Phoenix (Chapter 16)

ROBERT F. SPETZLER, M.D., Barrow Neurological Institute, Phoenix (Chapter 6)

BROOKE SWEARINGEN, M.D., Assistant Professor of Surgery, Harvard Medical School, Associate Visiting Neurosurgeon, Neurological Service, Massachusetts General Hospital, Boston (Chapter 2)

HARRY R. VAN LOVEREN, M.D., Department of Neurosurgery, University of Cincinnati College of Medicine, Cincinnati (Chapter 3)

MADHU VODDI, B.A., Division of Neurosurgery, University of Pennsylvania School of Medicine, Philadelphia (Chapter 15)

Biography of John A. Jane, M.D., Ph.D.

John Anthony Jane, M.D., Ph.D. FRCS(C), FACS, was born and raised in the Chicago area. He received his Bachelor of Arts degree *cum laude* from the University of Chicago in 1951 and attended the University of Chicago School of Medicine and graduated with an M.D. degree in 1956.

He did his internship at the Royal Victoria Hospital in Montreal and began his neurosurgical residency at the University of Chicago with Dr. Sean Mullan. During his residency he had a number of important research and clinical fellowships. He was a fellow in neurophysiology at the Montreal Neurological Institute in 1958 and a senior fellow and demonstrator in neuropathology in 1959 and 1960 at McGill University in Montreal. In 1961 he went to London to serve as a research assistant to Mr. Wylie McKissock at St. George's Hospital and the National Hospital at Queen Square. There he conducted his seminal work on the natural history of intracranial aneurysms. He subsequently returned to Duke University to study with Dr. Irving Diamond and in 1967 was awarded the Ph.D. degree from the University of Chicago, Division of Biological Sciences, Section of Biopsychology.

He completed his neurosurgical residency in 1963–1964 at the University of Illinois Neuropsychiatric Institute with Drs. Oscar Sugar and Eric Oldberg. In 1965 Dr. Jane became associated with Dr. Frank Nulsen at Case Western Reserve University. After 4 years he assumed his present position at the age of 37 as the Alumni Professor and Chairman of the Department of Neurological Surgery at the University of Virginia in Charlottesville, Virginia. He became the David D. Weaver Professor in 1987. Dr. Jane is especially proud of having participated in the programs at the Western Reserve and subsequently at the University of Virginia and in the training of 13 Professors of Neurosurgery, eleven of whom became Chairman, three Associate Professors, and five Assistant Professors. In 1992 Dr. Jane was elected as Editor of the *Journal of Neurosurgery.*

He has served as a Director of the American Board of Neurological Surgery and as Vice-President and President of the Society of Neurological Surgeons. In 1985 he received the Grass Award and was the Olivecrona Lecturer. He also received the Alumni Award for distinguished service from the University of Chicago. Dr. Jane has a unique perspective on neurosurgery. His initial work in comparative neuroanatomy and psychobiology of marsupials, reptiles, and teleost fish make him a veritable encyclopedia, reptiles, and telost fish make him a veritable encyclopedia of neuroanatomy and physiology. His clinical interests and research have been in the treatment of severe head injury and disorders of the spine. He has an active spine service operating on nearly 400 cases last year. He was one of the originators of modern techniques for the treatment of craniofacial disorders.

The residents who train with him respect his immense capacity for work, his surgical skill and judgment, his unselfish commitment to them, and his sense of humor. His bibliography lists over 250 publications.

He is married to the former Miss Noella Fortier of Montreal, Quebec, Canada. The Janes have four grown children (three daughters and one son), three grandsons, and one granddaughter.

Bibliography of John A. Jane, M.D., Ph.D.

PUBLICATIONS

JANE JA: A large aneurysm of the posterior inferior cerebellar artery in a 1-year-old child. **J Neurosurg** 18(2):245–247, 1961.

JANE JA, BERTRAND G: A cytological method for the diagnosis of tumor affecting the central nervous system. **J Neuropath Exp Neurol** 21:400–409, 1962.

JANE JA, SMIRNOV GD, JASPER HH: Effects of distraction upon simultaneous auditory and visual evoked potentials. **Electroencephalogr Clin Neurophysiol** 14:344–358, 1962.

JANE JA, MCKISSOCK W: Importance of failing vision in early diagnosis of suprasellar meningiomas. **Br Med J** 2:5–7, 1962.

WILHYDE DE, JANE JA, MULLAN S: Spinal epidural leukemia. **Am J Med** 34:281–287, 1963.

OLDBERG E, BAILEY OT, JANE JA: Spinal epidural granuloma. **Proc Inst Med Chicago** 25(4):94–95, 1964.

RICHARDSON AE, JANE JA, PAYNE PM: Assessment of the natural history of anterior communicating aneurysms. **J Neurosurg** 21: 266–274, 1964.

JANE JA: The prediction of mortality for operative and conservative management of aneurysms of the anterior communicating artery. **Proc Inst Med Chicago** 25(3):62–64, 1964.

YASHON D, JOHNSON AB, JANE JA: Bilateral internal carotid artery occlusion secondary to closed head injuries. **J Neurol Neurosurg Psychiatry** 27:547–552, 1964.

ERICKSON RP, JANE JA, WAITE R, DIAMOND IT: Single neuron investigation of sensory thalamus of the opossum. **J Neuro physiol** 27: 1026–1047, 1964.

JANE JA, EVANS JP, FISHER LE: An investigation concerning the restitution of motor function following injury to the spinal cord. **J Neurosurg** 21:167–171, 1964.

JANE JA, MASTERTON RB, DIAMOND IT: The function of the tectum for attention to auditory stimuli in the cat. **J Comp Neurol** 125: 165–192, 1965.

JANE JA, CAMPBELL CBG, YASHON D: Pyramidal tract: A comparison of two prosimian primates. **Science** 147:153–155, 1965.

YASHON D, JANE JA, SUGAR O: The course of severe untreated infantile hydrocephalus: Prognostic significance of the cerebral mantle. J Neurosurg 23:509–516, 1965.

JANE JA, YASHON D, SUGAR O: Cerebrovascular disease: An analysis of present knowledge and presentation of an investigative technique and attitude. Arch Intern Med 116:392–399, 1965.

BECKER DP, JANE JA, NULSEN FE: Investigation of sagittal sinus for venous shunt in hydrocephalus. Surg Forum 16:440–442, 1965.

YASHON D, SMALL E, JANE JA: Congenital hydrocephalus and chronic subdural hematoma in a dog. JAMA 147:832–836, 1965.

YASHON D, HILL BJ, JANE JA: Manual retrograde brachial angiography. Dis Nerv Syst 26:728–730, 1965.

YASHON D, JANE JA, JAVID H: Long-term results of carotid bifurcation endarterectomy. Surg Gynecol Obst 122:517–523, 1966.

RICHARDSON AE, JANE JA, YASHON D: Prognostic factors in the untreated course of posterior communicating aneurysms. Arch Neurol 14:172–176, 1966.

RICHARDSON AE, JANE JA, PAYNE PM: The prediction of morbidity and mortality in anterior communicating aneurysms treated by proximal anterior cerebral ligation. J Neurosurg 25:280–283, 1966.

CAMPBELL CBG, YASHON D, JANE JA: The origin, course and termination of corticospinal fibers in the slow loris, nycticebus coucang (Boddaert). J Comp Neurol 127:101–112, 1966.

YASHON D, JANE JA, GORDON M, HUBBARD JL, SUGAR O: Effects of methyl 2-cyanoacrylate adhesives on the somatic vessels and the central nervous systems of animals. J Neurosurg 24:883–888, 1966.

YASHON D, CAMPBELL CBG, JANE JA: Aspects of the evolution of the corticospinal tract. Proc Inst Med Chicago 26:54–55, 1966.

YASHON D, GRABER MR, JANE JA, SUGAR O: Prognostic indices in untreated hydrocephalus. Nature 212:709–710, 1966.

YASHON D, JANE JA, CASSEL S, CAMERON G, SUGAR O: Cerebrospinal fluid diversion in infantile hydrocephalus. Arch Neurol 15:541–544, 1966.

JANE JA, YASHON D, DEMYER W, BUCY PC: The contribution of the precentral gyrus to the pyramidal tract of man. J Neurosurg 26:244–248, 1967.

YASHON D, JANE JA: Subacute necrotizing encephalomyelopathy of infancy and childhood. J Clin Pathol 20:28–37, 1967.

MASTERTON RB, JANE JA, DIAMOND IT: Role of brain-stem auditory structures in sound localization. I. Trapezoid body, superior olive, and lateral lemniscus. J Neurophysiol 30:341–359, 1967.

MASTERTON RB, JANE JA, DIAMOND IT: Role of brain-stem auditory structures in sound localization. II. Inferior colliculus and brachium. **J Neurophysiol** 31:96–108, 1967.

CAMPBELL CBG, JANE JA, YASHON D: The retinal projections of the tree shrew and hedgehog. **Brain Res** 5:406–418, 1967.

WARREN KS, JANE JA: Comparative susceptibility to *Schistosoma mansoni* of the squirrel monkey, the slow loris, and the tree shrew. **Trans Soc Trop Med** 61:534–537, 1967.

ERICKSON RP, HALL WC, JANE JA, SNYDER M, DIAMOND IT: Organization of the posterior dorsal thalamus of the hedgehog. **J Comp Neurol** 131:103–130, 1967.

YOUNG HR, GREENBERG, PATON W, JANE JA: A reinvestigation of cognitive maps. **Psychol Sci** 9:589–590, 1967.

JANE JA: Role of auditory pathways in attention. University of Chicago, Ph.D. Dissertation, 1967.

YASHON D, JANE JA, WHITE RJ, SUGAR O: Traumatic subdural hematoma of infancy. **Arch Neurol** 18:370–377, 1968.

YASHON D, JANE JA, WHITE RJ: Arteriographic observation in craniocerebral bullet wounds. **J Trauma** 8:238–255, 1968.

YOUNG HR, BECKER DP, JANE JA, NULSEN FE: Mechanism of action of dimethyl sulfoxide. **Surg Forum** 19:439–440, 1968.

JANE JA, YASHON D, BECKER DP, BETTY R, SUGAR O: The effect of destruction of the corticospinal tract in the human cerebral peduncle upon motor function and involuntary movements. Report of 11 cases. **J Neurosurg** 29:581–585, 1968.

JANE JA, YASHON D, DIAMOND IT: An anatomic basis for multimodal thalamic units. **Exp Neurol** 22(3):464–471, 1968.

WEISS MH, JANE JA: Nocardia asteroides brain abscess successfully treated by enucleation. Case report. **J Neurosurg** 30:83–86, 1969.

GOLDEN PJ, JANE JA: Survival following profound hypovolemia: Role of heart, lung and brain. **J Trauma** 9:784–798, 1969.

BECKER DP, GLUCK H, NULSEN FE, JANE JA: An inquiry into the neurophysiological basis for pain. **J Neurosurg** 30:1–13, 1969.

BECKER DP, YOUNG HR, NULSEN FE, JANE JA: Physiological effects of dimethyl sulfoxide on peripheral nerves: Possible role in pain relief. **Exp Neurol** 24:272–276, 1969.

JANE JA, CAMPBELL CBG, YASHON D: The origin of the corticospinal tract of the tree shrew (*Tupaia glis*) with observations on its brain-stem and spinal terminations. **Brain Behav Evol** 2(2):160–182, 1969.

YASHON D, JANE JA, WHITE RJ: Prognosis and management of spinal cord and cauda equina bullet injuries in sixty-five civilians. **J Neurosurg** 32:163–170, 1970.

DIAMOND IT, SNYDER M, KILLACKEY H, JANE JA, HALL WC: Thalamo-cortical projections in the tree shrew (*Tupaia glis*). **J Comp Neurol** 139:273–306, 1970.

JANE JA, WARREN KS, VAN DEN NOORT S: Experimental cerebral schistosomiasis japonica in primates. **J Neurol Neurosurg Psychiatry** 33:426–430, 1970.

JANE JA, SCHROEDER DM: A comparison of dorsal column nuclei and spinal afferents in the European hedgehog (*Erinaceus europaeus*). **Exp Neurol** 30:1–17, 1971.

YASHON D, WHITE RJ, CROFT T, BECKER DP, JANE JA: Midline posterior fossa neoplasms without lateral ventricular enlargement. **JAMA** 215:89–93, 1971.

SCHROEDER DM, JANE JA: Projection of dorsal column nuclei and spinal cord to brainstem and thalamus in the tree shrew (*Tupaia glis*). **J Comp Neurol** 142:309–350, 1971.

SHUANGSHOTI S, NETSKY MG, JANE JA: Neoplasms of mixed mesenchymal and neuroepithelial type with consideration of the relationship between meningioma and neurilemmoma. **J Neurol Sci** 14:277–291, 1971.

LERNER PI, GOLDEN PF, JANE JA: Salmonella-infected subdural hematoma. **Pediatrics** 49:127–128, 1972.

EBBESSON SOE, JANE JA, SCHROEDER DM: A general overview of major interspecific variations in thalamic organization. **Brain Behav Evol** 6:92–130, 1972.

JANE JA, LEVEY N, CARLSON NJ: Tectal and cortical function of vision. **Exp Neurol** 35:61–77, 1972.

YASHON D, JANE JA, MARTONFFY D, WHITE RJ: Management of civilian craniocerebral bullet injuries. **Am Surg** 38:346–351, 1972.

LEVEY N, HARRIS J, JANE JA: Effects of visual cortical ablation on pattern discrimination in the ground squirrel (*Citellus tridecemlineatus*). **Exp Neurol** 39:270–276, 1973.

SADAR ES, JANE JA, LEWIS LW, ADELMAN LS: Traumatic aneurysms of the intracranial circulation. **Surg Gynecol Obstet** 137:59–67, 1973.

GRAEBER RC, EBBESSON SOE, JANE JA: Visual discrimination in sharks without optic tectum. **Science** 180:413–415, 1973.

NAUTA HJW, BUTLER AB, JANE JA: Some observations on axonal degeneration resulting from superficial lesions of the cerebral cortex. **J Comp Neurol** 150:349–360, 1973.

JANE JA, KAUFMAN B, NULSEN F, YASHON D, YOUNG H: The role of angiography and ventriculovenous shunting in the treatment of posterior fossa tumors. **Acta Neurochir (Wien)** 28:13–27, 1973.

GOLDEN PF, JANE JA: Experimental study of irreversible shock and the brain. **J Neurosurg** 39:434–441, 1973.

WINN HR, RICHARDSON AE, JANE JA: Late morbidity and mortality in cerebral aneurysms: A ten-year follow-up of 364 conservatively treated patients with a single cerebral aneurysm. **Trans Am Neur Assoc** 98:148–150, 1973.

ROSENTHAL JD, GOLDEN PF, SHAW CA, JANE JA: Intractable ascites. A complication of ventriculoperitoneal shunting with a silastic catheter. **Am J Surg** 127:613–614, 1974.

MARKS KE, JANE JA: Effects of visual cortical lesions upon ambulatory and static localization of light in space. **Exp Neurol** 42:707–710, 1974.

JANE JA. Letter: Acute paraplegia and leukemia. **J Neurosurg** 40:556–557, 1974.

EDGERTON MT, JANE JA, BERRY FA: Craniofacial osteotomies and reconstruction in infants and children. **Plast Reconstr Surg** 54:13–27, 1974.

EDGERTON MT, JANE JA, BERRY FA, FISHER JC: The feasibility of craniofacial osteotomies in infants and young children. **Scand J Plast Reconstr Surg** 8:164–168, 1974.

JANE JA, EDGERTON MT: Radical reconstruction of complex cranio-orbito-facial abnormalities. **MCV Q** 10:220–223, 1974.

ROSENTHAL J, JANE JA: Optic nerve meningioma: A potentially treatable form of progressive blindness in children and young adults. **Revista de Neurologia, Neurocircugia y Psiquiatria** 16:287–295, 1974.

LEVEY NH, JANE JA: Laminar thermocoagulation of the visual cortex of the rat. I. Interlaminar connections. **Brain Behav Evol** 11:257–274, 1975.

LEVEY NH, JANE JA: Laminar thermocoagulation of the visual cortex of the rat. II. Visual pattern discrimination. **Brain Behav Evol** 11:275–321, 1975.

EDGERTON MT, JANE JA, BERRY FA, MARSHALL KA: New surgical concepts resulting from cranio-orbito-facial surgery. **Ann Surg** 182:228–239, 1975.

THOMPSON RC, MORRIS JN JR, JANE JA: Current concepts in management of cervical spine fractures and dislocations. **J Sports Med** 3:159–167, 1975.

WEISS MH, JANE JA, APUZZO MLJ, HEIDEN JS, KURZE T: Ventriculogastrostomy, an alternative means for CSF diversion: A preliminary study. **Bull Los Angeles Neurol Soc** 40:140–144, 1975.

SCHROEDER DM, JANE JA: The intercollicular area of the inferior colliculus. **Brain Behav Evol** 13:125–141, 1976.

ROBBINS JB, FITZ-HUGH GS, JANE JA: Intracranial carotid catastrophies encountered by the otolaryngologist. **Laryngoscope** 86:893–902, 1976.

WINN HR, JANE JA, RODEHEAVER G, EDGERTON MT, EDLICH RF: Influence of subcuticular sutures on scar formation. **Am J Surg** 133:257–259, 1977.

BUTLER AB, JANE JA: Interlaminar connections of rat visual cortex: An ultrastructural study. **J Comp Neurol** 174:521–534, 1977.

KICLITER E, LOOP MS, JANE JA: Effects of posterior neocortical lesions on wavelength, light/dark and stripe orientation discrimination in ground squirrels. **Brain Res** 122:15–31, 1977.

WINN HR, RICHARDSON AE, JANE JA: The long-term prognosis in untreated cerebral aneurysms: I. The incidence of late hemorrhage in cerebral aneurysm: A 10-year evaluation of 364 patients. **Ann Neurol** 1:358–370, 1977.

WINN HR, DACEY RG, JANE JA: Intracranial subarachnoid pressure recording: Experience with 650 patients. **Surg Neurol** 8:41–47, 1977.

DUFF TA, ROSENTHAL J, JANE JA: Evaluation and revision of ventriculo-gastric shunts by gastroscopy. **Neurochirurgia (Stuttg)** 20:28–31, 1977.

JANE JA, WINN HR, RICHARDSON AE: The natural history of intracranial aneurysms: Rebleeding rates during the acute and long-term period and implication for surgical management. **Clin Neurosurg** 24:176–184, 1977.

WINN HR, RICHARDSON AE, JANE JA: Late morbidity and mortality of common carotid ligation for posterior communicating aneurysms. A comparison to conservative treatment. **J Neurosurg** 47:727–736, 1977.

POBERESKIN L, CABOT J, COHEN D, JANE JA, DACEY RG: Chronic systemic hypertension secondary to lesions in the nervous system. **Surg Forum** 28:477–479, 1977.

JANE JA, EDGERTON MT, FUTRELL JW, PARK TS: Immediate correction of sagittal synostosis. **J Neurosurg** 49:705–710, 1978.

GRAEBER RC, SCHROEDER DM, JANE JA, EBBESSON SOE: Visual discrimination following partial telencephalic ablations in nurse sharks (*Ginglymostoma cirratum*). **J Comp Neurol** 180:325–344, 1978.

HAHN JF, JANE JA: Craniosynostosis and related syndromes. Pathogenesis and treatment. **Cleve Clin Q** 45:213–217, 1978.

TYSON GW, JANE JA, STRACHAN WE: Intracerebral hemorrhage due to ruptured venous aneurysm. Report of two cases. **J Neurosurg** 49:739–743, 1978.

DACEY RG, WINN HR, JANE JA, BUTLER AB: Spinal subdural empyema: Report of two cases. **Neurosurgery** 3:400–403, 1978.

WINN HR, RICHARDSON AE, O'BRIEN W, JANE JA: The long-term prognosis in untreated cerebral aneurysms. II. Late morbidity and mortality. **Ann Neurol** 4:418–426, 1978.

RIMEL RW, TYSON GW, WINN HR, BUTLER AB, JANE JA: Acute management of head and spinal cord injured patients in the Emergency Room. Charlottesville, *University of Virginia Press,* 1978.

RIMEL RW, EDLICH RF, WINN HR, BUTLER AB, JANE JA: Acute care of the head and spinal cord injured patient at the site of injury. Charlottesville, *University of Virginia Press,* 1978.

DACEY RG, WELSH JE, SCHELD WM, WINN HR, JANE JA, SANDE MA: Alterations in cerebrospinal fluid outflow resistance in experimental bacterial meningitis. **Trans Am Neurol Assoc** 103:142–146, 1978.

BUTLER AB, JANE JA, FALK P: Interlaminar connections of tree shrew visual cortex. **Neurosci Lett** 11:107–110, 1979.

RIMEL RW, JANE JA, EDLICH RF: An injury severity scale for comprehensive management of central nervous system trauma. **JACEP** 8:64–67, 1979.

RIMEL RW, JANE JA, EDLICH RF: Care of central nervous system trauma at the site of injury. **Crit Care Q** 2:1–6, 1979.

TYSON, GW, RIMEL RW, WINN HR, BUTLER AB, JANE JA: Acute care of the head injured patient. **Crit Care Q** 2:23–44, 1979.

TYSON GW, RIMEL RW, WINN HR, BUTLER AB, JANE JA: Acute care of the spinal cord injured patient. **Crit Care Q** 2:45–60, 1979.

RIMEL RW, JANE JA, EDLICH RF: Assessment of recovery following head trauma. **Crit Care Q** 2:97–104, 1979.

SCHELD WM, PARK TS, DACEY RG, WINN HR, JANE JA, SANDE MA: Clearance of bacteria from cerebrospinal fluid to blood in experimental meningitis. **Infect Immunol** 24:102–105, 1979.

CAREY RM, DACEY RG, JANE JA, WINN HR, AYERS CR, TYSON GW: Production of sustained hypertension by lesions in the nucleus tractus solitarii of the American foxhound. **Hypertension** 1:246–254, 1979.

TYSON GW, WELSH, JE, BUTLER AB, JANE JA, WINN HR: Primary cerebellar nocardiosis. Report of two cases. **J Neurosurg** 51:408–414, 1979.

WELSH JE, TYSON GW, WINN HR, JANE JA: Chronic subdural hematoma presenting as transient neurologic deficits. **Stroke** 10:564–567, 1979.

RIMEL RW, WINN HR, RICE P, BUTLER AB, EDLICH RF, BUCK R, JANE JA: Prehospital treatment of the patient with spinal cord injury. **EMT J** 3:49–54, 1979.

PARK TS, DACEY RG, JANE JA, BUTLER AB, WINN HR: Donor artery changes following anastamosis. **Va Med** 107:108–112, 1980.

TYSON GW, CAIL WS, WELSH JE, MORRIS JL, JANE JA: Intraventricular extension of a ruptured basilar artery aneurysm. **Surg Neurol** 13:129–133, 1980.

DACEY RG, WELSH JE, SCHELD WM, WINN HR, SANDE MA, JANE JA: Bacterial meningitis: Changes in cerebrospinal fluid outflow resistance. **ICP** 4:350–353, 1980.

TYSON GW, STRACHAN WE, NEWMAN P, WINN HR, BUTLER AB, JANE JA: The role of craniectomy in the treatment of chronic subdural hematoma. **J Neurosurg** 52:776–781, 1980.

PERSING JA, PERSSON MK, ROY WB, BABLER WK, RODEHEAVER GT, WINN HR, JANE JA, EDGERTON MT, LANGMAN JS: Functional study of role of sutural tissue in regulating skull growth. **Am Coll Surg, Surg Forum** 31:463–465, 1980.

SCHELD WM, DACEY RG, WINN HR, WELSH JE, JANE JA, SANDE MA: Cerebrospinal fluid outflow resistance in rabbits with experimental meningitis: Alterations with penicillin and methylprednisolone. **J Clin Invest** 66:243–253, 1980.

WEAVER D, POBERESKIN L, JANE JA: Spontaneous resolution of epidural hematomas. Report of two cases. **J Neurosurg** 54: 248–251, 1981.

RIMEL RW, JANE JA, EDLICH RF: An educational training program for the care at the site of injury of trauma to the central nervous system. **Resuscitation** 9:23–28, 1981.

RIMEL RW, WINN HR, RICE P, BUTLER AB, EDLICH RF, BUCK R, JANE JA: Pre-hospital treatment of the spinal cord patient. **Resuscitation** 9:29–37, 1981.

EDGERTON MT, JANE JA: Vertical orbital dystopia: Surgical correction. **Plast Reconstr Surg** 67:121–138, 1981.

PERSING JA, BABLER W, WINN HR, JANE JA, RODEHEAVER G: Age as a critical factor in the success of surgical correction of craniosynostosis. **J Neurosurg** 54:601–606, 1981.

RIMEL RW, JANE JA, TYSON GW: Emergency management of head injuries. **Resuscitation** 9:75–97, 1981.

RIMEL RW, BUTLER AB, WINN HR, PARK TS, TYSON GW, JANE JA: Modified skull tongs for cervical traction: Technical note. **J Neurosurg** 55:848–849, 1981.

RIMEL RW, GIORDANI B, BARTH JT, BOLL TJ, JANE JA: Disability caused by minor head injury. **Neurosurgery** 9:221–228, 1981.

EDLICH RF, JANE JA, CROSBY IK, ROMANO TL, BOYD DR, KURTZ AB: Initial management of the multiple trauma patient. **Compr Ther** 7:31–48, 1981.

BABLER WJ, PERSING JA, PERSSON KM, WINN HR, JANE JA, RODE-HEAVER GT: Skull growth after coronal suturectomy, periostectomy, and dural transection. **J Neurosurg** 56:529–535, 1982.

BEDFORD RF, MORRIS L, JANE JA: Intracranial hypertension during surgery for supratentorial tumor: Correlation with preoperative computed tomography scans. **Anesth Analg** 61:430–433, 1982.

WEAVER DD, WINN HR, JANE JA: Differential intracranial pressure in patients with unilateral mass lesions. **J Neurosurg** 56:660–665, 1982.

GENNARELLI TA, SPIELMAN G, LANGFITT T, GILDENBERG P, HARRING-TON T, JANE JA, MARSHALL L, MILLER JD, PITTS L: Influence of the type of intracranial lesion on outcome from severe head injury. A multi-center study using a new classification system. **J Neurosurg** 56:26–32, 1982.

RIMEL RW, GIORDANI B, BARTH JT, JANE JA: Moderate head injury: Completing the clinical spectrum of brain trauma. **Neurosurgery** 11:344–351, 1982.

BABLER WJ, PERSING JA, WINN HR, JANE JA, RODEHEAVER GT: Compensatory growth following premature closure of the coronal suture in rabbits. **J Neurosurg** 57:535–542, 1982.

WINN HR, RICHARDSON AE, JANE JA: The late morbidity and mortality in ruptured single anterior circulation aneurysms treated by nonsurgical therapy. **Acta Neurochir** 63:71–81, 1982.

JANE JA, PARK TS, POBERESKIN LH, WINN HR, BUTLER AB: The supraorbital approach: Technical note. **Neurosurgery** 11:537–542, 1982.

HURT H, PARK TS, JANE JA: External hydrocephalus in the preterm infant. **Va Med** 109:840–842, 1982.

THORNER MO, PERRYMAN RL, CRONIN MJ, DRAZNIN MB, JOHANSON AJ, ROGOL AD, JANE JA, RUDOLF LE, HORVATH E, KOVACS K, VALE W. Somatotroph hyperplasia: Successful treatment of acromegaly by removal of a pancreatic islet tumor secreting a growth hormone-releasing factor. **Trans Assoc Am Phys** 95:177–187, 1982.

RIMEL RW, NELSON WE, PERSING JA, JANE JA: Epidural hematoma in lacrosse. **Phys Sports Med** 11(3), 1983.

JAGGER J, JANE JA, RIMEL RW: The Glasgow Coma Scale: "To sum or not to sum?" (letter) **Lancet** 2:97, 1983.

MARSHALL LF, BECKER DP, BOWERS SA, CAYARD C, EISENBERG H, GROSS CR, GROSSMAN RG, JANE JA, KUNITZ SC, RIMEL RW, TABADDOR K, WARREN J: The National Traumatic Coma Data Bank, Part 1: Design, purpose, goals, and results. **J Neurosurg** 59:276–284, 1983.

BARTH JT, MACCIOCCHI SN, GIORDANI B, RIMEL RW, JANE JA, BOLL TJ: Neuropsychological sequelae of minor head injury. **Neurosurgery** 13:529–533, 1983.

WINN HR, ALMAANI WS, BERGA SL, JANE JA, RICHARDSON AE: The long-term outcome in patients with multiple aneurysms: Incidence of later hemorrhage and implications for treatment of incidental aneurysms. **J Neurosurg** 59:642–651, 1983.

VERNBERG K, JAGGER J, JANE JA: The Glasgow Coma Scale: How do you rate? **Nurse Educ** 8:33–37, 1983.

WEAVER DD, CROSS DL, WINN HR, JANE JA: Computed tomographic findings in metastatic dural carcinomatosis. **Surg Neurol** 21:190–194, 1984.

JAGGER J, LEVINE JI, JANE JA, RIMEL RW: Epidemiologic features of head injury in a predominantly rural population. **J Trauma** 24:40–44, 1984.

JOHNS ME, KAPLAN MJ, JANE JA, PARK TS, CANTRELL RW: Supraorbital rim approach to the anterior skull base. **Laryngoscope** 94:1137–1139, 1984.

NELSON WE, JANE JA, GIECK JH: Minor head injury in sports: A new system of classification and management. **Phy Sports Med** 12:103–107, 1984.

JAGGER J, FIFE D, VERNBERG K, JANE JA: Effect of alcohol intoxication on the diagnosis and apparent severity of brain injury. **Neurosurgery** 15:303–306, 1984.

JANE JA, PARK TS, ZIDE BA, LAMBRUSCHI P, PERSING JA, EDGERTON MT: Alternative techniques in the treatment of unilateral coronal synostosis. **J Neurosurg** 61:550–556, 1984.

VOLLMER DG, JANE JA, PARK TS, PERSING JA: The variants of sagittal synostosis: Strategies for surgical correction. **J Neurosurg** 61:557–562, 1984.

NELSON WE, GIECK JH, JANE JA, HAWTHORNE P: Athletic head injuries. **J Natl Athletic Trainers Assoc.** 19:95–102, 1984.

WEAVER DD, VANDENBERG S, PARK TS, JANE JA: Selective peripancreatic sarcoma metastases from primary gliosarcoma: Case report. **J Neurosurg** 61:599–601, 1984.

HOROWITZ JH, PERSING JA, WINN HR, JANE JA, EDGERTON MT: The late treatment of vertical orbital dystopia resulting from an orbital roof fracture. **Ann Plast Surg** 13:519–524, 1984.

VOLLMER DG, PARK TS, CAIL WS, JANE JA: Hydromyelia complicating Apert's syndrome: A case report. **Neurosurgery** 17(1):70–74, 1985.

JANE JA, STEWARD O, GENNARELLI TA: Axonal degeneration induced by experimental non-invasive minor head injury. **J Neurosurg** 62:96–100, 1985.

JANE JA, KASSELL NF, TORNER JC, WINN HR: The natural history of aneurysms and arteriovenous malformations. **J Neurosurg** 62:321–323, 1985.

PARK TS, HAWORTH CS, JANE JA, BEDFORD RB, PERSING JA: Modified prone position for cranial remodeling procedures in children with craniofacial dysmorphism: A technical note. **Neurosurgery** 16:212–214, 1985.

PERSING JA, JANE JA: Surgical treatment of V_1 trigeminal neuralgia: Technical refinement. **Neurosurgery** 17:660–662, 1985.

COLOHAN ART, PERKINS NAK, BEDFORD RF, JANE JA: Intravenous fluid loading as prophylaxis for paradoxical air embolism. **J Neurosurg** 62:839–842, 1985.

COLOHAN ART, JANE JA, PARK TS, PERSING JA: Bifrontal osteoplastic craniotomy utilizing the anterior wall of the frontal sinus: Technical note. **Neurosurgery** 16(6):822–824, 1985.

COLOHAN ART, JANE JA, NEWMAN SA, MAGGIO WW: Frontal sinus approach to the orbit: Technical note. **J Neurosurgery** 63:811–813, 1985.

EDGERTON MT, PERSING JA, JANE JA: The surgical treatment of fibrous dysplasia with emphasis on recent contributions from craniomaxillo-facial surgery. **Ann Surg** 202(4):459–479, 1985.

GRADY MS, STEWARD O, JANE JA: Transplantation of embryonic chick spinal cord into transected adult chicken spinal cords: A useful model for transplantation research. **J Neurosci Res** 14:403–414, 1985.

GRADY MS, HOWARD MA, JANE JA, PERSING JA: Use of the Philadelphia collar as an alternative to the halo vest in patients with C2, C3 fractures. **Neurosurgery** 18:151–156, 1986.

GRADY MS, VANDENBERG SR, JANE JA: Long term survival of a patient with an intracranial ependymoma: Case Report. **Neurosurgery** 18:451–453, 1986.

JAGGER J, VERNBERG D, JANE JA: All-terrain vehicle injuries: by accident or by design (letter). **JAMA** 256:474, 1986.

PERSING JA, BABLER WJ, JANE JA, DUCKWORTH PF: Experimental unilateral coronal synostosis in rabbits. **Plast Reconstr Surg** 77(3): 369–377, 1986.

ALVES WM, COLOHAN ART, O'LEARY TJ, RIMEL RW, JANE JA: Understanding posttraumatic symptoms after minor head injury. **J Head Trauma Rehabil** 1(2):1–12, 1986.

COLOHAN ART, DACEY RG, ALVES WM, RIMEL RW, JANE JA: Neurological and neurosurgical implications of mild head injury. **J Head Trauma Rehabil** 1(2):13–21, 1986.

GLASER JA, WHITEHILL R, STAMP WG, JANE JA: Complications associated with the halo vest: A review of 245 cases. **J Neurosurg** 65:762–769, 1986.

EBBESSON SOE, BAZER GT, JANE JA: Some primary olfactory axons project to the contralateral olfactory bulb in *Xenopus laevis*. **Neurosci Lett** 65:234–238, 1986.

DELASHAW JB, PERSING JA, PARK TS, JANE JA: Surgical approaches for the correction of metopic synostosis. **Neurosurgery** 19(2): 228–234, 1986.

DACEY RG, ALVES WM, RIMEL RW, WINN HR, JANE JA: Neurosurgical complications after apparently minor head injury: Assessment of risk in a series of 610 patients. **J Neurosurg** 65:203–210, 1986.

GRADY MS, HOWARD MA, STEWARD O, JANE JA: The effects of embryonic rat hippocampus transplants on retrograde cell death following axotomy in the medial septal nucleus of adult rats. **Surg Forum** 37:498–500, 1986.

PERSING JA, BABLER WJ, NAGORSKY MJ, EDGERTON MT, JANE JA: Skull expansion in experimental craniosynostosis. **Plast Reconstr Surg** 78(5):594–603, 1986.

PERSING JA, NICHTER LS, JANE JA, EDGERTON MT: External cranial vault molding after craniofacial surgery. **Ann Plast Surg** 17(4): 274–283, 1986.

HINKLE JL, ALVES WM, RIMEL RW, JANE JA: Restoring social competence in minor head injury patients. **J Neurosci Nurs** 18:268–271, 1986.

BABLER WJ, PERSING JA, NAGORSKY MJ, JANE JA: Restricted growth at the frontonasal suture: Alterations in craniofacial growth in rabbits. **Am J Anat** 178:90–98, 1987.

JAGGER J, VERNBERG K, JANE JA: Air Bags: Reducing the toll of brain trauma. **Neurosurgery** 20(5):815–817, 1987.

COLOHAN ART, GRADY MS, BONNIN JM, THORNER MO, KOVACS K, JANE JA: Ectopic pituitary gland simulating a suprasellar tumor. **Neurosurgery** 20(1):43–48, 1987.

PERSING JA, EDGERTON MT, PARK TS, JANE JA: Barrel stave osteotomy for correction of turribrachycephaly craniosynostosis deformity. **Ann Plast Surg** 18(6):488–493, 1987.

MAGGIO WW, CAIL WS, BROOKEMAN JR, PERSING JA, JANE JA: Rathke's cleft cyst: Computed tomographic and magnetic resonance imaging appearances. **Neurosurgery** 21(1):60–62, 1987.

PERSING JA, CRONIN AJ, DELASHAW JB, EDGERTON MT, HENSON SL, JANE JA: Late surgical treatment of unilateral coronal synostosis using methyl methacrylate. **J Neurosurg** 66:793–799, 1987.

FARMER JP, COLOHAN ART, Y COMAIR, JANE JA: Less than severe head injury—an overview. **Acta Anaesthesiol Belg** 38:427–434, 1987.

ROOS KL, BRYAN JP, MAGGIO WW, JANE JA, SCHELD WM: Intracranial blastomycoma. **Medicine** 66(3):224–235, 1987.

WHITEHILL R, CICORIA AD, HOOPER WE, MAGGIO WW, JANE JA: Posterior cervical reconstruction with methyl methacrylate cement and wire: A clinical review. **J Neurosurg** 68:576–584, 1988.

DERDEYN CP, DELASHAW JB, BROADDUS WC, JANE JA: Detection of shunt-induced intracerebral hemorrhage by postoperative skull films: A report of two cases. **Neurosurgery** 22(4):755–757, 1988.

PERSING JA, DELASHAW JB, JANE JA, EDGERTON MT: Lambdoid synostosis: Surgical considerations. **Plast Reconstr Surg** 81:852–860, 1988.

GRADY MS, HOWARD MA, BROADDUS WC, WINN HR, JANE JA, RITTER RC, GILLIES GT, QUATE EG, MOLLOY JA: Initial experimental results of a new stereotaxic hyperthermia system. **Surg Forum** 39: 507–509, 1988.

DELASHAW JB, PERSING JA, BROADDUS WC, JANE JA: Cranial vault growth in craniosynostosis. **J Neurosurg** 70:159–165, 1989.

LEVINE PA, SCHER RL, JANE JA, PERSING JA, NEWMAN SA, MILLER J, CANTRELL RW: The craniofacial resection—eleven-year experience at the University of Virginia: Problems and solutions. **Otolaryngol Head Neck Surg** 101:665–669, 1989.

COLOHAN ART, ALVES WM, GROSS CR, TORNER JC, MEHTA VS, TANDON PN, JANE JA: Head injury mortality in two centers with different emergency medical services and intensive care. **J Neurosurg** 71:202–207, 1989.

GRADY MS, JANE JA, STEWARD O: Synaptic reorganization within the human central nervous system following injury. **J Neurosurg** 71:534–537, 1989.

PARK TS, BROADDUS WC, HARRIS M, PERSING JA, JANE JA: Vacuum-stiffened beanbag for cranial remodeling procedures in modified prone position: Technical note. **J Neurosurg** 71:623–625, 1989.

PERSING JA, JANE JA, SHAFFREY M, KNEUSEL R: Virchow and the pathogenesis of craniosynostosis: A translation of his original work. **Plast Reconstr Surg** 83:738–742, 1989.

JANE JA, HAWORTH CS, BROADDUS WC, LEE JH, MALIK J: A neurosurgical approach to far lateral disc herniation: Technical note. **J Neurosurg** 72:143–144, 1990.

PERSING JA, JANE JA, PARK TS, EDGERTON MT, DELASHAW JB: Floating C-shaped orbital osteotomy for orbital rim advancement in craniosynostosis: Preliminary report. **J Neurosurg** 72:22–26, 1990.

PERSING JA, JANE JA: Craniosynostosis. **Semin Neurol** 9(3):200–209, 1989 (Review article: 57 refs).

PERSING JA, JANE JA, DELASHAW JB: Treatment of bilateral coronal synostosis in infancy: A holistic approach. **J Neurosurg** 72:171–175, 1990.

SHAFFREY CI, SPOTNITZ WD, SHAFFREY ME, JANE JA: Neurosurgical applications of fibrin glue: Augmentation of dural closure in 134 patients. **Neurosurgery** 26:207–210, 1990.

PERSING JA, JANE JA, LEVINE PA, CANTRELL RW: The versatile frontal sinus approach to the floor of the anterior cranial fossa: Technical note. **J Neurosurg** 72:513–516, 1990.

DERDEYN C, PERSING JA, BROADDUS WC, DELASHAW JB, JANE JA, LEVINE PA, TORNER JC: Craniofacial trauma: An assessment of risk related to timing of surgery. **Plast Reconstr Surg** 86:238–245, 1990.

KASSELL NF, TORNER JC, HALEY EC JR, JANE JA, ADAMS HP, KONGABLE GL: The International Cooperative Study on the Timing of Aneurysm Surgery. Part 1: Overall management results. **J Neurosurg** 73(1):18–36, 1990.

KASSELL NF, TORNER JC, JANE JA, HALEY EC JR, ADAMS HP: The International Cooperative Study on the Timing of Aneurysm Surgery. Part 2: Surgical results. **J Neurosurg** 73(1):37–47, 1990.

RUFF RM, MARSHALL LF, KLAUBER MR, BLUNT BA, GRANT I, FOULKES MA, EISENBERG H, JANE JA, MARMAROU A: Alcohol abuse and neurological outcome of the severely head injured. **J Head Trauma Rehabil** 5:21–31, 1990.

EISENBERG HM, GARY HE JR, ALDRICH EF, SAYDJARI C, TURNER B, FOULKES MA, JANE JA, MARMAROU A, MARSHALL LF, YOUNG HF: Initial CT findings in 753 patients with severe head injury: A report from the NIH Traumatic Coma Data Bank. **J Neurosurg** 73(5): 688–698, 1990.

LEVIN HS, GARY HE JR, EISENBERG HM, RUFF RM, BARTH JT, KREUTZER J, HIGH WM JR, PORTMAN S, FOULKES MA, JANE JA, MARMAROU A, MARSHALL LF: Neurobehavioral outcome 1 year after severe head injury: Experience of the Traumatic Coma Data Bank. **J Neurosurg** 73(5):699–709, 1990.

BROADDUS WC, GRADY MS, DELASHAW JB JR, FERGUSON RDG, JANE JA: Preoperative superselective arteriolar embolization: A new approach to enhance resectability of spinal tumors. **Neurosurgery** 27(5):755–759, 1990.

MATTHEW TL, SPOTNITZ WD, GONIAS SL, ABBOTT RD, JANE JA: Increasing the life span of fibrin sealant: A comparison of three antifibrinolytic agents. **Surg Forum XLL** 504–506, 1990.

SHAFFREY ME, PERSING JA, FERGUSON RD, SHAFFREY CI, CANTRELL RW, JANE JA, NEWMAN SA: Vascular lesions involving the cranial base: A combined surgical and interventional radiologic approach. **J Craniofacial Surg** 1:106–111, 1990.

LEVIN HS, EISENBERG HM, GARY HE, MARMAROU A, FOULKES MA, JANE JA, MARSHALL LF, PORTMAN SM: Intracranial hypertension in relation to memory functioning during the first year after severe head injury. **Neurosurgery** 28(2):196–200, 1991.

LEE SI, PHILLIPS LH, JANE JA: Somato-somatic referred pain caused by suprasegmental spinal cord tumor. **Neurology** 41: 928–930, 1991.

LEVIN HS, SAYDJARI C, EISENBERG HM, FOULKES M, MARSHALL LF, RUFF RM, JANE JA, MARMAROU A: Vegetative state after closed head injury: A Traumatic Coma Data Bank Report. **Arch Neurol** 48: 580–585, 1991.

PERSING JA, JANE JA: Treatment of unilateral or bilateral coronal synostosis. **Neurosurg Operative Atlas,** Vol. 1, No. 2, 1991.

SHAFFREY ME, PERSING JA, ANGEL M, JANE JA, SHAFFREY CI: Age related technique modifications in the treatment of sagittal synostosis: Craniofacial Surgery, in **Proceedings of the Second International Congress of Cranio-Maxillofacial Surgery.** Bologna, Italy, Monduzzi Editore, 1991, pp. 237–242.

FOULKES MA, EISENBERG HM, JANE JA, MARMAROU A, MARSHALL LF, The Traumatic Coma Data Bank Research Group: The Traumatic Coma Data Bank: Design, methods, and baseline characteristics. **J Neurosurg** 75:S8–S13, 1991.

MARSHALL LF, MARSHALL SB, KLAUBER MR, CLARK MvB, EISENBERG HM, JANE JA, LUERSSEN TG, MARMAROU A, FOULKES MA: A new classification of head injury based on computerized tomography. **J Neurosurg** 75:S14–S20, 1991.

MARMAROU A, ANDERSON RL, WARD JD, CHOI SC, YOUNG HF, EISENBERG HM, FOULKES MA, MARSHALL LF, JANE JA: NINDS Traumatic Coma Data Bank: Intracranial pressure monitoring methodology. **J Neurosurg** 75:S21–S27, 1991.

MARSHALL LF, GAUTILLE T, KLAUBER MR, EISENBERG HM, JANE JA, LUERSSEN TG, MARMAROU A, FOULKES MA: The outcome of severe closed head injury. **J Neurosurg** 75:S28–S36, 1991.

VOLLMER DG, TORNER JC, JANE JA, SADOVNIC B, CHARLEBOIS D, EISENBERG HM, FOULKES MA, MARMAROU A, MARSHALL LF: Age and outcome following traumatic coma: Why do older patients fare worse? **J Neurosurg** 75:S37–S49, 1991.

RUFF RM, YOUNG D, GAUTILLE T, MARSHALL LF, BARTH J, JANE JA, KREUTZER J, MARMAROU A, LEVIN HS, EISENBERG HM, FOULKES MA: Verbal learning deficits following severe head injury: Heterogeneity in recovery over 1 year. **J Neurosurg** 75(S):S50–S58, 1991.

MARMAROU A, ANDERSON RL, WARD JD, CHOI SC, YOUNG HF, EISEN-
BERG HM, FOULKES MA, MARSHALL LF, JANE JA: Impact of ICP instability and hypotension on outcome in patients with severe head
trauma. **J Neurosurg** 75:S59–S66, 1991.

SHAFFREY ME, PERSING JA, SHAFFREY CI, JANE JA: Duraplasty in cranial base resection: Technical note. **J Craniofacial Surg** 2:152–
155, 1991.

SHAFFREY ME, POLIN RS, PHILLIPS CD, GERMANSON T, SHAFFREY CI,
JANE JA: Classification of civilian craniocerebral gunshot wounds: A
multivariate analysis predictive of mortality. **J Neurotrauma** 8(2):
253–260, 1991.

PRATT CB, JANE JA: Multiple colorectal carciniomas, polyposis-coli,
and neurofibromatosis, followed by multiple glioblastoma multi-
forme. **J Natl Cancer Inst** 83(12):880–881, 1991.

LARNER JM, KERSH CR, CONSTABLE WC, KLINE P, FERGUSON R, SHORT
R, JANE JA: Phase-I, II trial of superselective arterial 5-FU infusion
with concomitant external beam radiation for patients with either
anaplastic astrocytoma or glioblastoma multiforme. **Am J Clin On-
col-Cancer Clin Trials** 14(6):514–518, 1991.

EISENBERG HM, FOULKES MA, JANE JA, MARMAROU A, MARSHALL LF,
YOUNG HF: Report on the Traumatic Coma Data Bank: Preface. **J
Neurosurg** 75(S):US1–US1, 1991.

PIPAN CM, GLASHEEN WP, GONIAS SL, JANE JA, SPOTNITZ WD: The
lifespan of intraperitoneal fibrin sealant: The effects of three antifibrinolytic agents. **Surg Forum** XLII:519–521, 1991.

ALDRICH EF, EISENBERG HM, SAYDJARI C, LUERSSEN TG, FOULKES
MA, JANE JA, MARSHALL LF, MARMAROU A, YOUNG HF: Diffuse
brain swelling in severely-head injured children. **J Neurosurg**
76:450–454, 1992.

RIBAS GC, JANE JA: Traumatic contusions and intracerebral hematomas. **J Neurotrauma** 9(suppl 1):S265–S278, 1992.

SHAFFREY ME, JANE JA, PERSING JA, SHAFFREY CI, PHILLIPS LH: Surgeon's foot: A report of sural nerve palsy. **Neurosurgery** 30(6):
927–929, 1992.

SAGHER O, RIBAS GC, JANE JA: Nonoperative management of acute
epidural hematoma diagnosed by CT: The neuroradiologist's role.
AJNR 13:860–862, 1992.

PIPAN CM, GLASHEEN WP, MATTHEW TL, GONIAS SL, HWANG L-J,
JANE JA, SPOTNITZ WD: Effects of antifibrinolytic agents on the life
span of fibrin sealant. **J Surg Res** 53:1992.

LEVIN HS, ALDRICH EF, SAYDJARI C, EISENBERG HM, FOULKES MA,
BELLEFLEUR M, LUERSSEN TG, JANE JA, MARMAROU A, MARSHALL

LF, YOUNG HF: Severe head injury in children: Experience of the Traumatic Coma Data Bank. **Neurosurgery** 31(3):435–444, 1992.

MARSHALL LF, MARSHALL SB, KLAUBER MR, CLARK MVB, EISENBERG H, JANE JA, LUERSSEN TG, MARMAROU A, FOULKES MA: The diagnosis of head injury requires a classification based on computed axial tomography. **J Neurotrauma** 9(1):S287–S292, 1992.

PIEK J, CHESNUT RM, MARSHALL LF, VAN BERKUM-CLARK M, KLAUBER MR, BLUNT BA, EISENBERG, HM, JANE JA, MARMAROU A, FOULKES, MA: Extracranial complications of severe head injury. **J Neurosurgery** 77:901–907, 1992.

CLIFTON GL, KREUTZER JS, CHOI SC, DEVANY CW, EISENBERG HM, FOULKES MA, JANE JA, MARMAROU A, MARSHALL LF: Relationship between Glasgow Outcome Scale and neurophysiological measures after brain injury. **Neurosurgery** 33(1):34–38; discussion 38–39, 1993.

CHESNUT RM, MARSHALL LF, KLAUBER MR, BLUNT BA, BALDWIN N, EISENBERG HM, JANE JA, MARMAROU A, FOULKES MA: The role of secondary brain injury in determining outcome from severe head injury. **J Trauma** 34(2):216–222, 1993.

SAGHER O, MALIK JM, LEE JH, SHAFFREY CI, SHAFFREY ME, SZABO TA, JANE JA: Fusion with occipital bone for atlantoaxial instability: Technical note. **Neurosurgery** 33(5):926–928; discussion 928–929, 1993.

FRANCEL PC, LONG BA, MALIK JM, TRIBBLE C, JANE JA, KRON IL: Limiting ischemic spinal cord injury using a free radical scavenger 21-aminosteroid and/or cerebrospinal fluid drainage, **J Neurosurgery** 79:742–751, 1993.

DELASHAW JB JR, JANE JA, KASSELL NF, LUCE C: Supraorbital craniotomy by fracture of the anterior orbital roof: Technical note. **J Neurosurg** 79(4):615–618, 1993.

SIMMONS NE, HELM GA, CAIL WS, BENNETT JP, JANE JA: Magnetic Resonance Imaging of neuronal grafts in the primate. **Exp Neurol** 125:52–57, 1994.

FRANCEL PC, BELL A, JANE JA: Operative positioning for patients undergoing repair of craniosynostosis. **Neurosurgery** 35(2):304–306, 1994.

JANE JA: The golden anniversary celebration of the *Journal* (Editorial Comment). **J Neurosurg** 80:1–2, 1994.

LARNER JM, PHILLIPS CD, DION JE, JENSEN ME, NEWMAN SA, JANE JA: A phase 1-2 trial of superselective carboplatin, low-dose infusional 5-fluorouracil and concurrent radiation for high-grade gliomas. **Am J Clin Oncol** 18(1):1–7, 1995.

DANISA OA, SHAFFREY CI, JANE JA, WHITEHILL R, WANG GJ, SZABO TA, HANSEN CA, SHAFFREY MA, CHAN DPK: Surgical approaches for the correction of unstable thoracolumbar burst fractures: A retrospective analysis of treatment outcomes. **J Neurosurg** 83, In press, 1995.

DIPIERRO CG, HELM GA, SHAFFREY CI, CHADDUCK JB, HENSON SL, MALIK JM, SZABO TA, SIMMONS NA, JANE JA: Treatment of lumbar spinal stenosis by extensive unilateral decompression and contralateral autologous bone fusion: Operative technique and results. **J Neurosurg** 84, in press, 1996.

BOOKS AND CHAPTERS IN BOOKS

Books

JANE JA, YASHON D: *Cytology of Tumors Affecting the Nervous System.* Springfield, IL, Charles C Thomas, 1969.

JANE JA, RIMEL RW, ALVES W, DACEY RG JR, WINN HR, COLOHAN AR (eds): *Seminars in Neurological Surgery: Trauma of the Central Nervous System.* New York, Raven Press, 1985.

PERSING JA, EDGERTON MT, JANE JA (eds): *Scientific Foundations and Surgical Treatment of Craniosynostosis.* Baltimore, Williams & Wilkins, 1989.

Chapters in Books

Pathophysiology of head injury, in Tansill BC (ed): *Pathophysiology of Shock, Anoxia, and Ischemia.* Baltimore, Williams & Wilkins.

The natural history of saccular aneurysm, in *Textbook of Cerebrovascular Surgery.* New York, Springer-Verlag.

PEARSON OH, THOMAS CH, KAUFMAN B, SHEALY CN, COLLINS WF, JANE JA, JACKSON CCR: Pituitary ablation in the treatment of diabetic retinopathy, in Goldberg MF, Find SL (eds): *Symposium on Treatment of Diabetic Retinopathy.* Airlie House, Warrenton, VA, 9-29/10-1-68. Arlington, VA, Public Health Service Publication No. 1890, pp 331–339.

JACKSON CCR, JANE JA: Transseptal sphenoidal hypophysectomy, in *Otolaryngology.* Hagerstown, MD, Harper & Row, 1971, vol. 3.

YASHON D, JANE JA: Central nervous system tissue cytology, in Homburger F (ed): *Recent Advances in Brain Tumor Research: Progress in Experimental Tumor Research.* Basel, Karger, 1972, vol. 17, pp 346–362.

JACKSON CC ROE, JANE JA: Transseptal-sphenoidal hypophysectomy, in *Otolaryngology.* Hagerstown, MD, Harper & Row, 1974, vol. 3.

GOSSMAN HH, SADAR ES, JANE JA: Intracranial infection, in Buske KA, Spoerri O, Shaw J (eds): *Progress in Paediatric Neurosurgery.* Stuttgart, Hippokrates-Verlag, 1974, pp 224–228.

JANE JA: Radical reconstruction of complex cranioorbitofacial abnormalities, in Bergsma D (ed): *Birth Defects: Original Article Series. Morphogenesis and Malformation of Face and Brain.* The National Foundation, 1975, vol. 11, pp 341–347.

EDGERTON MT, MARSHALL KA, JANE JA, WINN HR: New surgical techniques in major orbito-cranio-facial reconstruction, in Marchac D (ed): *Transactions of the Sixth International Congress of Plastic and Reconstructive Surgery.* Paris, Masson, 1976, pp 166–171.

FUTRELL JW, EDGERTON MT, JANE JA: Bones and joints, in Gellis, Kagan (eds): *Current Pediatric Therapy.* 1978, pp 426–431.

BEDFORD RF, WINN HR, TYSON GW, PARK TS, JANE JA: Lidocaine prevents increased ICP after endotracheal intubation, in Shulman K, Marmarou A, Miller JD, Becker DP, Hochwald GM, Brock M (eds): *Intracranial Pressure IV.* Berlin, Springer-Verlag, 1980, pp 595–598.

WINN HR, RICHARDSON AE, JANE JA: The assessment of the natural history of single cerebral aneurysms which have ruptured, in Hopkins LN, Long DM (eds): *Clinical Management of Intracranial Aneurysms.* New York: Raven Press, 1981, pp 1–11.

WINN HR, BERGA SL, RICHARDSON AE, WALDMAN MT, O'BRIEN WM, JANE JA: Long-term evaluation of patients with multiple cerebral aneurysms, in Duvoisin RC (ed): *Trans Am Neurol Association* New York, Springer, 1981, pp 365–367.

WINN HR, RICHARDSON AE, JANE JA: The natural history of cerebral aneurysms: The rate of late rebleeding, in Brock M (ed): *Modern Neurosurgery.* Berlin, Springer-Verlag, 1982, pp 417–423.

JANE JA, RIMEL RW, POBERESKIN LH, TYSON GW, STEWARD O, GENNARELLI TA: Outcome and pathology of head injury, in Grossman RG, Gildenberg PL (eds): *Head Injury: Basic and Clinical Aspects.* New York, Raven Press, 1982, pp 229–237.

JANE JA, RIMEL RW: Prognosis in head injury, in Grossman RG, Gildenberg PL (eds): *Clinical Neurosurgery: Proceedings of the Congress of Neurological Surgeons. Los Angeles, CA. 1981.* Baltimore: Williams & Wilkins, 1982, vol 29, pp 346–352.

GENNARELLI TA, JANE JA, THIBAULT L, STEWARD O: Axonal damage in mild head injury demonstrated by the Nauta method, in Villani R, Papl I, Giovanelli M, Gaini SM, Tomei G: (eds): *Advances in Neurotraumatology,* Proc Intl. Symposium, Milan, Oct. 11–13. Amsterdam, Excerpta Medica, 1982, pp 37–39.

BOND MA, JENNETT B (eds): *The Characteristics of the Head Injured Patient.* Philadelphia, F.A. Davis, 1983.

RIMEL RW, TYSON GW, JANE JA: Head injuries, in Kravis TC, Warner CG (eds): *Emergency Medicine: A Comprehensive Review.* Rockville MD, Aspen Publications, 1983, pp 597–613.

DACEY RG, SCHELD WM, WINN HR, JANE JA, SANDE MA: Bacterial meningitis: Selected aspects of cerebrospinal fluid pathophysiology, in Wood JW (ed): *Neurobiology of Cerebrospinal Fluid II.* New York, Plenum Press, 1983, pp 727–738.

DACEY RG, JANE JA: Craniocerebral trauma, in BAKER AB, BAKER LH (eds): *Clinical Neurology.* Hagerstown, MD, Harper & Row, 1984, vol 3, pp 1–61.

ALVES WM, JANE JA: Mild brain injury: Damage and outcome, in Becker DP, Povlishock JT (eds): *Central Nervous System Trauma Status Report—1985.* Bethesda, MD, National Institutes of Health, National Institutes of Neurological and Communicative Diseases and Stroke, 1985, pp 255–270.

JANE JA, RIMEL RW, ALVES WM, DACEY RG, WINN HR, COLOHAN ART: Minor and moderate head injury: model systems, in Dacey RG Jr, Winn HR, Rimel RW, Jane JA (eds): *Seminars in Neurological Surgery: Trauma to the Central Nervous System.* New York, Raven Press, 1985, pp 27–34.

PERSING JA, JANE JA: Craniosynostosis, in Long D (ed): *Current Therapy in Neurological Surgery.* Grand Junction, CT, B.C. Decker, 1985, pp 214–219.

JANE JA, JOHNS ME, CANTRELL RW, COLOHAN ART, KAPLAN M: Supraorbital rim approach to lesions of the craniofacial junction, in Chretien PB, Johns ME, Shedd DP, Strong WE, Ward PH (eds): *Head and Neck Cancer: Proceedings of the International Conference.* Baltimore, MD, July 22–27, 1984. Philadelphia, B.C. Decker, 1985, vol 1, pp 272–274.

WINN HR, RICHARDSON AE, JANE JA: The natural history of intracranial aneurysms, in Fein JM, Flamm ES (eds): *Cerebrovascular Surgery.* New York, Springer-Verlag, 1985, vol 3, pp 667–678.

RIMEL RW, JANE JA: Minor head injury: Management and outcome, in Wilkins, Rengachary (eds): *Neurosurgery.* New York, McGraw-Hill, 1985, pp 1608–1611.

PERSING JA, EDGERTON MT, PARK TS, JANE JA: Barrel stoave osteotomy for correction of turribrachycephaly craniosynostosis deformity, in Marchac D (ed): *Transactions of the First International Congress of Cranio-maxillofacial Surgeons.* Boston, Little Brown, 1985, pp 145–150.

PERSING JA, KASSELL NF, JANE JA: Neurosurgical perspectives of special perioperative consideration, in Cummings CW, Frederickson JM, Harker LA, Krause CJ, Schuller DE (eds): *Otolaryngology—Head and Neck Surgery*. St. Louis, C. V. Mosby, 1986, pp 3377–3388.

JANE JA, PERSING JA: Neurosurgical treatment of craniosynostosis, in Cohen MM (ed): *Craniosynostosis: Diagnosis, Evaluation, and Management*. New York, Raven Press, 1986, pp 249–320.

KASSELL NF, TORNER JC, JANE JA: Studio cooperativo internazionale sul timing chirurgico degli aneurismi cerebrali, in Da Pian R, Pasqualin A, Scienza R: *Aneurismi e Angiomi Cerebrali*. Verona, Italy, Cortina Verona, 1986, pp 141–146.

BABLER WJ, PERSING JA, WINN HR, JANE JA, RODEHEAVER GT: Compensating growth following premature closure of the ocronal sutute in rabbits, in Moyers R (ed): *Year Book of Dentistry*. 1986.

Characteristics of the Patient with Head Injury, in Becker DA, Gudeman SE (eds): *Head Injury*. Philadelphia, W.B. Saunders, in press.

COLOHAN ART, JANE JA, ALVES WM, RIMEL RW: Less-than-severe head injury: Pathology and outcome, in Miner ME, Wagner KA (eds): *Neurotrauma: Treatment, Rehabilitation, and Related Issues, No. 2*. Proceedings of the Second Houston Conference on Neurotrauma, held in May 1985. Boston, Butterworths, 1987, pp 3–14.

Neurosurgical aspects of craniosynostosis, in *Comprehensive Handbook of Craniosynostosis,* New York, Raven Press.

COLOHAN ART, JANE JA, PERSING JA: Encephaloceles, in Mustarde, Jackson (eds): *Plastic Surgery in Infancy and Childhood*. London, Churchill Livingstone, ed 3, 1988, pp 165–179.

HALEY EC, TORNER JC, KASSELL NF, VERNBERG KK, KONGABLE GL, JANE JA: Design of clinical trial to evaluate vasospasm treatment, in Wilkins RH (ed): *Cerebral Vasospasm*. New York, Raven Press, 1988, pp 503–507.

EISENBERG HM, GARY HE JR, TURNER B, JANE JA, MARMAROU A, MARSHALL LF, YOUNG H: NIH TCDB Writing Group: CT scan findings in 683 patients with severe (Glasgow Coma Scale Score) closed head injury: A report from the NIH Traumatic Coma Data Bank, in Hoff JT (ed): *Intracranial Pressure VII (Proceedings of the 7th International Symposium)*, Berlin, Springer-Verlag, 1988.

PERSING JA, JANE JA, EDGERTON MT: Surgical treatment of craniosynostosis, in Persing JA, Edgerton MT, Jane JA (eds): *Scientific Foundations and Surgical Treatment of Craniosynostosis*. Baltimore, Williams & Wilkins, 1989, pp 117–238.

BARTH JT, ALVES WA, REIN, MACHIOCHI, RIMEL RW, JANE JA, NELSON: Neuropsychological sequelae and recovery of function, in Levin,

Eisenberg, Burton (eds): *Mild Head Injury in Sports*. New York, Oxford Press, 1989, pp 257–275.

ALVES WA, ET AL.: Post-traumatic syndrome, in Youmans (ed): *Neurological Surgery*, Philadelphia, W. B. Saunders, 1990, ed 3, pp 2230–2242.

JANE JA: Definitions. Mild to moderate head injury, in Hoff, Anderson, Cole (eds): *Contemporary Issues in Neurological Surgery*. Boston, Blackwell Science Publications, 1989.

BROADDUS WC, PENDLETON GA, DELASHAW JB, SHORT RV, KASSELL NF, GRADY MS, JANE JA: Differential intracranial pressure recordings in patients with dual ipsilateral monitors, in Hoff JT, Betz AL (eds): *Intracranial Pressure VII*. Berlin, Springer-Verlag, 1989, pp 41–44.

JANE JA: Left parietal lobe after nodular melanoma, in Wanebo HJ (ed): *Common Problems in Cancer Surgery*. Chicago, IL, Year Book Medical Publishers, 1989.

VOLLMER DG, DACEY RG, JANE JA: Craniocerebral trauma, in Joynt R (ed): *Clinical Neurology*. Philadelphia, J. B. Lippincott, 1991.

PERSING JA, JANE JA: Preface, in Persing JA, Jane JA (Guest Editors): *Neurosurgery Clinics of North America. Vol. 2. Craniofacial Disorders*. Philadelphia, W. B. Saunders, 1991, p xiii.

DELASHAW JB, PERSING JA, JANE JA: Cranial deformation in craniosynostosis: A new explanation, in Persing JA, Jane JA (eds): *Neurosurgery Clinics of North America. Vol 2. Craniofacial Disorders*. Philadelphia, W. B. Saunders, 1991, pp 611–620.

SHAFFREY ME, PERSING JA, DELASHAW JB, SHAFFREY CI, JANE JA: Surgical treatment of metopic synostosis, in Persing JA, Jane JA (eds): *Neurosurgery Clinics of North America, Vol 2, Craniofacial Disorders*. Philadelphia, W. B. Saunders, 1991, pp 621–627.

PERSING JA, JANE JA: Treatment of syndromic and nonsyndromic bilateral coronal synostosis in infancy and childhood, in Persing JA, Jane JA (eds): *Neurosurgery Clinics of North America, Vol 2. Craniofacial Disorders*. Philadelphia, W. B. Saunders, 1991, pp 655–663.

SHAFFREY ME, PERSING JA, ANGEL M, SHAFFREY CI, JANE JA: Age related technique modifications in the treatment of sagittal synostosis, in Monduzzi (ed): *Craniofacial Surgery: Proceedings of the Second International Congress of Cranio-Maxillofacial Surgery*. Bologna, Italy, 1991, pp 237–242.

SHAFFREY ME, PERSING JA, SHAFFREY CI, DELASHAW JB, HENNESSY RJ, JANE JA: Craniofacial reconstruction, in Apuzzo M (ed): *Brain Surgery: Complication Avoidance and Management*. New York, Churchill Livingstone, 1993, pp 1373–1393.

SHAFFREY ME, PERSING JA, SHAFFREY CI, JANE JA: Craniosynostosis, in Rengachary SS, Wilkins RH (eds): *Principles of Neurosurgery.* London, Wolfe Publishing, 1994, pp 8.1–8.16.

FRANCEL PC, JANE JA: Age and outcome from head injury, in Narayan RK, Wilberger JE, Povlishock JT (eds): *Neurotrauma,* New York, McGraw Hill, 1995.

PERSING J, JANE JA: Craniosynostosis, in Youmans JR (ed): *Neurological Surgery.* Philadelphia, W. B. Saunders, ed 4, 1995.

FRANCEL PC, ALVES W, JANE JA: Mild head injuries in adults, in Youmans JR (ed): *Neurological Surgery.* Philadelphia, W. B. Saunders, 1995, ed 4.

FRANCEL PC, JANE JA: Diagnosis and treatment of moderate and severe head injuries in infants and children, in Youmans JR (ed): *Neurological Surgery.* Philadelphia, W. B. Saunders, 1995, ed 4.

PERSING JA, JANE JA: Coronal synostosis: Unilateral and bilateral, in *Atlas of Surgery AANS,* in press.

PERSING JA, JANE JA:Craniofacial Surgery, in *Atlas of Surgery AANS,* in press

WOLCOTT WP, MALIK JM, SHAFFREY CI, SHAFFREY ME, JANE JA: Differential diagnosis of surgical disorders of the spine, in *Spine Surgery Techniques, Complication Avoidance & Management.* New York, Churchill Livingstone, in press, 1996.

Professional Societies and Activities

Director, American Board of Neurological Surgeons	1989–1996
Editor, *Journal of Neurosurgery*	1992–present
Associate Editor, *Journal of Neurosurgery*	1991–1992
Chairman, Editorial Board, *Journal of Neurosurgery*	1990–1991
Member, Editorial Board, *Journal of Neurosurgery*	1984–1990
Member, Editorial Board, *Journal of Neurotrauma*	
Member, Editorial Board, *Brain Injury*	1987–present
Vice President, Society of Neurological Surgeons	1988
Vice President, American Academy of Neurological Surgeons	1988
Chairman, Van Wagenen Fellowship Committee	1990
AOA University of Virginia School of Medicine	1992
Board of Directors, National Head Injury Foundation	1992
President-elect, Senior Society of Neurological Surgeons	1992
Albemarle County Medical Society	
American Academy of Neurological Surgery	
American Association of Anatomists	

American Association of Neurological Surgeons
American Medical Association
American Physiological Society
The Cajal Club
The Canadian Neurosurgical Society
Medical Society of Virginia
Neurosurgical Society of the Virginias
Neurosurgical Society of America
Pavlovian Society
Research Society of Neurological Surgeons
Royal College of Physicians and Surgeons of Canada
Society of British Neurological Surgeons
Society of Neurological Surgeons
Society of University Surgeons
Society for Neuroscience (Chairman, Membership Committee)
Southern Neurosurgical Society

National Institutes of Health
1. Neurology B Study Section   1971–1974
2. Neurological Disorders Program
   Project Review B Committee   1979–1983
3. Special Study Section on Interdisciplinary Studies of
   the Role of the Central Nervous System in Hypertension   1979
4. Scientific Advisory Committee Office
   of Biometry and Field Studies
5. Review Committee of the National Committee for
   Research on Neurological and Communicative
   Disorders (NCR)   December 1981

TEACHING AND RESEARCH APPOINTMENTS PREVIOUSLY HELD

1951–1952: Department of Psychology
            Division of Biological Sciences University of Chicago
1953–1956: Research Assistant, Department of Psychology
            University of Chicago
1956–1957: Intern, Royal Victoria Hospital, McGill University
1957:   Junior Assistant Resident in Neurosurgery
            University of Chicago Clinics
1957–1958: Junior Assistant Resident in Surgery
            Royal Victoria Hospital, McGill University
1958–1959: Fellow in Neurophysiology
            Montreal Neurological Institute, NIH
1959–1960: Senior Fellow in Neuropathology and
            Demonstrator in Neuropathology
            McGill University, Montreal

1961:	Research Assistant in Neurosurgery to Mr. Wylie McKissock, St. George's Hospital and The National Hospital, Queen Square, London, England
1962:	Research Associate, Department of Psychology Duke University
1963–1964:	Senior Resident in Neurosurgery; Assistant in Neurology and Neurosurgery University of Illinois Research and Educational Hospital and the Illinois Neuropsychiatric Institute
1965–1966:	Senior Instructor in Neurosurgery Case Western Reserve University School of Medicine Assistant Neurosurgeon, University Hospital of Cleveland Chief, Neurosurgical Division Cleveland Veteran's Administration Hospital
1967–1968:	Assistant Professor of Neurosurgery Case Western Reserve University School of Medicine Assistant Neurosurgeon, University Hospital of Cleveland Chief, Neurosurgical Division Cleveland Veteran's Administration Hospital
1969–1987:	Alumni Professor and Chairman Department of Neurological Surgery University of Virginia School of Medicine Charlottesville, Virginia
1987– Present	David D. Weaver Professor of Neurosurgery Chairman, Department of Neurological Surgery University of Virginia Health Sciences Center Charlottesville, Virginia

Awards

Harry Wilkins Lectureship, University of Oklahoma	1983
Samuel Snodgrass Lectureship University of Texas, Galveston	1983
Grass Prize and Medal of the Society of Neurological Surgeons for Meritorious Research	1985
Herbert Olivecrona Lectureship of the Karolinska Institute of Stockholm, Sweden	1985
29th Annual Fellows Day Lecture, Montreal Neurological Institute, Montreal, Quebec, Canada	1986
Arthur A. Ward Lectureship University of Washington, Seattle	1986
The First Stuart Rowe Lectureship in Neurosurgery University of Pittsburgh, Pittsburgh, Pennsylvania	1987
E. S. Gurdjian Lectureship Wayne State University, Detroit, Michigan	1987

Alumni Award for Distinguished Service
  University of Chicago, Chicago, Illinois   1988
John E. Adams Visiting Professor
  University of California at San Francisco   1989
Guest of Honor Georgia Neurosurgical Society   1990
Honored Guest Neurosurgical Society of the Virginias   1991
Gardner Lecture Cleveland Clinic, Cleveland, Ohio   1991
Campbell Lecture Albany Medical College   1994
Charles Elsburg Lecture Albany Medical College   1994
Klüver Lecture University of Chicago, Chicago, Illinois   1994

Abstracts

ERICKSON RP, JANE JA, WAITE R, DIAMOND IT: Single neuron investigation of somesthetic thalamus of the opossum. **Physiologist** 6:177, 1963.

YASHON D, JANE JA: A cytologic method for rapid diagnosis of neoplasms affecting the nervous system. **Proc Inst Med Chicago** 25:318, 1965.

JANE JA, CAMPBELL CBG, YASHON D: Some aspects of the evolution of the pyramidal tract. **Neurology** 16:318, 1966.

CAMPBELL CBG, JANE JA, YASHON D: The retinal projections of tree shrews and hedgehog. **Anat Rec** 154:326, 1966.

HALL WC, ERICKSON RP, JANE JA, SNYDER M, DIAMOND IT: Sensory thalamus in hedgehog. **Physiologist** 9:3, 1966.

BECKER DP, GLUCK H, JANE JA, ECKSTEIN RW: Single neuron response pattern in paramedial mesencephalic reticular formation to large fiber (A beta) and small fiber (A-gamma-delta and C) peripheral nerve stimulation. **Fed Proc** 26:491, 1967.

BECKER DP, GLUCK H, JANE JA: Response pattern of single paramedial mesencephalic neurons in relation to noxious and non-noxious stimuli and peripheral nerve fiber diameter. **Anat Rec** 157:211, 1967.

YOUNG H, JANE JA, NULSEN FE, WHITE RJ, YASHON D, BECKER DP: Treatment of posterior communicating aneurysms. **Neurology** 17: 313, 1967.

SCHROEDER D, YASHON D, BECKER DP, JANE JA: The evolution of the primate medial lemniscus. **Anat Rec** 160:424, 1968.

JANE JA, LEVEY N, CARLSON NJ: Vision following cortex and midbrain lesions in the tree shrew. **Fed Proc** 28:2, 1969.

VONEIDA T, NAUTA HJW, JANE JA: Interhemispheric connections in the European hedgehog (*Erinaceus europaeus*). *Anat Rec* 163:280, 1969.

JANE JA, CARLSON NJ, LEVEY N: A comparison of the effects of lesions of striate cortex and superior colliculus on vision in the Malayan tree shrew (*Tupaia glis*). **Anat Rec** 163:306, 1969.

SCHROEDER DM, JANE JA, NAUTA HJW: Thalamic projections from the dorsal column and cerebellar nuclei and tectum in the hedgehog (*Erinaceus europaeus*). **Anat Rec** 166:374, 1970.

LEVEY N, HARRIS J, WINN HR, JANE JA: Anatomical and behavioral studies of the visual system of the ground squirrel (*Citellus tridecemlineatus*). **Anat Rec** 169:367, 1971.

MARKS KE, JANE JA: Functions of the visual cortex for localization of light in space. **Fed Proc** 30:1329, 1971.

BUTLER AB, JANE JA: An ultrastructural study of interlaminar connections of rat supragranular visual cortex. **Anat Rec** 175:282, 1973.

SCHROEDER DM, JANE JA: Somatosensory afferents to the external nucleus of the inferior colliculus. **Soc Neurosci** 1973.

WATKINS DW, BUTLER AB, SHERMAN SM, JANE JA: Supragranular laminar lesions of cat striate cortex: Effects on visual receptive fields. **Soc Neurosc** 1974.

WINN HR, RICHARDSON A, JANE JA: Late mortality and morbidity of common carotid ligation for posterior communicating artery aneurysms. A comparison with conservative treatment. **J Neurol Neurosurg Psychiatry** 38:406, 1975.

JANE JA: Surgery of craniofacial deformities. **J Neurol Neurosurg Psychiatry** 38:409, 1975.

JANE JA, SCOVILLE S: The effect of bilateral neonatal eyelid suture on visual discrimination in the rat. **Neuroscience Abstracts,** Vol II, Parts 1 & 2, 1976.

BUTLER AB, JANE JA: An ultrastructural study of supragranular to infragranular connections in the visual cortex of normal and visually deprived rats. **Anat Rec** 190:353, 1978.

WINN HR, RICHARDSON AE, JANE JA: 15-year evaluation of 258 patients with a single anterior communicating artery aneurysm. **Neurosurgery** 2:165, 1978.

DACEY RG, WELSH JE, SCHELD WM, WINN HR, SANDE MA, JANE JA: Alterations of cerebrospinal fluid outflow resistance in experimental bacterial meningitis. **Ann Neurol** 4:173, 1978.

JANE JA, POBERESKIN LH, PARK TS, WINN HR, BUTLER AB: A new approach to the orbit and subfrontal region. **Proc AANS 1980,** pp 179–180.

PERSING JA, BABLER W, PERSSON KM, RODEHEAVER G, WINN HR, ROY W, JANE JA, EDGERTON MT, LANGMAN J: The effect of the timing of surgery in experimental craniosynostosis. **Proc AANS 1980** pp 63–65.

TYSON GW, JANE JA, RIMEL RW, BUTLER AB, WINN HR, JAGGER J, LEVINE J: Comparison of results of multi-modality medical therapy with bi-modality therapy in a minimally selected population of patients with severe head injury. **Proc AANS, 1980**, pp 131–132.

WINN HR, BERGA SL, RICHARDSON AE, JANE JA, WALDMAN MT, O'BRIEN WM: The natural history of vertebral basilar aneurysms. **Proc AANS (Plenary Session)**, 1980, pp 58–60.

WINN HR, BERGA SL, RICHARDSON AE, JANE JA, WALDMAN MT, O'BRIEN WM: The natural history of vertebral basilar aneurysms (VBA). **Stroke** 12:120, 1981.

WINN HR, RICHARDSON AE, JANE JA: The natural history of ruptured cerebral aneurysms. World Fed Neurosurg Soc, **Intl Congress of Neurol Surg**, 1981.

WINN HR, BERGA SL, RICHARDSON AE, WALDMAN MT, O'BRIEN WM, JANE JA: Long-term evaluation of patients with multiple cerebral aneurysms. **Ann Neurol** 10:106, 1981.

PERSING JA, BABLER W, PERSSON M, RODEHEAVER G, WINN HR, JANE JA: Timing of surgery in experimental craniosynostosis. **Child's Brain** 8:70–71, 1981.

JANE JA, PERSING JA, WINN HR, BUTLER AB, EDGERTON M: Metopic synostosis. **Child's Brain** 8:68, 1981.

JANE JA, PERSING JA, LAMBRUSCHI P, EDGERTON J, WINN HR: Unilateral coronal synostosis: A new approach. **Child's Brain** 8:71–72, 1981

GRADY MS, HOWARD MA, JANE JA, STEWARD O: the effects of embryonic rat hippocampus transplant on retrograde cell death following axotomy on the medial septal nucleus of adult rats. **Am Coll Surg Abstr**, 1986.

Contents

———————————— I ————————————

GENERAL SCIENTIFIC SESSION I
INNOVATIONS IN CRANIAL APPROACHES AND EXPOSURES

———————————— II ————————————

GENERAL SCIENTIFIC SESSION II
INNOVATIONS IN THE TREATMENT OF CRANIOFACIAL
DISORDERS AND SPINAL DYSRAPHISMS

———————————— III ————————————

GENERAL SCIENTIFIC SESSION III
LUMBAR DISC DISEASE: CURRENT TRENDS
IN MANAGEMENT

IV
GENERAL SCIENTIFIC SESSION IV
INNOVATIONS IN MINIMALISM

1

Managed Care and Managed Golf: Lessons for Neurosurgery in 1995*

RALPH G. DACEY, JR., M.D.

It's been a great honor for me to serve as the president of the Congress of Neurological Surgeons for this past year. The friendships that have developed as a result of my work in the Congress has meant a great deal to me, and the opportunity to work with such a talented and energetic bunch of people, not only in the Congress, but also in the AANS, has been one of the most rewarding experiences of my life. I am very grateful to you, the members of the Congress, for allowing me to serve in this capacity.

What I would like to do this morning is make some observations about the practice environment for neurosurgery and medicine in 1995. I am going to discuss the way managed care is changing our ability to care for our patients. I would then like to describe to you how I think our specialty should rededicate itself to the scientific principles of continuous improvement of patient care and technology that have made our specialty so great.

Before I discuss these serious issues however, I'd like to tell you about a nightmare that I had a couple of weeks ago. The nightmare was that the same executives who are running America's managed care companies extended their reach into another American institution—golf. You see, in my dream a group of key policymakers got together in Jackson Hole, Wyoming and decided that the country was spending too much of its gross domestic product on golf, and that if something was not done to halt the skyrocketing cost of the sport, eventually we wouldn't have enough money to pay for other important national priorities. These policymakers came up with the concept of managed golf. Under this plan, costs would be controlled by limiting the number of golf balls that a golfer would have access to. All the golf balls were divided up and distributed by individuals called primary recreationalists.

Presidential Address delivered at the 43rd Annual Meeting of the Congress of Neurological Surgeons, San Francisco, California, October 14–19, 1995.

These individuals didn't know much about golf and couldn't play golf, but they were the gatekeepers for the system. In my dream golfers would spend a lot of time sitting around on the tee, waiting for the primary recreationalists to give them access to a golf ball. When a ball finally became available, the golfer would have to call in to a central location and ask permission to tee off. The clerks that he or she would speak to on the phone would usually know very little about the game of golf, but they had golf guidelines available to them. In one case, the golfer was somewhat upset with the managed golf clerk, because he wanted to use a driver. He was there on the tee and he knew the conditions and felt that this was the best club to use. The managed golf clerk, however, told him that the guidelines called for a three-wood. You'll notice here that the equipment was not state of the art. Equipment manufacturers had to get out of the business because of cost pressures and, hence, the high-tech clubs that had been so prevalent were replaced with suboptimal technology and equipment. Another thing that became very noticeable around golf courses in my dream was that the golfers came to be outnumbered by people walking around the course in suits. These people were lawyers, golf course administrators, and managed golf company executives. Initially, they allowed the golfers about 12 minutes to play each hole, but gradually, over time, the number went down to 11, then 10, and then finally ended up at about 8 minutes. If you took longer than 8 minutes, they took the ball away from you. The whole emphasis in the world of managed golf was on controlling resource utilization. For example, a shot such as this, where sand is knocked out of the bunker, was perceived as a very negative occurrence, because they would have to pay someone to rake the bunker. Similarly, if a golfer ever took a divot, it would be entered into his computerized profile and he would be penalized. This became known as divot credentialing, and it led to some fundamental differences in the way the game was played. Golfers would never consider using a wedge under these circumstances, because it might hurt the golf course and drive up costs. As a result, scores changed dramatically and the quality of play suffered. Eventually, society became critical of what had happened to the game. Golfers were again brought back into the system in a meaningful way. They reminded the managed golf executives that what really counts is how many strokes it takes to hole the ball, and that occasionally it might be necessary to take a divot or use other resources to achieve the desired goal. They gradually were given more direct access to golf balls, and the role of the primary recreationalists diminished. In retrospect, the whole thing turned around only when the golfers became more effective at proving that they could lower scores by playing their best golf. Eventually, the fact that they knew the most about the game and were the most sophisticated about exactly what the score was led society to again accept their authority.

Obviously, the analogy I've drawn in describing this nightmare is a great oversimplification, but neurosurgeons, like golfers, are problem solvers, and they are being removed from the process of patient care in the name of reducing cost. The managed care system today removes the most knowledgable players, emphasizes only resource utilization, and, despite much talk to the contrary, ignores outcomes.

Now let me emphasize that I am not suggesting that we don't have a big problem in our society with the cost of care. Dr. Kenneth Shine (7), the President of the Institute of Medicine, recently observed that the current rate of increase in the cost of medical care simply cannot continue (Fig. 1). Legitimate arguments can be made that national health care expenditures should be 7 or 12% or even 15% of our gross domestic product, but I think that no one would argue that the rate of increase we have seen in the last 25 years can be sustained. Data from a variety of sources, including most recently the RBRVS Volume Performance Standards, indicate that the cost of surgical care has increased at a slower rate, when compared to overall health care expenditures. Nonetheless, because of the observations of Newhouse (6), indicating that at least half of the current inflation rate for medical care is due to the diffusion of new technology, neurosurgeons and other surgical subspecialists are cited as a major cause of this increase in the cost of care.

National Health Expenditures (In Billions of Dollars)

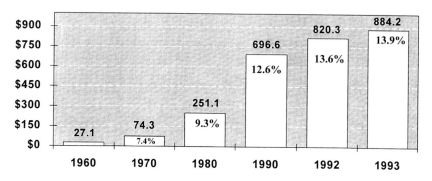

FIG. 1 National health expenditures and percentage of gross domestic product. [Reproduced with permission from: *Socio-Economic Factbook for Surgery 1995*. Chicago, Socioeconomic Affairs Department, American College of Surgeons.]

The corporatization of medicine began many years ago. In the western United States in the 19th century, mining, railroad, and forestry corporations had to provide health care for their employees in rural locations. The rise of Kaiser and other prepaid health-care plans immediately after World War II was at first held in check in the 1970s and 1980s; however, costs rose significantly and the stage was clearly set for managed care to come in and control health care costs when no other element in the private or public sector could do so. As Rhinehart (personal communication) has observed, the managed care companies are like the bounty hunters employed in the 19th century to catch animals who could not be caught by conventional law enforcement. The services of the managed care corporations are engaged by society for the purpose of restraining health care costs.

Recent data indicate that the managed care companies may be meeting with some success. Health insurance premiums in California, for example, appear to be decreasing for the first time in recent memory, and reports from the Congressional Budget Office (2) and other sources indicate that most elderly and employer-based subscribers to managed care plans are happy with the care that they get (although there is evidence that sicker patients are less pleased with their managed care plans). So at least for now, it appears that managed care is firmly entrenched in our health-care system and that no amount of nostalgia for the halcyon days of the '60s, '70s, and early '80s will dislodge it from its position.

Despite the successes that managed care has experienced so far, however, there are a few cracks showing up in the edifice. There is a growing impression that decisions are increasingly being made by the wrong people for the wrong reasons. Recent articles in the *Wall Street Journal* and the *New York Times* (3) have pointed to the increasingly large portion of the health-care dollar that is siphoned to administrative cost and profits in most large, for-profit, HMOs. At U.S. Healthcare, this number approaches 30% of the premiums collected (Fig. 2). The CEO of U.S. Healthcare, Mr. Leonard Abramson, last year earned $9.8 million in salary, bonuses, and options, and his yearly stock dividends accounted for another $11.4 million. The recent novel by John Grisham, *The Rainmaker* (4), describes in detail the inherent conflict between corporate profits and medical loss ratios in a large managed care organization. A group of employers in Minneapolis has recently indicated that they want to get the huge HMOs out of the middle of the relationship between patients and physicians and are trying to contract directly with groups of physicians and hospitals to provide care at a reasonable price. Finally, executives at the Glaxo Corporation, not-

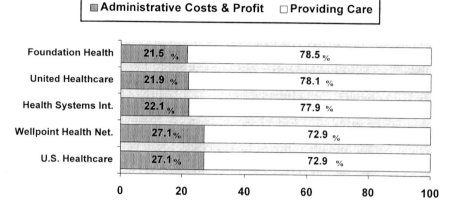

FIG. 2 Premium revenue allocation managed care plans. [Reproduced with permission from (3).]

ing decreased returns on their flagship products, Zantac and Imetrex, have suggested that corporate belt tightening, produced by managed care, may result in decreased corporate investment in research and development, raising the specter of diminished availability of innovations and pharmaceutical treatment for disease. All of these trends indicate that the weakness of the managed care juggernaut is increasingly being recognized by society at large.

Neurosurgeons, therefore, must do two things: (1) realize that managed care is here to stay and (2) devise strategies that will allow us to continue to improve our ability to care for patients within the context of managed care. Changes in the organization and financing of health care have always been difficult for practicing physicians, as this quote from an AMA leader in 1943 illustrates: "The AMA hierarchy was unalterably opposed to Blue Cross and Blue Shield." Our predecessors learned to adapt and thrive with Blue Cross and Blue Shield and, although times are very different now, we must also learn to change. Accepting the need for cost containment does not mean, however, that we must accept the techniques that managed care organizations are using to drive down costs (9). Specifically, neurosurgeons should fight against the tendency of managed care plans to have primary care physicians manage neurosurgical diseases. This simply represents rationing by ignorance. We should also fight the progressive substitution of low-tech, symptomatic treatment in cases in which scientifically based treatments are clearly superior.

Increasingly, fully integrated health care systems and managed care systems will be concerned about the quality of patient care. Pricing is the current battlefield; quality is the next battlefield. Right now, we are at a stage in which managed care companies can vigorously compete on price and be successful in enhancing their market share because of the huge transition that is occurring in health care. Eventually, however, the savings that can be gotten out of this system, even given proportional reductions in cost, will lead to a smaller absolute dollar savings, and plans will no longer be able to discriminate themselves based on cost alone. This stage will rapidly come upon us. Neurosurgery needs to be prepared to demonstrate quantitatively the effectiveness of our interventions and the superiority of a scientifically based approach to patient management and technological improvement.

Our specialty's renewed concentration on its scientific and technical foundation must occur on several levels. First, we must continue to improve our capabilities to care for individual patients. In some ways, we are better off than other specialties. There is a huge reservoir of basic neuroscience information that is waiting for practical application in the treatment of nervous system disease. Right now, only a trickle of this information is flowing into patient care—we need to decrease that flow so that patients can benefit from basic research. I believe that recent advances in the treatment of Parkinson's disease by neurosurgeons will be supplemented by advances in the treatment of neurodegenerative disease, craniospinal trauma, and malignant gliomas. All of this will be possible as a result of collaboration with basic neuroscience and the expansion of our capabilities to deal with nervous system disease. In this regard, I think it is appropriate for the Residency Review Committee in Neurosurgery to significantly enhance the standards of the neurosurgical residency training programs at this time to improve the clinical and research training that our residents receive. The time is right for changes to be made in this area. This will enhance the scientific basis of our discipline.

Such an enhancement of the scientific activities in neurosurgical residency training programs will come at a difficult time, however. Academic centers are being threatened by a multitude of factors. Clinical neurosurgical research supported by patient care revenues will be increasingly difficult, but we must continue to invest in the intellectual and technical infrastructure of our specialty. Organized neurosurgery should also vigorously lobby for continued generous support of basic neuroscience research and *augmented support* of patient-oriented research from the National Institutes of Health. This recommendation is in concert with the new director of the National

Institute of Health, Dr. Varmis, to increase patient-oriented research, despite an overall leveling off of NIH funding as bimedical research enters a steady state.

Another level on which neurosurgery must work to improve its scientific foundation is at the level of defining populations that can benefit from neurosurgical care. I believe that the main reason that neurosurgery and other scientifically based specialties in medicine have been marginalized with the development of managed care is that we have not been rigorous in providing the data to determine the value of what we do. Neurosurgeons must become much more skilled at quantitatively defining the financial cost and clinical benefit of our interventions. It is absolutely imperative, and I cannot emphasize this too much, that neurosurgeons in academic and community practice start to examine patient outcome using modern outcomes assessment and cost benefit analysis techniques. Notable progress has been made in this area by a few neurosurgeons but much, much more needs to be done on this, and it needs to be done rapidly.

Let me give you an example of where I think our lack of participation in population-based outcome studies has hurt us. Last week, an article concerning care for low back pain appeared in the *New England Journal of Medicine*[1]. The authors compared the outcomes among approximately 1500 patients with low back pain seen by primary care physicians, chiropractors, and orthopaedic surgeons. (Neurosurgeons were not included.) They found that the outcomes among all of these patients were essentially the same, no matter what group of practitioners evaluated them. Only about one fifth of the patients had any leg pain, and only in about 30% of the whole group of patients did the duration of the episode of pain last for longer than 2 weeks. Within hours this paper was picked up by the lay press and inappropriately generalized to all patients with back pain.

I believe that studies such as this one suffer from what I call the *High-Altitude Problem*. That is, if you get far enough away from two things they invariably will look the same, no matter how different they are. I recently looked at a photograph of St. Louis taken from the space shuttle. It looks like most of the eastern United States and Europe from this altitude. Similarly, if you look at the entire universe of patients with all types of back pain, no matter how minor or short lived, the positive effects of a careful specialist's evaluation and treatment will be hard to discern. This is the problem with looking at neurosurgical illness through the perspective of an epidemiologist or primary care physician. Neurosurgeons have generally not participated in studies such as this, because they suffer from another problem, the *Low-Al-*

titude Problem. a photograph taken through the operative microscope represents the usual level of perspective we have as neurosurgeons. We are generally so focused on the details of microsurgery, skull base surgery, and biomechanics that we have not taken the time to conduct enough studies that demonstrate our worth in taking care of patients in the context of a defined population. We simply must do more sophisticated assessments of clinical outcomes in our patients.

To handle the volume of data that will result from such studies, neurosurgery must also become much more skilled as a specialty at medical informatics. This will probably be done on a variety of levels in universities, in large integrated health plans, and in individual community practices. *Neurosurgery On Call* has recently been proposed by Dr. Sidney Tolchin, President of the AANS, to enhance outcomes assessment and information transfer between neurosurgeons. This project will be jointly sponsored by the AANS and CNS over the next few years. It is crucial that neurosurgeons take the time to become familiar with information management systems as they impact our specialty. This is the tremendous advantage that the managed care plans have over us at the present time, and we need to change that.

Finally, I believe that we need to continue to vigorously support our journals and major neurosurgical meetings. Over the past few years, attendance at the meetings of the Congress of Neurological Surgeons and the AANS has progressively increased. I believe that this is a logical response to the pressures that are upon us as a specialty. Recently, I have heard a number of opinions indicating that perhaps we cannot have two meetings a year. I do not believe that this is the case. The clinical demands in many practices make it impossible for coverage to be obtained for one meeting, and if neurosurgeons are only able to go to one major meeting every 2 to 3 years, the scientific foundations of our specialty will be eroded. Our meetings represent an extremely important function within our specialty. I believe that our meetings should increasingly concentrate on information technology and outcomes assessment to supplement their traditional emphasis on improvements in neurosurgical diagnosis and technique. It is only through such continuous improvement that our specialty will survive and thrive in the coming years.

Let me finish with some observations on the role of the specialist in today's health care. We have all seen the opinions expressed from multiple sources that there are too many neurosurgeons practicing in the United States. Despite the relative constancy of surgical subspecialists (Fig. 3), Weiner (11), in his study of medical manpower, has predicted that there will be a surplus of 150,000 physicians in the year 2000, and

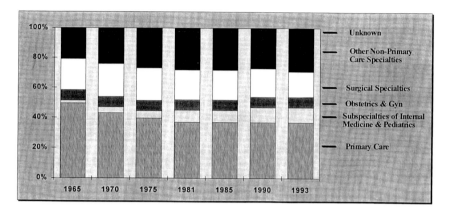

FIG. 3   Fully trained specialists. [Reproduced with permission from (2).]

almost all of these will be in specialties. He has estimated, based on staffing patterns at Kaiser and Group Health of Puget Sound, that about half the number of neurosurgeons that is currently practicing will be needed in the future. It's interesting to note that recent data has indicated that there will also probably be a surplus of primary care physicians (10).

These data have been extrapolated by many in the health policy establishment to suggest that care provided by specialists is somehow irrelevant or even bad. Yet, this concept runs counter to history and common sense. Adam Smith indicated, in the *Wealth of Nations* (8), that the division of labor—that is, specialization—inexorably increases as markets expand. The specialist inevitably concentrates his activities in the areas that enhance his ability to produce a better product. The rise of scientifically based medicine in Europe and the United States, especially within the past 100 years, has been founded on the focused scholarship and progress that characterized specialization. There is perhaps no other field in human endeavor that illustrates this better than our profession, neurosurgery. Cushing and others realized the fundamental principle that effective care for surgical diseases of the nervous system can only be provided by concentrated effort based on a coherent scientific knowledge base and a set of technical principles that are unique to the specialty. Biomedical science in the United States— which is unquestionably the best in the world—did not achieve its present greatness as the result of efforts by generalists. I agree that more generalists and fewer specialists need to be trained. We should probably be turning out fewer, but better trained, neurosurgeons. However, none of us should accept the propaganda that has emanated from the health policy establishment to suggest that neurosurgical diseases can be treated more effectively by generalists than by neurosurgeons. Such propaganda is widespread today and suggests that prevention and continuity of care can make up for a lack of knowledge and experience in the treatment of nervous system disease. Yet, our practical experience runs counter to these theoretical advantages of generalism. There is hardly any continuity of care in the current managed care maelstrom, and the few treatments that can prevent nervous system disease, such as carotid endarterectomy and clipping of unruptured aneurysms and resection of arteriovenous malformations, are largely administered not by generalists but by neurosurgeons.

Neurosurgery must press for easy access of patients with neurosurgical disease to the neurosurgeon. This is because primary care physicians are simply not equipped to deal with neurosurgical illnesses, as a result of their education and knowledge base. As the work of Ralph Lehman, et al. (5) has shown, students at medical schools in the United States have on average 1 to 2 weeks of exposure to neurosurgery and neurosurgery patients during their third-year clerkship. For most primary care physicians, this constitutes the entirety of exposure to neurosurgical diseases throughout their career. Recently, at Barnes Hospital and Washington University in St. Louis, neurology was removed as a rotation from the Pgy 1 year in the internal medicine training program to make space for more ambulatory care. It is extremely unlikely that any changes in training or CME would ever allow primary care physicians to be even marginally competent at dealing with neurosurgical illnesses. I know this from direct personal experience, having been trained in internal medicine years ago. It is remarkable that most training programs in internal medicine go to some length to inculcate residents with a feeling of confidence that they can deal with almost any problem simply because they are internists. How often have each of us witnessed that peculiar sense of confidence as subarachnoid hemorrhages are missed and intracranial mass lesions are mismanaged. Organized neurosurgery must press for early and easy access to patients with neurosurgical illnesses. I am confident that we can provide more cost-effective care with greater patient satisfaction, if patients can see us earlier in the course of their illness.

In summary, if neurosurgery's future is to be as distinguished as it's past, we must adapt to the new practice environment and conclusively document the effectiveness of our scientifically based treatments. We must jump into the fray and battle with the primary care health policy establishment to prove, in appropriately designed outcome studies, that the care we deliver is superior. Only if we do this will we shed the dysphoria that afflicts all specialists at this time. Neurosurgery's scientific and technical foundation has never been stronger; it's up to us to exploit this opportunity for the benefit of our patients.

REFERENCES

1. Carey TS, Garrett J, Jackman A, *et al.* The outcomes and costs of care for acute low back pain among patients seen by primary care practitioners, chiropractors, and orthopedic surgeons. **N Engl J Med** 333(14):913–917, 1995.
2. Congress of the United States Congressional Budget Office: *Medicare and Graduate Medical Education,* Washington, DC. U.S. Government Printing Office, 1995.
3. Freudenheim M: A bitter pill for the H.M.O.'s—swallow hard and cut your costs, customers say. *The New York Times,* April 28, 1995.
4. Grisham J: *The Rainmaker.* New York, Doubleday, 1995.
5. Lehman RAW, Brodner RA, Greenblatt SH, *et al.*: Clinical clerkships in neurosurgery and neurology at United States medical schools. **Neurosurgery** 29(4): 624–628, 1991.
6. Newhouse JP: An inconoclastic view of health cost containment. Health Aff (Millwood) 12(suppl):152–171, 1993.
7. Shine K: Making choices: for patients and physicians. **Bull Am Coll Surg** April: 1995.
8. Smith A: *The Wealth of Nations.*
9. Starr P: *The Social Transformation of American Medicine—the rise of a Sovereign Profession and the Making of a Vast Industry.* New York, Basic Books. 1982.
10. US Department of Health and Human Services, Public Health Service, Health Resources and Services Administration: Council on Graduate Medical Education, Sixth Report, *Managed Health Care: Implications for the Physician Workforce and Medical Education,* June 15, 1995.
11. Weiner JP: Forecasting the effects of health reform on US physician workforce requirement—evidence from HMO staffing patterns. **JAMA** 272(3):220–230, 1994.

I

General Scientific Session I—Innovations in Cranial Approaches and Exposures

2

Anterior Midline Approaches to the Central Skull Base

GRIFFITH R. HARSH IV, M.D., MICHAEL P. JOSEPH, M.D.,
BROOKE SWEARINGEN, M.D., AND ROBERT G. OJEMANN, M.D.

The central skull base presents a substantial challenge to surgical access. Problems are posed by the critical neurovascular structures that lesions in the region involve, by the depth of surgical field required, and the obstruction of operative exposure by important soft tissue structures of the head and neck and by bone that is structurally important, dense, and irregular and that itself invests crucial neural and vascular entities. Given these problems, surgical treatment of lesions of the central cranial base should be undertaken only with unequivocal necessity and extensive forethought and preparation. The goal of skull base surgery is usually exposure adequate for resection or repair of the lesion, avoidance of neural and vascular injury, prevention of CSF leakage, avoidance of infection, and satisfactory cosmesis. The basic principle guiding such surgery is maximizing exposure of the interface of pathologic lesion and critical neurovascular structure while minimizing brain retraction, usually by removing bone. This chapter will provide a brief review of the anatomy and pathology of the central cranial base as an introduction to a section of six chapters that present six directions of approach to this region; it will review more extensively recent innovations in anterior midline approaches to the central skull base; and it will present the authors' recent experience with one such approach, pedicled rhinotomy, to tumors in this region.

ANATOMY

The central skull base extends from the anterior inferior aspect of the frontal bone to the posterior clinoid processes and then down the clivus to the foramen magnum. It encompasses the frontal air sinuses anteriorly, the nasion, and paranasal air sinuses between the orbits, the foramen cecum, crista galli, cribriform plates, planum sphenoidale, tuberculum sellae, sella, and clivus from posterior clinoid processes through the foramen magnum. The roof of the ethmoid sinus begins in the midline just behind the foramen cecum. It contains the crista galli in the midline and cribriform plates bilaterally. The anterior and posterior ethmoidal arteries and olfactory nerves pass through foramina in the cribriform plates. The roof of the sphenoid sinus, the planum sphenoidale, begins just behind the cribriform plate and extends to the tuberculum sellae. Lateral to the cribriform plate and planum sphenoidale, the orbital processes of the frontal base, the plana orbitale, form the orbital roofs that converge posteromedially to the optic canals and the anterior clinoid processes. The anterior clinoid processes, extending laterally as the superior aspects of the lesser wings of the sphenoid bones, define the posterior margin of the ACF. The greater wing of the sphenoid bone forms part of the posterolateral wall of the orbit and contains the foramen rotundum and foramen ovale. Extending interiorly from the greater sphenoid wing between the foramen rotundum and the foramen ovale are the pterygoid plates.

The clivus extends from dorsum sellae to foramen magnum (Fig. 1). It can be divided into three parts. (a) The superior third from the dorsum sellae and posterior clinoid processes to the petrous apices is sphenoidal in origin: anteriorly lie the sella turcica and sphenoid sinus; laterally, the intracavernous internal carotid artery (ICA), cavernous sinus, tentorial notch, and temporal lobe; and posteriorly, the basilar

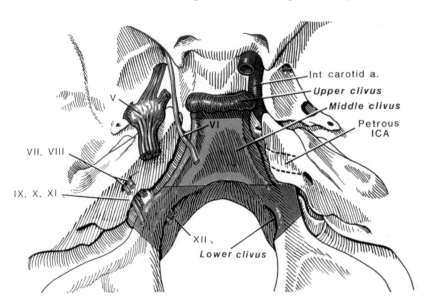

FIG. 1 Posterior view of the clivus and adjacent structures. The clivus can be divided into three parts. [Reproduced with permission from (36).]

artery, its branches, and the midbrain. (b) The middle third, between the petrous apex at Dorello's canal and the pars nervosa of the jugular foramen, is the superior extension of the basiocciput; anteriorly lie the nasopharynx and retropharyngeal tissue; laterally, the inferior petrosal sinus, the anterior petrous face, and seventh and eighth cranial nerves; and posteriorly, the basilar artery and its branches, the vertebrobasilar junction, and the pons. (b) The lower third, between the pars nervosa of the jugular foramen and the foramen magnum, includes the occipital condyles and hypoglossal canals of the basiocciput; anteriorly lie the nasopharynx and retropharyngeal tissues; laterally, the sigmoid sinus, jugular bulb, and hypoglossal nerve; and posteriorly, the vertebral artery, pontomedullary junction, medulla, and cervicomedullary junction (37).

PATHOLOGY

Four basic types of lesions of the central skull may warrant surgery: (a) bony anomalies, such as rheumatoid arthritis requiring resection of the odontoid process; occipital and upper cervical fractures or ligamentous injury requiring repair; basilar invagination and other craniospinal malformations requiring decompression; and meningocele; (b) tumors that may be either intracranial, intraosseous, or intranasal in origin: Intracranial tumors include meningioma, pituitary adenoma, schwannoma, hemangiopericytoma, and nasal glioma; intraosseous tumors include the benign osteoma, osteoblastoma, osteochrondroma, hemangioma, ossifying fibroma, and fibrous dysplasia; malignant varieties include metastases, chordoma, chondrosarcoma, chondroma, and osteogenic sarcoma; nasal and paranasal sinus tumors include benign lesions, such as nasopharyngeal angiofibroma and inverted papilloma, and malignant head and neck cancers, such as squamous cell carcinoma, adenocystic carcinoma, adenocarcinoma, esthesioneuroblastoma, sarcoma, and rhabdomyosarcoma; (c) infections of bone or soft tissues of the skull base, such as fungal or bacterial osteomyelitis; and (d) vascular lesions, such as vertebrobasilar aneurysms (20, 25, 31, 35, 36).

SURGICAL APPROACHES

Surgical approaches to these lesions of the central skull base can be organized from anterior midline to posterolateral. In that the skull base falls off from superior to inferior as one moves from foramen cecum to foramen magnum, the area of the skull base exposed by these various approaches moves from anterior superior to posterior inferior. For the purposes of this review, they have been divided into midline anterior cranial fossa (ACF), ACF oblique, middle cranial fossa (MCF)

TABLE 1
Surgical Routes to the Central Skull Base

Approach	Bones Traversed	Limiting Structures
ACF midline	Frontal, ethmoid, sphenoid maxilla	Orbits and optic nerves Cavernous, petrous ICA Vertebral arteries
ACF oblique	Frontal (orbital), sphenoid (lesser wing)	Paranasal air sinuses Optic nerves Contents of superior orbital fissure
MCF anterior	Frontal, temporal (squamous), sphenoid (lesser, greater wing)	Optic nerve Intracavernous ICA
MCF posterior	Temporal (squamous), temporal (anterior petrous)	Petrous ICA, V3, VII, VIII
PCF superior	Temporal (posterior petrous)	VII, VIII, sigmoid sinus
PCF inferior	Occipital (lateral)	Sigmoid sinus, vertebral arteries, VI, IX-XII

anterior, MCF posterior, posterior cranial fossa (PCF) superior, and PCF inferior. The area of the skull base exposed and the bones removed in achieving this exposure are listed in Table 1.

ANTERIOR MIDLINE APPROACHES TO THE SKULL BASE

An anterior approach is usually preferred for lesions of the anterior skull base. It should achieve full exposure of the tumor, permit repair of dural defects, and be cosmetically acceptable. Lateral barriers to the central skull base include the orbits and optic nerves, cavernous sinus, both cavernous and petrous segments of the ICA, cranial nerves III to XII, maxilla, mandible, and vertebral artery. Midline anterior approaches have anatomic and physiologic advantages. The face is a bilaterally symmetric structure, formed from the midline fusion of paranasal, frontal, maxillary, and mandibular processes during embryogenesis (17). This midline plane of fusion provides an optimal plane of surgical cleavage. Division of facial soft tissues and bone along this plane is less traumatic and more easily repaired than is the case with paramedian or lateral approaches. In that the neural and vascular supply to these paired processes pass to the midline from each side, a midline cleavage plane is usually less vascular and risks injury to distal rather than proximal vessels and nerves. Expansion of midline tumors will often displace the structures that limit lateral exposure. The lateral origin of the blood supply also provides perfusion of pedicled flaps based laterally. Reconstruction of midline dissections recapitulates embryogenesis and thus is more likely to be functionally and esthetically satisfactory (18).

Most anterior approaches utilize the cavities of the nose, paranasal sinuses, mouth, and pharynx as portals through which posterior structures can be viewed. Placing retractors within these cavities opens a wide surgical approach with a more shallow depth of field than would otherwise be obtained. Working through air-filled cavities avoids the more extensive dissection and blood loss concomitant to traverse of solid bone or soft tissue. Retraction of brain is either unnecessary or minimized by removal of bone; cerebral swelling does not occur; the facial swelling that can occur is well tolerated and without permanent sequelae (17). Traverse of the face and these nasal and oropharyngeal cavities, however, has distinct disadvantages as well. The contaminated field risks soft-tissue infections, osteomyelitis, and brain abscess or meningitis. Facial incisions and osteotomies of the facial skeleton risk contracting scar and disfigurement that may be cosmetically and psychologically injurious. Visceral functions of speech, swallowing, and airway management are also vulnerable. In general, two basic principles (at times in conflict with one another) should be kept in mind: (a) pathology ventral to the brainstem and spinal cord should be approached from an anterior route because of the risk of retraction of these structures. (b) Intradural extension is a strong relative contraindication to a transnasal or transoral route because of the difficulty of dural repair and the high risk of meningitis. If the tumor extends from anteriorly into the dura, however, the need to repair the dura and the risk of meningitis are present with all directions of approach.

There are two basic anterior midline routes to the central skull base: transnasal and transoral. The nasal cavity and associated paranasal air sinuses are limited superiorly by the floor of the ACF and interiorly by the hard palate of the maxilla. The oral cavity is limited superiorly by the hard palate and inferiorly by the tongue and mandible. Each basic approach can be extended, both superiorly and interiorly: (a) the transnasal route, superiorly by combination with a frontal craniotomy in a transbasal or craniofacial approach (27) and inferiorly by combination with a maxillotomy that divides the hard palate (21); and (b) the transoral route, superiorly by division of the soft palate and removal of part of the hard palate (1) and inferiorly by combination with division of the tongue, floor of mouth, and mandible (11). The two exposures at the superior and inferior extremes of transnasal and transoral routes, in their simplest forms, avoid traverse of contaminated cavities: (a) A frontal craniotomy through the lower frontal bone does open the frontal air sinus, but this can be permanently obliterated prior to opening of the dura and poses relatively little risk to intracranial contamination. A standard low bifrontal craniotomy is adequate for removal of many basal ACF tumors, closure of CSF fistulae, and repair of encephaloceles. Extension of tumors to the ethmoid or sphenoid sinuses, sella, or clivus requires combining frontal craniotomy with traverse of other paranasal sinuses (4, 27, 33). (b) A transcervical approach takes an extraoral, retropharyngeal route to the upper cervical spine (39). It is useful for decompression and stabilization at the C1-C2 level, particularly when bone grafting is used. Cranial exposure is limited to the most caudal tip of the clivus. Tumors extending across the anterior craniovertebral junction will require an oropharyngeal route (3, 8, 25).

The clivus is the defining osseous component of the central cranial base. Anterior midface approaches to the central skull base have transclival exposure of dura as their final common pathway. Consideration of various anterior routes is simplified by the realization that, in the axial planes, the clivus lies behind the nose (Fig. 2). Each extends superiorly to inferiorly for 4 to 5 cm. The superior third of the clivus involving the posterior clinoid process and dorsum sellae down to the level of the petrous apex lies behind the upper third of the nose, the ethmoid and sphenoid sinuses, and the sella. The middle third of the clivus extending from the petrous apex to the jugular foramen lies be-

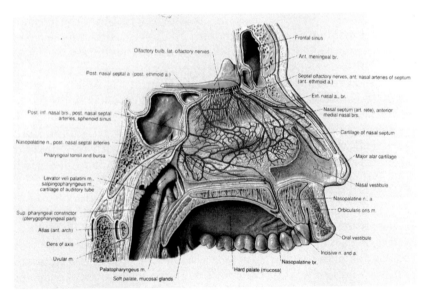

FIG. 2 Midsagittal view of the nose and clivus. The nose and clivus are coextensive superiorly and inferiorly. [Reproduced with permission from (28).]

hind the middle third of the nose, the nasal cartilage, and the superior nasopharynx. The lower third of the clivus extending from the jugular foramen to the foramen magnum lies behind the lower third of the nose, the vomer, the soft palate, and the inferior nasopharynx. All aspects of the clivus can be accessed through the nose, and nasal traverse is key to most transfacial approaches to the clivus (29). The superior limit of the clivus is the floor of the ACF. Expansion of a transnasal exposure superiorly is achieved by craniotomy in a transbasal approach (12). The inferior limit of the nose is the hard palate. Extension of exposure below the clivus to the anterior cervical region can be achieved by adding maxillotomy in a transpalatal approach (2, 5, 15, 21) or shifting beneath the maxilla in a transoral approach (3, 8). The various anterior midface approaches can thus be considered in terms of their ability to enlarge the nasal cavity. In that their superior and inferior limits of exposure are similar, the anterior midface approaches differ primarily in the extent of lateral exposure they provide. Increased lateral exposure has two benefits: (a) access is provided to progressively more lateral structures of the skull base and (b) surgical instruments and the surgeon's fingertips can be moved closer to the skull base pathology as the surgical corridor is widened. The depth of the surgical field can be diminished substantially.

Anterior midface approaches through the nose encounter the maxilla on each side. The nose is bounded by the ascending maxillary processes and the medial wall of the maxillary sinuses on each side and the hard plate of the maxilla below. Transnasal and midface approaches can be widened by expanding into the maxilla: (a) Medial maxillotomy is an opening in the medial maxillary wall; the bone can be pushed laterally or removed (9, 13, 22). (b) Medial maxillectomy is the removal of the entire medial maxillary wall; the medial inferior orbital rim may also be removed (35). (c) Transverse maxillotomy separates the hard palate from the maxillary sinuses so that it can be displaced downward into the oral cavity (5, 33). (d) Sagittal maxillotomy is a midline division of the hard palate; when transverse and sagittal maxillotomy are combined, the palate can be displaced downward, and each half can be moved laterally (2, 15). (e) Extended subtotal maxillotomy detaches and rotates a segment of maxilla that includes the inferior orbital rim, palate, and sinus walls (7). (f) Extended subtotal maxillectomy completely removes such a segment (7). (g) Facial translocation frees medial maxillary units to permit their lateral rotation (17, 18). With these different techniques, progressively greater exposure of the skull base can be obtained by removing progressively greater amounts of the maxilla (Fig. 3).

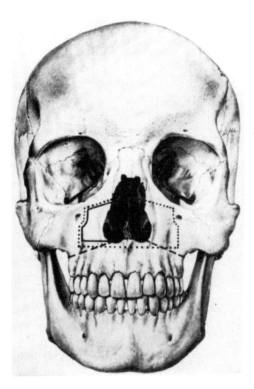

FIG. 3 Maxillotomies. Osteotomies of the maxilla: unilateral (*solid line*), bilateral (*dotted line*), and transverse (LeFort I, *dashed line*) enlarge the transnasal route. [Reproduced with permission from (13).]

Two basic categories of incision are used in these midface approaches: mucosal incisions and facial incisions. Mucosal incisions are of three types: (a) septal transfixion, which exposes the cartilaginous septum, vomer, and sphenoid sinus; (b) sublabial, which exposes the midline anterior maxilla laterally to the foramen of the infraorbital nerve; and (c) midface degloving, a combination of septal transfixion and sublabial incisions that extends exposure as far as the maxillary buttresses bilaterally (6, 24, 30). Similarly, facial incisions can be characterized by their extent and the subsequent lateral exposure of the maxilla achieved: (a) A simple lateral rhinal incision through the lateral superior aspect of the nasal skin permits a transethmosphenoid exposure of the superior and midclivus (9, 22). (b) A lateral and inferolateral incision opens a full transnasal exposure that permits medial maxillotomy or maxillectomy and a transmaxillary, as well as a transethmosphenoid, approach (34). (c) Further inferior extension through the philtrum divides the upper lip and exposes the nose and complete maxilla on one side (7). (d) Bilateral face incisions permit opening of the nose and both maxillae (17). As the length of these facial incisions and the extent of soft-tissue mobilization accompanying them increase, greater lateral exposure of the maxilla is accomplished, but the risk of unsightly deformity increases as well.

Recent innovative modifications of transfacial approaches that will prove most useful include the following: (a) medial maxillotomy added to a transnasal, transsphenoid, or transethmosphenoid approach; this extends the standard exposure of the sella laterally to include the inferomedial aspect of the cavernous sinus (Fig. 4) (13); (b) medial maxillectomy; this exposes cranial base lesions extending well lateral to the clivus (Fig. 5) (35); (c) the extended frontal modification of the trans-

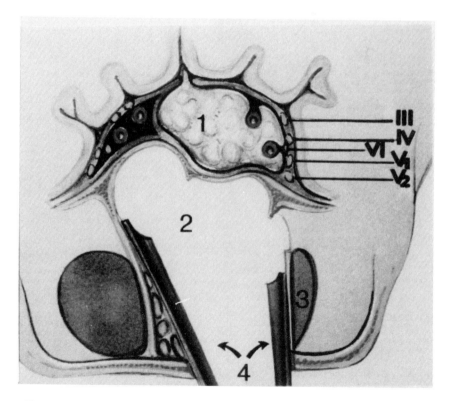

FIG. 4   Medial maxillotomy. The transnasal (4)-transsphenoidal (2) approach to a sellar tumor (1), extending into the cavernous sinus, is enlarged by lateral displacement of the medial wall of the maxillary sinus (3) to provide better exposure of lateral extensions of tumor. [Reproduced with permission from (13).]

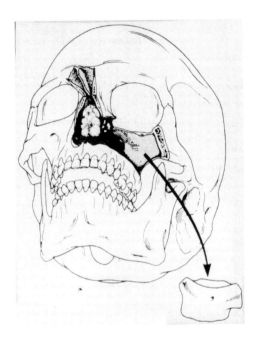

FIG. 5 Medial maxillotomy. The transnasal route is expanded laterally by midface degloving and osteotomies of the nasal and maxillary bones. The anterior maxilla and attached orbital floor are replaced in closure. [Reproduced with permission from (34).]

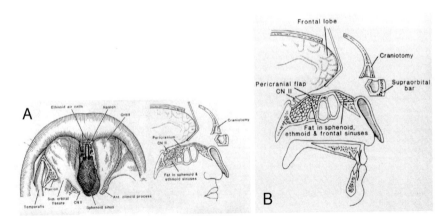

FIG. 6 The extended frontal transbasal approach. Removal of both superior orbital
rims (*supraorbital bar*) and opening into ethmoid and sphenoid sinuses permits a more
oblique view of the clivus with less frontal lobe retraction. In closure, opened ethmoid air
cells are packed with fat and covered with a pericranial flap. [Reproduced with permission from (35).]

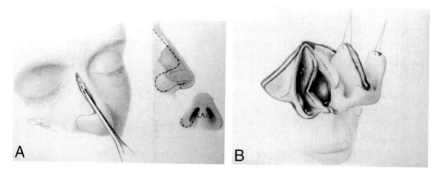

FIG. 7 (A and B) Pedicled rhinotomy: incision and nasal dissection. The lateral rhino-tomy incision passes down the nasofacial line around the right ala nasi and across the columella. Nasal osteotomies and removal of the nasal septum develop a small ipsilateral flap and a large nasal flap pedicled contralaterally. [Reproduced with permission from (19)].

basal approach; this expands superior exposure posteriorly by opening the paranasal cavities from above (Fig. 6) (36); (d) inferior maxillotomy, the combination of transverse release and sagittal division of the maxilla; this extends the transnasal approach inferiorly (Fig. 3) (2, 15); and (e) pedicled rhinotomy; this provides access to the entire clivus and craniovertebral junction down to the body of C2 without the need for extended maxillotomy or maxillectomy (Fig. 7) (10, 20, 40).

Medial Maxillotomy in Transnasal-Transsphenoid and Transethmosphenoid Approaches

The standard transseptal, transsphenoidal route to the sella provides excellent exposure of the sphenoid sinus, sella, and immediately subadjacent clivus. Lateral exposure at the level of the sella, particularly of the adjacent cavernous sinuses, is limited by the orthogonal midline orientation of the nasal speculum. This orientation results from the restrictions posed by the medial maxillary walls on either side. Lateral extensions of sellar tumors into the posterolateral sphenoid and inferomedial cavernous sinus require more laterally directed exposure. This can be achieved either by placing the speculum more laterally after lateral displacement of the medial wall of the maxillary sinus (in a transnasal-transsphenoid approach with medial maxillotomy) or by orienting the speculum obliquely (in a transethmosphenoid approach with medial maxillotomy).

The transseptal-transsphenoidal route to the sella begins with either a transnasal septal transfixion incision or a sublabial superior alveolar mucosal incision (23). Both attain the nasal septal midline, expose the sphenoid rostrum, and permit wide opening of the sphenoid sinus. The rostrum, the anterior aspects of the lateral walls, and the mucosal lining of the sphenoid are removed. When aeration of the sphenoid sinus is deficient, the route must be enlarged by drilling away the walls of the sinus. The anterior face of the sella, its floor back to the clivus, and the clivus from the sella floor to the inferior aspect of the sphenoid sinus can be removed. Exposure extends from the tuberculum sellae through the clivus at the level of the sphenoid sinus floor. Usually, lateral exposure extends only to the medial walls of the cavernous sinuses. This exposure is adequate for small tumors of the sphenoid sinus, sella, and upper third of the clivus with only limited lateral extension. Larger intrasellar tumors can be removed through a wide sphenoid and sellar opening if they have expanded the sella and pushed the medial walls of the cavernous sinus laterally; suprasellar tumor is accessed if the tumor has extended superiorly and posteriorly in the line of transseptal approach.

Tumors extending laterally into the cavernous sinus can be exposed by extending removal of the bone of the anterior wall and floor of the sella laterally out over the cavernous sinus (14). Removal of bone from the superior posterolateral aspect of the sphenoid sinus and inferomedial cavernous sinus, however, risks injury to the underlying intracavernous ICA and warrants a more direct view. A direct view of more lateral posterior structures is achieved by opening the maxillary sinus more anteriorly. As the transnasal speculum is being placed, the medial wall of the maxillary sinus is fractured and displaced laterally toward its lateral wall (Fig. 4). This more lateral fenestration proximally opens a more direct view of the superior posterolateral sphenoid sinus. After the anterior wall and floor of the sella are removed, the posterolateral sphenoid sinus wall is thinned with a drill as needed and removed with microcurettes to expose the dura of the inferomedial cavernous sinus. The sellar dura is opened in the normal fashion, and the tumor is resected. The opening in the sellar dura is then extended laterally into the dura of the inferior aspect of the cavernous sinus. As tumor is gently removed, bleeding is controlled with Surgicel packing. Tumor removal exposes to direct vision the intracavernous ICA. Because the cavernous sinus is approached by an inferomedial route, the cranial nerves, which are lateral and superior, are preserved (13).

An alternative means of achieving this lateral exposure is the transethmosphenoid approach (9, 22). It exposes the entire sphenoid sinus, the sella, the superior half of the clivus, and the prepontine space through a paramedian approach. A curvilinear incision is extended inferiorly from just beneath the medial aspect of the eyebrow down between the inner canthus of the eye and the dorsum of the nose. Periosteum of the nasal dorsum and the anterior half of the lamina papyracea is elevated, and the orbital contents are retracted laterally. The lacrimal sac is elevated, and the underlying ethmoid cells are entered. The lamina papyracea is removed past the foramen of the anterior ethmoidal artery to that of the posterior ethmoidal artery lying just anterior to the distal optic canal. The bony labyrinth of the ethmoid is removed, and the sphenoid sinus is entered. The rostrum, floor, and septations of the sphenoid sinus are removed. If required to expose the contralateral sphenoclival area, the posterior 2 cm of the vomer is removed. After retractors are placed, exposure extends from the tuberculum sellae above to the midclival area below. Lateral exposure is limited by the cavernous and petrous ICAs to a total of 2 cm. This exposure is obtained at a depth of field that is more shallow than is the case with a more inferior transnasal approach. It involves less soft-tissue dissection than facial degloving, and the extent of facial incision is really quite limited.

This exposure can be expanded in a number of ways. Transsellar exposure of the suprasellar region is limited by the more orthogonal approach to the sella face. For tumors that extend intracranially, this transethmosphenoid approach is combined with bilateral frontal craniotomy in an anterior craniofacial resection (4, 27). Asymmetric extension of the tumor beyond the ICA on one side, particularly posterolaterally, warrants an approach through the contralateral side of the nose, the posterior nasal septum, and the ethmoid sinus (22). This provides an oblique view with improved exposure of the posterosuperior lateral wall of the sphenoid sinus covering the ICA above and of the midclivus out to Dorello's canals below. Should the tumor extend posterolateral to the ICA on both sides, then bilateral transsphenoethmoid routes may be needed. As with the transnasal-transseptal approach, inferolateral exposure of posterior structures can be increased by opening into the maxillary sinus anteriorly (13). This requires extending the paranasal incision inferiorly and then removing the medial wall of the maxillary sinus (medial maxillotomy) and the middle and inferior nasal turbinates (Fig. 3). Exposure then includes the lower half of the clivus, almost to the foramen magnum. If the tumor extends below the craniocervical junction, an inferior maxillotomy or a transoral approach may be needed.

In summary, the predominant advantage of these laterally directed modifications of the transnasal-transsphenoid and transethmoid approaches is better exposure of the inferomedial cavernous sinus. Risks include bleeding from the cavernous sinus, injury to the intracavernous and intrapetrous internal carotid artery (ICA), and sixth nerve palsies.

Medial Maxillectomy

The exposure resulting from the addition of medial maxillotomy to the transethmosphenoid approach is limited by its unilaterality and by constraints of soft tissue on exposure of the lateral aspects of the maxillary face. These limits are overcome by midface degloving that exposes the full medial-to-lateral extent of both anterior maxillae (6, 24). The maxillary bone and sinus thus exposed can be removed either in pieces by rongeuring away the walls of the sinus or en bloc as maxillary segment consisting of maxillary bone about the sinus and the anterior orbital floor (35). Both maneuvers extend the transnasal-transethmosphenoid exposure laterally in attempts to resect nasal and craniofacial malignant tumors, such as large invasive pituitary adenomas, chordomas, and sinus carcinomas, in the posterior sphenoid and clival region with significant lateral extension.

Midface degloving, mobilization of the soft tissues from the midface skeleton, allows extensive bilateral medial maxillotomy, as well as ethmoidectomy and sphenoidectomy (6, 24). Midface degloving involves a combination of intranasal and sublabial incisions: intranasal incisions include a complete transfixion incision (between the columella and septum), bilateral circumferential piriform aperture incisions within the vestibule at the mucoperiosteal junction, and bilateral intercartilaginous incisions between the upper and lower lateral nasal cartilages (30). The nasal tip and its lower lateral cartilaginous skeleton are then separated from the septum, upper lateral cartilage, and nasal dorsum. Mucosa is mobilized from the nasal floor. Soft tissues of the nasal dorsum are widely elevated in the subperiosteal plane through intercartilaginous incisions bilaterally from nasal supertip up to the maxillary nasal suture at the glabella. A bilateral sublabial incision extends between the two first molars and permits elevation of the soft tissues covering the anterior maxilla. Dissection in the subperiosteal plane is carried from the nasal elevation medially to the zygomatic buttresses bilaterally. The soft tissues of the face, including the lips, cheeks, nasal tip, columella, and nasal skin, are then elevated superiorly to the infraorbital rim, sparing the infraorbital nerve. This exposes the anterior walls of the maxillary sinuses bilaterally up to the infraorbital rim. A midface degloving is repaired by replacing the nasal tip and other soft tissues of the face. The vestibular and then the sublabial incisions are closed, and the nose is taped and splinted.

Medial maxillectomy is begun by breaking through the anterior wall of the maxillary sinus and resecting the anterior wall from its junction with the nasal bone medially, the zygomatic buttress laterally, the infraorbital rim superiorly, and the maxillary sinus floor interiorly (30).

Osteotomy cuts release bone from the superior and inferior margins of the piriform fossa, and the frontal process of the maxilla is removed. Both ethmoid sinuses and the sphenoid sinus are entered by opening the medial wall of the maxillary sinus. Ethmoidectomy and sphenoidectomy are performed by removing their walls. The nasal septum is displaced contralaterally, and the anterior skull base is exposed. The posterior maxillary wall and the ascending palatine process are removed to expose the clivus. Excessive bleeding from the greater palatine and sphenopalatine arteries needs to be avoided (30). The resulting exposure thus includes nasal, ethmoid, and sphenoid cavities; the nasopharynx; the clivus and posterior bone; and the medial pterygoid region. The floor of the ACF and the palate pose limits superiorly and inferiorly, respectively.

Medial en bloc maxillectomy involves removal and subsequent replacement of the anterior maxilla and orbital floor on one or both sides (35). Midface degloving incisions and a short midline incision at the nasion permit subperiosteal elevation of the soft tissues over the maxillae. Bilateral superior nasal and transverse nasion osteotomies permit elevation of the nasal bridge and completion of the midface degloving. The nose is retracted superiorly after the septum is cut. The exposed anterior maxilla is divided by osteotomies through the frontal process of the maxilla; the anterior, inferior, and posterior wall of the maxillary sinus; and the malar process, such that the anterior maxillary wall, infraorbital rim, and anterior half of the orbital floor can be removed (Fig. 5). Ethmoidectomy, sphenoidectomy, and removal of the posterior maxillary wall and ascending palantine processes provide exposure of the cribriform plate, inferomedial orbital apex, sella, and clivus. The limits of the exposure are as follows: (a) the ACF floor and frontal air sinus, best exposed in combination with a transbasal approach; (b) the medial canthal and lacrimal region that requires medial orbital exploration; (c) the ICA within the petrous apex that is best approached laterally; (d) the far lateral maxilla, accessible through a lateral rhinotomy and unilateral facial flap; and (e) the upper cervical spine below C2. The maxillary segment is replaced using titanium miniplates for fixation.

In summary, this extensive exposure of the anterior middle skull base bilaterally is achieved without the risk of palatal necrosis inherent in transpalatal approaches and without significant facial incision. The predominant risks are necrosis of the maxillary segment and damage to overlying soft tissue that might deform the face, sinusitis, osteomyelitis, bleeding, crusting, facial paresthesias, excessive tearing, and diplopia. Even more lateral exposure requires the longer facial incisions and greater facial disassembly of extended maxillotomy (7), extended subtotal maxillectomy (7), and facial translocations (17, 18).

The Transbasal Approach

Transfacial exposure is extended superiorly for pathology of the median ACF by combining bifrontal craniotomy with opening of the frontal, ethmoid, and sphenoid sinuses. The osteotomies for combined craniofacial exposure were initially used for repair of developmental anomalies (41). They were subsequently incorporated into the transbasal approach to tumors of the anterior skull base (12). The combination of bifrontal craniotomy and superior ethmosphenoidectomy exposes the floor of the ACF from inferior frontal bone to the tuberculum sellae and from the sella down the clivus beyond the foramen magnum to the C2 level. It permits en bloc resection of tumors of the median anterior skull and their extensions into the cranial cavity, the ethmoid and sphenoid sinuses, and the clivus.

Attempts at en bloc resection are appropriate for tumors limited to midline structures that are resectable, such as the frontal, ethmoid, and sphenoid sinuses; the lamina papyracea; the perpendicular plate of the ethmoid; the nasal septum; and the superior and middle turbinates (4, 27, 28). Tumors involving these structures may be sarcoma, adenocarcinoma, squamous cell carcinoma, esthesioneuroblastoma, or neuroendocrine cancers. The transbasal approach is inadequate for tumors invading the inferior orbit or maxillary sinuses. Such lateral extension requires transmaxillary exposure. When tumors extend laterally into the parasellar or petrous apex regions, the transbasal approach should be combined with a more lateral route, such as the subtemporal preauricular infratemporal or the anterior transpetrous approach (37). If intracranial extension is limited and involvement of the skull base is anterior and superior, a simple transbasal approach is appropriate. Deep subfrontal exposure is not needed. Simultaneous opening of the dura and paranasal sinuses can be avoided by a two-stage approach (4). A bifrontal craniotomy permits initial removal of subfrontal and intraparenchymal tumor. The frontal air sinuses should be repaired by removing their posterior wall and plugging their ostia with muscle, bone dust, or fat before the dura is opened. After intracranial tumor is removed, the dura is closed and reinforced before the more inferior resection that involves opening for paranasal sinus cavities. The dural opening should be repaired primarily. Small tears about the cribiform plate and crista galli should be covered with a free graft of pericranium or fascia lata. This dural repair is subsequently reinforced by a pedicled pericranial graft (32, 38).

Tumor involving the nose and paranasal air sinuses is then removed. Paranasal facial incisions expose nasal bone and cartilage and permit entry into the ethmoid, sphenoid, and maxillary sinuses, as described above. Periorbita is dissected from the medial orbital wall, and the anterior and posterior ethmoidal arteries are identified and coagulated. Horizontal osteotomies are carried through the medial wall of each orbit at its junction with the orbital floor. Posteriorly, vertical cuts are extended from above at the level of the posterior ethmoidal foramina. Anteriorly, similar vertical cuts are made from the lacrimal fossae to the nasion. The vomer is transected through the nasopharynx. The posterior cuts are completed by extension from the posterior sphenoid sinus to the nasopharynx. When en bloc resection is needed, paramedian cuts lateral to the tumor are carried through the medial roof of the orbit and turned medially into the planum sphenoidale posterior to the posterior margin of the tumor (4, 12, 27). This releases tumor of the ACF to be removed along with tumor from the paranasal sinus. This creates a defect with margins consisting of the posterior portion of the planum sphenoidale or the tuberculum sellae and optic nerves posteriorly, the periorbita bilaterally, and the nasopharynx inferiorly. Repair of this defect prevents CSF leak.

Tumors that involve more of the ACF floor and extend down the clivus require more posterior exposure. The extended frontal modification of the transbasal approach provides this; osteotomies of the nasion and both superior orbital rims permit a more basal approach that minimizes the need for frontal lobe retraction (Fig. 6) (31, 36). It begins with a bicoronal incision extending from the temporal region just anterior to the origin of the zygomatic arch on one side to that on the other. Scalp, including the pericranium, is elevated over the frontal bone and supraorbital ridges down to the nasion medially and the frontozygomatic suture bilaterally. Temporalis muscle and fascia are divided from their anterior and superior attachments and reflected laterally. A bifrontal craniotomy extending to within 1 cm of the orbital rim is opened. Basal frontal dura is dissected from the crista galli, cribriform plates, planum sphenoidale, and orbital roofs bilaterally. The olfactory nerves are divided at the cribriform plate. The ACF floor back to the base of the anterior clinoid processes, the tuberculum sellae, and the posterior edge of the left wing of the sphenoid is exposed extradurally. Periorbita is stripped form the orbital roof and medial and lateral walls. The anterior and posterior ethmoidal arteries are coagulated and divided, using the posterior ethmoid foramen as a limit of posterior exposure to avoid injury to the optic nerve in the distal optic canal. A supraorbital bar, which includes the nasion and supraorbital rims bilaterally, is separated by osteotomies that divide both frontozy-gomatic sutures laterally and pass lateral to medial across each orbital roof (approximately 2 cm behind the orbital rim) to just anterior to the cribriform plates (36). A horizontal cut through the frontonasal suture frees the supraorbital bar. This removal of supraorbital rims opens a path to the ACF floor that requires less retraction of the frontal lobes (16, 19). The orbital roofs are removed by drilling from anterior to posterior toward the optic canal. The sphenoid sinus is entered through the planum sphenoidale at the posterior aspect of the resection. Both optic nerves can be decompressed as needed. The ethmoid air cells are unroofed, and the medial wall of each orbit is removed back to the posterior ethmoidal foramen.

The cribriform plate and planum sphenoidale of the ACF floor, the upper walls of the ethmoid and sphenoid sinuses, and the anterior wall and floor of the sella are resected. This provides excellent exposure of the clivus from the tuberculum sellae to the foramen magnum. Hidden from direct view are the dorsum sellae and posterior clinoid processes (36). Removal of additional ethmoid air cells permits a more orthogonal inferior view, extending the range of exposure to the C1-C2 level (Fig. 6). Pharyngeal mucosa may be dissected from the anterior arch of C1 and C2. Although the anterior petrous apices can be seen, the ICA defines the lateral limit of exposure inferiorly, just as the optic nerves do superiorly.

Closure begins with the dural repair described above. Opened ethmoid air cells are then plugged with fat and Surgicel. The anteriorly pedicled pericranial flap supplied by supraorbital and supratrochlear arteries is passed over the exposed superior orbits and remaining orbital roofs (32, 38). Its posterior margin is sutured to the basal dura as far posteriorly as possible (Fig. 6). Reconstruction of the base is required if the orbital floor and the medial walls of both orbits have been removed. Large osseous defects in the floor can be repaired with split calvarial bone placed between the pericranial flap and dura; this, however, is not usually necessary (36). If the anterior frontal base above the nasion has been resected, it is reconstructed with bone graft to avoid midline meningocele or encephalocele, enophthalmos or pulsatile exophthalmus, CSF leak, and an unsatisfactory appearance.

Potential complications include the following: (a) CSF leakage associated with pneumocranium, pneumocephalus, meningitis, and epidural, subdural, or intracranial abscess; (b) frontal lobe contusion, edema, or seizures; (c) cranial nerve loss, especially cranial nerves I through VI; (d) injury to the ICA carotid artery; (e) unsatisfactory cosmesis secondary to facial incisions, bone deformities, or resorption of the cranial plate; (f) retraction of the globe; (g) mucocele of the paranasal sinuses; and (h) palatal dysfunction.

In summary, advantages of the extended frontal transbasal approach include reduction of the frontal lobe retraction needed and facilitation of early interruption of the tumor's blood supply. Disadvantages of this approach include its time-consuming, technically challenging nature, the depth of the field, particularly in its inferior extent, the possibility of frontal lobe injury, and the risk of meningitis.

Inferior Maxillotomy

Inferior maxillotomy combines transverse and sagittal maxillotomies to create hemimaxillotomy flaps (2, 15). It expands the transnasal-transmaxillary exposures inferiorly into the oropharynx by temporarily mobilizing and downwardly displacing a sagitally divided hard palate. The transverse maxillotomy alone extends transnasal exposure to near the foramen magnum; palatal split extends exposure to the C2-C3 disk.

Inferior maxillotomy requires tracheostomy. A sublabial superior alveolar mucosal incision is extended bilaterally from midline to beyond the upper molars. Mucosa and periosteum are elevated to expose the floor of the nasal cavity and the anterior and lateral walls of the maxilla to the maxillary buttress bilaterally. Maxillary mucoperiosteum, upper lip, and anterior nasal soft tissue are retracted superiorly. The mucoperiosteum of the nasal floor is reflected from the piriform aperture to the level of the soft palate. The nasal septum is sectioned horizontally at its junction with the maxilla. The maxillary tuberosities are separated from the pterygoid plates. Oblique maxillary osteotomies are planned through the maxillary buttress, and holes for fixation plates are drilled to ensure alignment before the cuts are made (15). The cuts are carried through the maxilla at an angle to avoid the dental roots, the infraorbital nerve, and the palatine artery and nerve (Fig. 3). The mobilized maxilla, including the hard palate, is downfractured into the oral cavity. If sagittal maxillotomy is not needed, nasal mucosa is dissected, the nasal septum is displaced, and the vomer is removed. The transoral retractor with the transmaxillary plate adaptor is placed in the expanded nasal cavity. The sphenoid sinus is opened, and the sella and superior clivus are exposed. The sphenoid floor and midclivus are exposed by incising and elevating the overlying pharyngeal mucosa and constrictor muscles. The floor of the sphenoid sinus is removed as needed, and the clivus is drilled open. Exposure from this transverse (LeFort) osteotomy alone extends from tuberculum to lower clivus (5, 33).

Midsagittal division of the downwardly displaced hard and soft palates significantly extends exposure superiorly and inferiorly, as well as laterally (2, 15). After the dissection and LeFort osteotomy described above, a midsagittal incision is placed in the mucoperiosteum of the hard palate. A midsagittal cut is taken through the hard palate and between the medial incisors. Median section is completed by dividing the soft palate in the midline down to the base of the uvula and then turning obliquely so as to leave the uvula intact. This allows a hemimaxillary flap to swing laterally to each side. The vomer can be removed to expose the roof of the nasopharynx, sphenoid sinus, and clivus. The pharyngeal mucosa, longus capitis, and longus colli are dissected. The resultant exposure extends from the floor of the sphenoid sinus to the tip of the clivus and across the craniovertebral junction to the C2-C3 disk. Lateral exposure can be further increased by lateral fracture of the pterygoid plates, which permits greater lateral displacement of the maxillary flaps (15). After resection of the neoplastic or osseous lesion, maxillary osteotomies are repaired with titanium fixation plates.

In summary, the combined inferior maxillotomy is indicated for tumors that extend below the foramen magnum and for the correction of bony anomalies of osteogenesis imperfecta, such as severe basilar impression combined with maxillary hypoplasia and palatal deformity (15). It is a lengthy, complicated procedure that requires precise reapproximation of palatal and maxillary segments to prevent malocclusion and palatal dysfunction.

PEDICLED RHINOTOMY

The pedicled rhinotomy is a transnasal approach involving lateral rotation of the nose (Fig. 7). It provides relatively shallow field exposure of the midline anterior skull base. It has five major components: (a) a modified lateral rhinotomy incision that avoids the glabella and philtrum; (b) osteotomies of nasal bones and cartilage that free the nose and the ascending processes of the maxilla; (c) removal of the nasal septum and medial walls of the maxilla; (d) opening of ethmoid and sphenoid sinuses; and (e) dissection of nasopharynx and oropharynx to explose the clivus and craniovertebral junction (10, 20, 40). This permits exposure from the tuberculum sellae to the junction of the dens with the body of C2. Lateral limits are set by the intracavernous and intrapetrous ICAs (Fig. 8). It is indicated for medial sella and clival tumors, such as chordomas, macroadenomas, and metastases, for repair of vertebrobasilar aneurysms and for removal of craniovertebral junction osseous anomalies (Fig. 8).

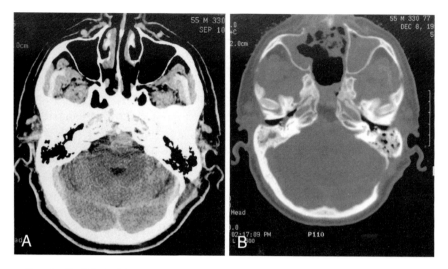

FIG. 8 Pedicled rhinotomy: clival opening and tumor resection. A preoperative gadolinium-enhanced axial MR image (*A*) shows transdural extension of a clival chordoma whose predominantly midline location permitted its removal by pedicled rhinotomy. A bone-windowed postoperative axial CT scan (*B*) shows a midline opening in the clivus that extends laterally to the distal petrous ICA on each side.

Details of the Procedure

PREPARATION

The patient is in a supine, semisitting position. Mayfield-Keyes tongs hold the head rotated to the right, facing the surgeon standing on the patient's right, and slightly flexed or extended, depending on whether inferior or superior exposure, respectively, is more crucial for a particular lesion. An orotracheal tube is used. Rarely, when palatal and pharyngeal function is compromised by tumor, tracheostomy and gastrostomy are needed. A lumbar drain is placed if opening of the dura is anticipated. Tarsorrhaphy is performed. The hypopharynx and oropharynx are packed with moist gauze, and 0.05% oxymetazoline HCl (Afrin) is applied to the nasal mucosa. The face is washed with 10% povidone iodine (Betadine) solution. The face, the right lower quadrant of the abdomen (for a subcutaneous fat graft), and the right thigh (for a split-thickness skin graft or fascia lata graft) are prepared and draped.

INCISION

The nasal incision is marked after superficial Doppler imaging locates and verifies the patency of the contralateral facial artery that will supply the pedicled nasal flap. The incision is infiltrated with 1% lido-caine (Xylocaine) with 1:100,000 epinephrine solution. The incision is carried through skin, subcutaneous tissue, and periosteum. It begins over the nasal bone at the upper one-third of the nose along its side at the break point between the dorsum and lateral wall of the nose. It does not extend across the glabella but rather passes inferiorly over the up-per and then the lower lateral cartilage. It is curved into the nasal sill along the base of the right alae nasi and columella at the base of the piriform aperture (Fig. 7). The lip is not divided.

NASAL DISSECTION

Lateral nasal osteotomies are performed bilaterally at the junction between the nasal bones and the ascending processes of the maxilla. The nasal bone is separated from the base of the frontal base. The up-per lateral cartilage is separated from the cartilaginous nasal septum, and the septum is disarticulated from the vomer and separated from the ethmoid bone. The ipsilateral nasal bone is not elevated with the flap. The nasal process of the frontal bone is detached at its base. The lower lateral cartilages are separated from the nasal spine by a transcolumellar cut through the medial crus of each lateral cartilage. The anterior cartilaginous septum is divided from the maxillary crest by a cut that passes along the nasal floor for 2 cm and then turns ver-tically. It thus remains part of the nasal pedicle.

A stab incision just anterior to the inferior turbinates permits a sub-periosteal dissection that preserves both the facial artery and the at-tachment of the nasal bone to the maxilla after the osteotomies. The ipsilateral lateral nasal bone and the upper lateral cartilage are re-tracted laterally as the ipsilateral flap. The contralateral nasal flap comprised of the contralateral lateral nasal bone, upper lateral nasal cartilage, and the nose with the septum and both lower lateral carti-lages attached, is rotated to the side opposite the incision (Fig. 7). The contralateral nasal flap is pedicled on a nasal branch of the facial artery. Compromise of this vascular supply is avoided by placing a rolled sponge beneath the fold and returning both flaps to their anatomic position for 5 minutes every hour.

SINUS OPENING

Remnants of the nasal septum are removed, except for a narrow strip containing olfactory epithelium along the roof of the nasal cavity. The posterolaterally directed exposure of the medial cavernous sinus and ICA rostrally down to the jugular foramen and lower cranial nerves cau-dally is enhanced by removing the inferior turbinates and medial walls of the maxillary sinuses. The middle turbinates are resected, and the ethmoid air cells are opened widely. The medial walls of the maxillary sinuses, including the inferior turbinates, are then removed. The medial maxillotomy requires division of the lacrimal ducts. Maxillotomy is extended ipsilaterally by removing the anterior wall of the sinus as far laterally as the foramen of the infraorbital nerve. The opening into the contralateral maxillary sinus is enlarged as needed. The soft palate is retracted inferiorly by a Penrose drain passed through the mouth. The rostrum and anterior face of the sphenoid sinus are removed.

Clival Exposure and Opening. The tuberculum sellae and the anterior wall and floor of the sella are identified and cleaned of mucosa. The septations of the sphenoid sinus serve as a guide to medial-to-lateral orientation before their removal. The posterior pharyngeal mucosa and musculature are incised in the midline and elevated from underlying clivus or tumor out to the lateral gutter just medial to the carotid canal. If the lesion extends below the foramen magnum, the atlantoaxial joint is removed. After resection of the anterior arch of C1, the dens, and associated ligaments, exposure extends inferiorly to the top of the body of C2 (Fig. 9).

The anterior clivus is opened with a high-speed drill. Orientation in depth is best obtained by exposing normal dura both superior and inferior to the tumor. Clival bone is then removed first in the midline and

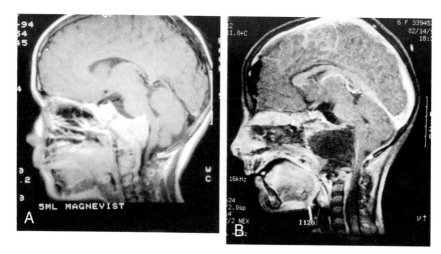

FIG. 9 Pedicled rhinotomy for clival chordoma. Preoperative (*A*) and postoperative (*B*) midsagittal MR images with gadolinium contrast demonstrate the superior (tuberculum sellae) to inferior (mid-C2) extent of the exposure provided by pedicled rhinotomy.

then as widely as is possible on each side. Definition of lateral limits is critical. Superiorly, the intracavernous ICAs are separated by approximately 2 cm. They can be identified by the carotid prominences in the superior posterolateral wall of the sphenoid sinus. These lie in parallel on each side just inferior and slightly lateral to the medial wall of the cavernous sinus. In that overlying sphenoid wall bone may be deficient, one should palpate for soft tissue and be observant for pulsations while removing bone or tumor from this area. In the midclivus at the level of junction of petrous and cavernous carotid segments, the more apical half of the petroclival junction, and Dorello's canal, this intercarotid corridor remains approximately 2 cm (Fig. 8). Dense attachment of preclival periosteum to the anterolateral aspect of the clivus and the curvature of the clivus as it falls away from its midline convexity help define this lateral limit of resection. More inferiorly, at the level of the jugular tubercle, the junction of middle and lower thirds of the clivus, the surgical corridor widens as a result of the obliquity of the horizontal petrous segment of the ICA. Here, the foramina laceri are separated by 5 cm, but the width of exposure is limited to approximately 3 cm by the combination of inferior petrosal sinus, jugular bulb, and cranial nerves IX through XII. More inferiorly, the separation of the vertebral arteries lateral to C1 and C2 defines the width of exposure. At each level, the actual width of exposure that can be obtained will vary with individual differences of head size and shape. Lateral displacement of limiting neurovascular structures by tumor can widen surgical access (Fig. 10). Comparison of intraoperative anatomy and preoperative magnetic resonance imaging (MRI) and computerized tomographic (CT) studies will help guide bone and tumor removal.

TUMOR RESECTION

After clival opening, the exposed dura can be opened as needed. Basal venous sinuses are avoided if possible. Bleeding from them can be controlled by using a right-angled bipolar forceps or by packing them with oxidized cellulose (Surgicel). Exposed tumor can then undergo biopsy for frozen section pathologic analysis and then resected. Central debulking using morselization with bipolar cautery and suction helps mobilize into direct view lobules of tumor that extend beyond the limits of exposure. Cautious curettage with small ring curettes and microdissectors can help remove tumor extending superiorly toward the dorsum sellae and inferiorly behind the body of C2. As the tumor is debulked centrally and its circumferential margin dissected, the extent of dural involvement can be assessed. If dura is not transgressed, attached tumor can be stripped from it. If tumor extends intradurally

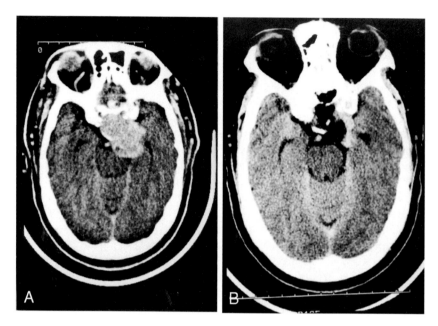

FIG. 10. Pedicled rhinotomy for pituitary macroadenoma. Preoperative (*A*) and post-operative (*B*) CT axial images demonstrate the medial to lateral extent of the surgical field of a pedicled rhinotomy. Lateral exposure is increased by medial maxillotomy that permits angulation of the retractor posterolaterally and by tumors that displace the ICAs laterally.

and needs to be removed, the margins of dural involvement should be defined. If possible, dura should be opened longitudinally and both dural and intradural tumor resected. In that removal of bone extends from tuberculum sellae to the body of C2—with the exception of the top of the dorsum sellae and posterior clinoid processes hidden behind the pituitary gland—exposure of the medulla, pons, and upper segment of the spinal cord, including the vertebral arteries bilaterally, the vertebrobasilar junction, and the inferior half of the basilar artery, is achieved.

CLOSURE

Closure begins with repair of any dural defect. Primary suture is preferred but is often precluded by tumor disruption of the dura. A patch of fascia lata can be sewn to superior and inferior dural edges. Exposed dura and the dural graft are then covered with layers of Surgicel, abdominal fat, and fascia lata. A split-thickness (0.12-inch) skin graft is placed over the opening in the clivus. This is held in place by packing the posterior pharynx with Bacitracin-impregnated iodoform gauze. The lacrimal duct is repaired with Silastic tubing. Gauze packed within a finger cot is placed along the soft palate. The pedicled nasal flap is rotated back into position. The cartilaginous nasal septum is sutured to the remnant of septal cartilage along the maxillary crest. The external incisions are closed in two layers with 5-0 clear polydioxanone suture subcutaneously and 6-0 nylon suture in skin. The transcolumellar incision is closed with 6-0 nylon suture. The medial crus is reapproximated, and a columellar strut is positioned behind it. Clear polydiaxonone sutures (5-0) and Surgicel impregnated with Bacitracin are used to stabilize the anterior cartilaginous complex and nasal bone. An external cast is applied, and the tarsorrhaphy sutures are removed. Postoperatively the lumbar drain, nasal splint, and nylon sutures are removed on the 5th postoperative day. Nasal packing is removed on the 14th day, after which intravenous antibiotics are discontinued. The lacrimal tube is removed after 2 months. The patient irrigates the nasal cavity daily to prevent crusting and the collection of mucus.

In summary, the upper third of the clivus is best approached by a transseptal-transsphenoid or transethmosphenoid route that avoids the facial incision of a pedicled rhinotomy. The lower third of the clivus and the C1-C2 junction are often best approached by a transoral route that also avoids facial incisions. Pedicled rhinotomy achieves, by means of a single transfacial route, exposure of the midline anterior skull base, from tuberculum to C2, similar to that from the combination of transnasal, transsphenoid, and transoral routes. Exposure and closure each take approximately 1 hour. The average blood loss during opening and closing is approximately 200 ml. The risks of pedicled rhinotomy include CSF leakage and subsequent meningitis, injury to the ICA, and dysfunction of cranial nerves III through VI and IX to XI. In comparison with the transpalatal approach, there is no risk of palatal dysfunction. Disadvantages include the use of a facial incision, even though the cosmetic outcome is highly acceptable. The risk of loss of the nasal flap is quite low, although intranasal crusting and at least partial loss of smell can be frequent. Inferior maxillotomy and extensive maxillectomy, maxillotomy, or facial translocation can provide similar exposure, but division of the palate and extensive facial osteotomies are required. Lesions lateral to the ICA or in the medial petrous bone require a lateral, as well as an anterior, approach.

Pedicled Rhinotomy Case Series

From December of 1990 to May of 1995, we have used pedicled rhinotomy in 13 cases of tumor, some of which have previously been reported

(26, 40). This includes 10 clival chordomas, 1 ethmosphenoid chondrosarcoma, 1 ethmosphenoid schwannoma, and 1 pituitary macroadenoma. Five of the 13 cases were reoperations. Complications in these 13 cases have included a tear in the palate in 1, dehiscence of the columellar incision in 1, and a lacrimal sac infection in 1. There have been three instances of CSF leakage and meningitis, two of which were fungal and one of which was bacterial. One patient with fungal meningitis died; the other developed a hemiparesis that resolved. In each case, the preoperative goal of either gross total removal or resection sufficient to relieve brainstem compression in anticipation of high-dose proton therapy was achieved.

SUMMARY

Anterior midline approaches are safe and appropriate for extradural lesions of the central skull base. They are occasionally warranted for intradural lesions as well. Transnasal routes expose the clivus well. They are readily expanded superiorly, inferiorly, and laterally. Recent innovations are reductive; they expand exposure with less facial disassembly. Lateral and most intradural extensions of lesions warrant more lateral approaches.

ACKNOWLEDGMENTS

The authors thank Dr. Mack Cheney for his assistance in performing pedicled rhinotomy and Ms. Arline Broberg for her help in preparing the manuscript.

REFERENCES

1. Alonso WA, Black P, Connor GH, et al. Transoral transpalatal approach for resection of clival chordoma. **Laryngoscope** 81:1626–1631, 1971.
2. Anand VK, Harkey HL, Al-Mefty O: Open-door maxillotomy approach for lesions of the clivus. **Skull Base Surg** *1:217–225, 1991.*
3. Apuzzo MLJ, Weiss MH, Heiden JS: Transoral exposure of atlanto-axial region. **Neurosurgery** 3:201–207, 1978.
4. Blacklock JB, Weber RS, Lee YY, et al. Transcranial resection of tumors of the paranasal sinuses and nasal cavity. **J Neurosurg** 71:10–15, 1989.
5. Brown DH: The LeFort 1 maxillary osteotomy approach to surgery of the skull base. **Otolaryngology** 18:289–292. 1989.
6. Casson PR, Bonanno PC, Converse JM: The midfacial degloving procedure. **Plast Reconstr Surg** 53:102–103, 1974.
7. Cocke EW Jr, Robertson JH, Robertson JT, et al. The extended maxillotomy and subtotal maxillectomy for excision of skull base tumors. **Arch Otolaryngol Head Neck Surg** 116:92–104, 1990.
8. Crockard AH: Transoral approach to intra/extradural tumors, in: Sekhar L, Janecka IP (eds): *Surgery of Cranial Base Tumors.* New York, Raven Press, 1993, pp. 225–234.

9. Crumley RL, Gutin PH: Surgical access for clivus chordoma. **Arch Otolaryngol Head Neck Surg** 115:295–300, 1989.

10. deFries HO, Deeb ZE, Hudkins CP: A transfacial approach to the nasal paranasal cavities and anterior skull base. **Arch Otolaryngol Head Neck Surg** 114:766–769, 1988.

11. Delgado, TE, Garrido E, Harwick RD: Labiomandibular, transoral approach to chordomas of the clivus and upper cervical spine. **Neurosurgery** 8:675–679, 1981.

12. Derome PJ: Surgical management of tumours invading the skull base. **Neurol. Sci.** 12:345–347, 1985.

13. Fraioli B, Esposito V, Santoro A, *et al.*: Transmaxillosphenoidal approach to tumors invading the medial compartment of the cavernous sinus. **J Neurosurg** 82:63–69, 1995.

14. Inoue T, Rhoton AL, Theele D, *et al.*: Surgical approaches to the cavernous sinus: A microsurgical study. **Neurosurgery** 26:903–932, 1990.

15. James D, Crockard HA: Surgical access to the base of skull and upper cervical spine by extended maxillotomy. **Neurosurgery** 29:411–416, 1991.

16. Jane JA, Park TS, Pobereskin LH, *et al.*: The supraorbital approach: Technical note. *Neurosurgery* 11:537–542, 1982.

17. Janecka IP: Classification of facial translocation approach to the skull base. **Otolaryngol Head Neck Surg** 112:579–585.

18. Janecka IP, Sen CN, Sekhar LN, *et al.*: Facial translocation: A new approach to the cranial base. **Otolaryngol Head Neck Surg** 103:414–419, 1990.

19. Johns ME, Kaplan MJ, Park TS, *et al.*: Supraorbital rim approach to the anterior skull base. **Laryngoscope** 94:1137–1139, 1984.

20. Joseph M: Pedicled rhinotomy for exposure of the clivus, in: Schmidek HH, Sweet WH (eds). Philadelphia, WB Saunders, 1995, pp. 469–475.

21. Kennedy DW, Papel ID, Holliday MJ: Transpalatal approach to the skull base. **Ear Nose Throat J** 65:125, 127–133, 1986.

22. Lalwani AK, Kaplan MJ, Gutin PH: The transsphenoethmoid approach to the sphenoid sinus and clinus. **Neurosurgery** 31:1009–1014, 1992.

23. Laws ER Jr: Transsphenoidal surgery for tumors of the clivus. **Otolaryngol Head Neck Surg** 92:100–101, 1984.

24. Maniglia AJ: Indications and techniques of midfacial degloving. **Arch Otolaryngol Head Neck Surg** 112:750–752, 1986.

25. Menezes AH, VanGilder JC, Graf CJ, *et al.*: Cranocervical abnormalities: Comprehensive surgical approach. **Neurosurgery** 53:444–455, 1980.

26. Ojemann RG, Thornton AC, Harsh GR IV: Management of anterior cranial base and cavernous sinus neoplasms with conservative surgery alone or in combination with fractionated photon or stereotactic proton radiotherapy. **Clin Neurosurg** 42:71–98, 1995.

27. Panje WE, Dohrmann GJ, Pitchock JK, *et al.*: The transfacial approach for combined anterior craniofacial tumor ablation. **Arch Otolaryngol Head Neck Surg** 115:301–307, 1989.

28. Pinsolle J, San-Galli F, Siberchicot F, *et al.*: Modified approach for ethmoid and anterior skull base surgery. **Arch Otolaryngol Head Neck Surg** 117:779–782, 1991.

29. Platzer, W: *Pernkopf's Anatomy*, Vol I, *Head and Neck*. Baltimore, Urban & Schwarzenberg, 1989.

30. Price JC: The midfacial degloving approach to the central skull base. **Ear Nose Throat J** 65:46–53, 1986.

31. Raveh J, Turk JB, Ladrach K, *et al.:* Extended anterior subcranial approach for skull base tumors: Long-term results. **J Neurosurg** 82:1002–1010, 1995.
32. Rinehart, GC, Jackson IT, Potparic Z, *et al.:* Management of locally aggressive sinus disease using craniofacial exposure and the galeal frontalis fascia-muscle flap. **Plast Reconstr Surg** 92:1219–1225, 1993.
33. Sasaki CT, Lowlicht RA, Astrachan DI, *et al.:* LeFort 1 osteotomy approach to the skull base. **Laryngoscopy** 100:1073–1076, 1990.
34. Schramm VL Jr, Myers EN, Maroon JC: Anterior skull base surgery for benign and malignant disease. **Laryngoscope** 89:1077–1091, 1979.
35. Schuller DE, Goodman JH, Brown BL, *et al.:* Maxillary removal and reinsertion for improved access to anterior cranial base tumors. **Laryngoscope** 102:203–212, 1992.
36. Sekhar LN, Nanda A, Sen CN, *et al.:* The extended frontal approach to tumors of the anterior middle, and posterior skull base. **J Neurosurg** 76:198–206, 1992.
37. Sekhar LN, Sen C, Snyderman C, *et al.:* Anterior, anterolateral, and lateral approaches to extradural petroclival tumors, in: Sekhar LN, Janecka IP (eds): *Surgery of Cranial Base Tumors.* New York, Raven Press, 1993, pp. 157–173.
38. Snyderman, C, Janecka IP, Selchar LN, *et al.:* Anterior cranial base reconstruction: Role of galeal and pericranial flaps. **Laryngoscope** 100:607–614, 1990.
39. Stevenson GC, Stoney RJ, Perkins RK, *et al.:* A transcervical transsclival approach to the ventral surface of the brainstem for removal of a clivus chordoma. **J Neurosurg** 24:544–551, 1966.
40. Swearingen B, Joseph M, Cheney M, *et al.:* A modified transfacial approach to the clivus. **Neurosurgery** 36:101–105, 1995.
41. Tessier P, Guiot G, Rougerie J: Osteotomies cranio-nasa-orbito-faciales. Hypertelorisme. **Ann Chir Plast** 12:103–118, 1967.

CHAPTER

3

Innovations in Cranial Approaches and Exposures: Anterolateral Approaches

HARRY R. VAN LOVEREN, M.D., ASIM MAHMOOD, M.D.,
SHIH SING LIU M.D., AND DAVID GRUBER, M.D.

Similar to any social movement, skull base surgery has evolved through the common phases of development: early *skepticism; fanaticism* with over-application; *reconciliation,* with reports of morbidity and recurrence; and *maturation,* in which reasonable goals and expectations translate into reasonable application (Fig. 1).

ANTEROLATERAL SKULL BASE APPROACHES

Anterolateral skull base approaches are essentially modifications of the pterional approach, perhaps the most widely used route of exposure for cranial neurosurgery. In essence, neurosurgeons in search of a route to the cavernous sinus discovered the sphenoid bone and its attachments. Previously, the greater and lesser wing of the sphenoid bone and the bony orbit remained as impediments to intracranial exposure. Anterolateral approaches are now applied to more ordinary tumors and aneurysms than those extraordinary lesions usually presented by skull base surgeons to mobilize or resect the greater and lesser wing of the sphenoid bone, orbital roof, optic canal, anterior clinoid process, lateral wall of the superior orbital fissure, and middle fossa floor. Bone resection is performed instead of brain retraction, resulting in wide-field superficial exposure, decreased depth of surgical field, increased deep exposure and, consequently, better surgical outcome. This is only achieved if the anatomy for each approach is well understood and the steps of the approach are properly executed (23).

Orbitozygomatic Osteotomy

The orbitozygomatic osteotomy is the most useful modification of the pterional approach (Fig. 2, **A** and **B**). The neurosurgical literature is inundated with descriptions of modifications of the orbitozygomatic osteotomy (Table 1). Each variation has specific usefulness; however, the number of variations reported confounds the reader. Until the surgeon

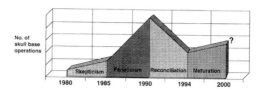

FIG. 1 Skull base surgery: a movement within neurosurgery. Nonstatistical chart characterizing skull base surgery as evolving through the same stages of development as social movements.

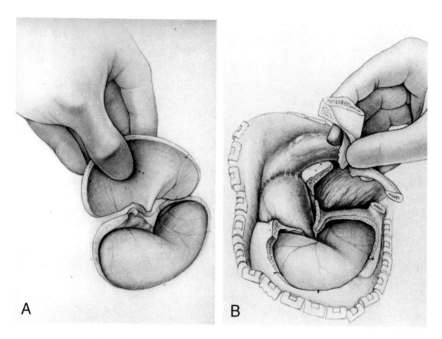

FIG. 2 Modification of pterional craniotomy. (**A**) Pterional craniotomy. Frontotemporal bone flap is elevated, exposing the sphenoid ridge, frontal lobe, and temporal lobe. (**B**) Total orbitozygomatic osteotomy. The orbitozygomatic osteotomy is removed after a standard pterional craniotomy through a key burr hole. Currently, the osteotomy is left attached to the masseter muscle as a vascularized osteoplastic construct. [Reproduced with permission from (23).]

is familiar enough with the approach to improvise, we recommend four variations for an osteotomy: frontal orbitozygomatic, temporal orbitozygomatic, total orbitozygomatic, and zygomatic arch (Fig. 3).

Although these four variations were primarily developed to approach complex skull base lesions, they improve exposure of more ordinary

TABLE 1
Proposed Nomenclature for Variations of the Orbitozygomatic
Osteotomy Reported in the Literature

Previous Nomenclature	Author	Proposed Nomenclature
Supraorbital	Jane et al. (14)	Frontal orbitozygomatic
Two-step supraorbital	Delfini *et al.* (5)	Frontal orbitozygomatic
Supraorbital pterional	Al-Mefty (1)	Frontal orbitozygomatic
Combined frontotemporal and lateral infra-temporal fossa	Mickey *et al.* (17)	Temporal orbitozygomatic
Zygomatico temporal	Neil-Dwyer *et al.* (18)	Temporal orbitozygomatic
Orbitozygomatic osteotomy	Jackson *et al.* (13)	Temporal orbitozygomatic
Transzygomatic	Gerber *et al.* (9)	Temporal orbitozygomatic
Frontozygomatic	Uttley *et al.* (25)	Temporal orbitozygomatic
Zygomatic	Fujitsu and Kuwabara (8)	Temporal orbitozygomatic
Orbitofrontomalar	Pellerin *et al.* (20)	Total orbitozygomatic
Orbitozygomatic infratemporal	Hakuba *et al.* (10)	Total orbitozygomatic
Orbitozygomatic temporopolar	Ikeda *et al.* (12)	Total orbitozygomatic
Combined frontotemporal orbitozygomatic	McDermott *et al.* (16)	Total orbitozygomatic
Modified supraorbital craniotomy	Delashaw *et al.* (4)	Total orbitozygomatic
Orbitomaxillary osteotomy	Jackson *et al.* (13)	Total orbitozygomatic
Zygomatic temporopolar	Shiokawa *et al.* (22)	Zygomatic arch
Subtemporal approach with section of zygomatic arch	Pitelli *et al.* (21)	Zygomatic arch

tumors and vascular lesions encountered by the general cranial neuro-surgeon.

Sphenoid Wing Meningioma

For example, consider the approach to sphenoid wing meningiomas. One of the authors (HRVL) titled a lecture, "Everything I Ever Wanted to Know about Meningiomas, I Learned on the Convexity." Convexity meningiomas are generally resected with low morbidity, because their vascular supply is eliminated early in the procedure by a craniotomy, their dural base of attachment is circumferentially resected, which also eliminates most of the remaining blood supply, and the tumor-brain interface is dissected late in the procedure. With the total orbitozygomatic osteotomy, the sphenoid wing meningioma becomes an upside down convexity meningioma (Fig. 4).

By adding several smaller components of bone resection (*i.e.,* orbital osteotomy, anterior clinoidectomy, resection of the lateral bony wall of the superior orbital fissure) to a pterional approach, it is possible to mo-

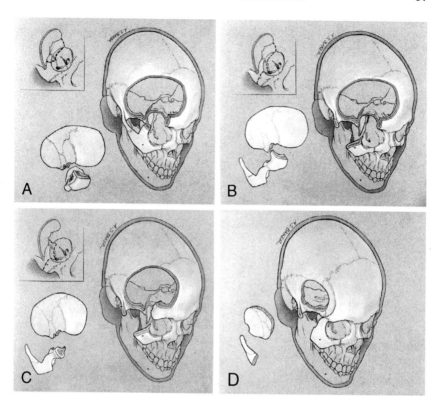

FIG. 3 Variations on orbitozygomatic osteotomies. (A) Frontal orbitozygomatic osteotomy. Osteotomies are made at the supraorbital notch, across the orbital roof, and at the frontozygomatic suture. (B) Total orbitozygomatic osteotomy. Osteotomies are performed at the supraorbital foramen or notch, across the zygomatic lateral to zygomaticofacial foramen through the inferior orbital fissure, across the zygomatic process anterior to the articular eminence and across orbital roof and lateral wall of orbit into inferior orbital fissure. (C) Temporal orbitozygomatic osteotomy. Osteotomies are made at the frontozygomatic suture, lateral wall of the orbit, across the zygoma into inferior orbital fissure lateral to zygomaticofacial foramen, and anterior to the articular eminence. (D) Zygomatic arch osteotomy. Periosteum of zygomatic arch is incised anterior to the articular eminence posteriorly and at temporozygomatic suture anteriorly. The zygomatic arch with the masseter muscle is reflected inferiorly. [Reproduced with permission from Mayfield Neurological Institute.]

bilize and/or resect the lateral wall of the cavernous sinus (26). This allows resection of the portion of a medial sphenoid wing meningioma that occasionally attaches to the lateral cavernous wall or invades the lateral compartment of the cavernous sinus. This presentation intentionally does not address holocavernous meningiomas that encase the

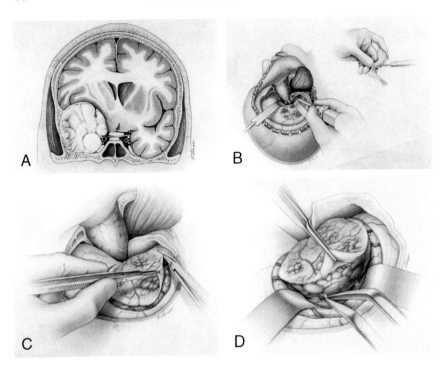

FIG. 4 Sphenoid wing meningioma: coronal section and operative technique. (A) Coronal section demonstrates compression of the cavernous sinus with attachment to lateral wall of cavernous sinus and encasement of the middle cerebral artery within an arachnoid cleavage plane in the tumor. Note hyperostosis. (B) Pterional bone flap is elevated, and the orbitozygomatic osteotomy is fractured out of position. *Inset* shows drilling away of the hyperostotic sphenoid bone. (C) A dural incision is made around the tumor, maintaining a 1 to 2 cm margin, thus eliminating the dural base and vascular supply of the tumor. (D) Circumferential dissection of the tumor cap margins from adhesions to the brain. (Reproduced with permission from Tew JM Jr, van Loveren HR, Keller JT: *Atlas of Operative Microneurosurgery* 2, Philadelphia, W.B. Saunders Company, in press, 1996.)

internal carotid artery, because those tumors are more complex in terms of resectability and surgical indications. We believe that the removal of meningioma "extension" confined to the lateral cavernous wall or lateral compartment of the cavernous sinus, in young or middle-aged patients without physiologic compromise, is feasible, advisable, and a challenge to current standards of care.

Ophthalmic Segment Aneurysms

Ophthalmic segment aneurysms represent a common vascular lesion that has benefited from application of the modifications of the an-

terolateral approach (3). An aneurysm clipping is considered successful if the following goals are achieved: proximal control, exposure of the
entire aneurysm neck, and clip application parallel to the course of the
parent artery. The standard approach of partial intradural anterior clinoid resection is often not sufficient to achieve these goals in proximal,
complex, or giant ophthalmic segment aneurysms, especially those
that involve and dilate the distal dural carotid ring. Orbital osteotomy,
anterior clinoidectomy, mobilization of the optic nerve, and section of
the distal ring captures the clinoid (C5) arterial segment and achieves
these goals (2) (Fig. 5, **A** and **B**). This strategy should reduce the morbidity and mortality associated with clipping of ophthalmic segment

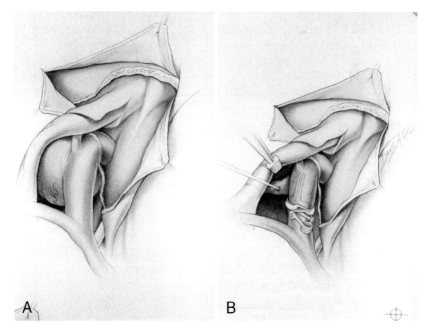

A   B

FIG. 5 Ophthalmic segment aneurysm: operative technique. (**A**) An incision is made
through the medial dural flap across the distal ring to expose the origin of the ophthalmic
artery, the base of the medially directed aneurysm, and the proximal dural ring. A parallel incision is made in the optic sheath to permit medial displacement of the nerve. (**B**)
The optic nerve is retracted medially. The internal carotid artery (ICA) is temporarily
occluded to decrease intra-aneurysmal pressure. The aneurysm is punctured with a 22-
gauge needle. While the aneurysm is aspirated, a right-angle fenestrated clip closes the
aneurysm base. Intraoperative angiography is performed to document the effective closure of the aneurysm and preservation of patency of the ICA. [Reproduced with permission from (23).]

aneurysm to a level comparable with aneurysms of the posterior communicating segment.

Cavernous Sinus

As previously stated, anterolateral approaches have been used to aid the resection of cavernous sinus lesions. The once impossible task of cavernous sinus exploration is becoming routine. The pioneers of surgery in this area should be properly credited, including Parkinson (19), Hakuba *et al.* (11), and Dolenc (6). Through their heroic efforts and the courage of their patients, we now realize the anatomic basis for successful and safe cavernous exploration. The cavernous sinus is neither cavernous nor a sinus. It is a parasellar epidural venous plexus in continuity with the basilar epidural venous plexus. The lateral wall of the cavernous sinus is the medial temporal lobe dura. Therefore, the lateral wall of the cavernous sinus continues past, rather than continuing with, the superior orbital fissure. Additionally, the lateral wall of the cavernous sinus can be mobilized most often without permanent damage to the cranial nerves (7). The sinusoidal channels of the cavernous sinus (since true veins have not been well-identified) remain largely protected by the periosteal dural layer and the inner membranous layer, which is formed from the epineurium of the cranial nerves (24).

Holocavernous Meningioma

Although the original objective of treatment was the extirpation of holocavernous meningiomas, that particular objective remains controversial. As we detail in another report, the surgical "cure" rate of holocavernous meningiomas is approximately 20%, is associated with significant new cranial nerve morbidity, and depends largely on the degree of internal carotid artery encasement (O'Sullivan MG, Park K, Ernst R, *et al.*: The surgical resectability of cavernous sinus meningiomas. **Neurosurgery,** submitted for publication). Additional limits on resectability relate to possible cranial nerve invasion by meningioma and cranial nerve infarction caused by sacrifice of cranial nerve arterial supply during tumor resection (15).

CONCLUSION

Standards of care are becoming global rather than regional. As the time delay to dissemination of information shortens, advantages available to patients in one location in the world will be expected for all patients worldwide. Skull base surgery is now in the maturation phase of development, a phase in which the application of skull base techniques and the modifications of the anterolateral approach to the conventional pterional approach challenge the existing standards of care and may some day constitute a new standard. We recommend that young neurosurgeons study these techniques as part of their general training.

ACKNOWLEDGMENTS

The authors thank Kathy Brady, Department of Neurosurgery Editorial Office, for editorial review and Tony Hines, Medical Illustration and Photography, for preparation of the figures.

REFERENCES

1. Al-Mefty O: Supraorbital-pterional approach to skull base lesions. **Neurosurgery** 21:474–477, 1987.
2. Bouthillier A, van Loveren HR, Keller JT: Segments of the internal carotid artery: A new classification. **Neurosurgery** 38, in press, 1996.
3. Day AL: Aneurysms of ophthalmic segment: A clinical and anatomical analysis. **J Neurosurg** 72:677–691, 1990.
4. Delashaw JB, Tedeschi H, Rhoton AL: Modified supraorbital craniotomy: Technical note. **Neurosurgery** 30:954–956, 1992.
5. Delfini R, Raco A, Artico M, *et al.:* A two-step supraorbital approach to lesions of the orbital apex. **J Neurosurg** 77:959–961, 1992.
6. Dolenc VV (ed): *The Cavernous Sinus.* New York, Springer-Verlag, 1987.
7. El-Kalliny M, van Loveren HR, Keller JT, *et al.:* Tumors of the lateral wall of the cavernous sinus. **J Neurosurg** 77:508–514, 1992.
8. Fujitsu K, Kuwabara T: Zygomatic approach for lesions in the interpeduncular cistern. **J Neurosurg** 62:340–343, 1985.
9. Gerber CJ, Neil-Dwyer G, Evans BT: An alternative surgical approach to aneurysms of the posterior cerebral artery. **Neurosurgery** 32:928–931, 1993.
10. Hakuba A, Liu SS, Nishimura S: The orbitozygomatic infratemporal approach: A new surgical technique. **Surg Neurol** 26:271–276, 1986.
11. Hakuba A, Tanaka K, Suzuki T, *et al.:* A combined orbitozygomatic infratemporal epidural and subdural approach for lesions involving the entire cavernous sinus. **J Neurosurg** 71:699–704, 1989.
12. Ikeda K, Yamashita J, Hashimoto M, *et al.:* Orbitozygomatic temporopolar approach for a high basilar tip aneurysm associated with a short intracranial internal carotid artery: A new surgical approach. **Neurosurgery** 28:105–110, 1991.
13. Jackson IT, Marsh WR, Bite U, *et al.:* Craniofacial osteotomies to facilitate skull base tumour resection. **Br J Plastic Surg** 39:153–160, 1986.
14. Jane JA, Park TS, Pobereskin LH, *et al.:* The supraorbital approach: Technical note. **Neurosurgery** 11:537–542, 1982.
15. Larson JJ, von Loveren HR, Balko MG, *et al.:* Evidence of meningioma invasion into cranial nerves: Clinical implications for cavernous sinus meningiomas. **J Neurosurg** 83:596–599, 1995.
16. McDermott MW, Durity FA, Rootman J, *et al.:* Combined frontotemporal-orbitozygomatic approach for tumors of the sphenoid wing and orbit. **Neurosurgery** 26:107–116, 1990.
17. Mickey B, Close L, Schaefer S, *et al.:* A combined frontotemporal and lateral infratemporal fossa approach to the skull base. **J Neurosurg** 68:678–683, 1988.

18. Neil-Dwyer G, Sharr M, Haskell R, *et al.:* Zygomaticotemporal approach to the basis cranii and basilar artery. **Neurosurgery** 23:20–22, 1988.
19. Parkinson D: A surgical approach to the cavernous portion of the carotid artery: Anatomical studies and case report. **J Neurosurg** 23:474–483, 1965.
20. Pellerin P, Lesoin F, Dhellemmes P, *et al.:* Usefulness of the orbitofrontomalar approach associated with bone reconstruction for frontotemporosphenoid meningiomas. **Neurosurgery** 15:715–718, 1984.
21. Pitelli SD, Almeida GGM, Nakagawa EJ, *et al.:* Basilar aneurysm surgery: The subtemporal approach with section of the zygomatic arch. **Neurosurgery** 18:125–128, 1986.
22. Shiokawa Y, Saito I, Aoki N, *et al.:* Zygomatic temporopolar approach for basilar artery aneurysms. **Neurosurgery** 25:793–797, 1989.
23. Tew JM Jr, van Loveren HR: *Atlas of Operative Microneurosurgery.* Philadelphia, W.B. Saunders, 1994, vol 1.
24. Umansky F, Nathan H: The lateral wall of the cavernous sinus: With special reference to the nerves related to it. **J Neurosurg** 56:228–234, 1982.
25. Uttley D, Archer DJ, Marsh HT, *et al.:* Improved access to lesions of the central skull base by mobilization of the zygoma: Experience with 54 cases. **Neurosurgery** 28:99–104, 1991.
26. van Loveren HR, Keller JT, El-Kalliny M, *et al.:* The Dolenc technique for cavernous sinus exploration (cadaveric prosection): Technical note. *J Neurosurg* 74:837–844, 1991.

4

Transcranial Orbital Surgery

JOHN A. JANE, SR., M.D., PH.D. AND STEVEN A. NEWMAN, M.D.

HISTORICAL REVIEW

Although recognized since antiquity, the pathology affecting the orbit was not within the general expertise of early barber surgeons. Prior to the latter half of the 19th century, the surgical approaches to the orbit designed by ophthalmologists were timid at best. In 1888 Krönlein (11) described the lateral orbit approach in which the lateral orbital wall was removed so that ophthalmic surgeons could access pathology deeper within the orbit. Despite this and other advances, three basic problems remained: (*a*) the lateral orbital approach often left a disfiguring scar on the face; (*b*) both anterior and lateral approaches could potentially damage important intraorbital structures including the extraocular muscles and the optic nerve; and (*c*) lesions that extended beyond the confines of the orbit could be only partially resected. Although modifications by Berke (3), Wright (19), Birch-Hirschfeld (5), and Leone (12) improved the cosmetic aspects of the lateral orbitotomy, the advances of ophthalmologic surgeons remained limited.

The timidity of most ophthalmic surgeons provided an invitation for early neurosurgeons to become interested in orbital pathology. At the Johns Hopkins Hospital in 1934, all patients with pathology that was believed to be deep within the orbit were routinely seen in consultation by both the ophthalmological and neurological neurosurgery divisions. In 1918, Walter Dandy first became interested in tumors of the orbit. He subsequently gained extensive experience in dealing with these lesions, which he reported in the 1941 monograph, *Orbital Tumors* (8). It is fitting that the preface was written by Dr. Alan C. Woods (18), then chairman of the Department of Ophthalmology.

This early collegial team division of labor was a model for our later multidisciplinary approach to tumors of the skull base. Three years earlier, Cushing and Eisenhardt (7) suggested in their monograph, *Meningiomas,* that ophthalmologists and neurosurgeons could meet in harmony and not competition at the orbital apex; Alan Woods (18) would also write that "ophthalmologists have therefore long realized that conventional methods of approach to the orbit are often totally inadequate, and so have turned to the neurosurgeon for assistance."

Neurosurgeons responded by providing new approaches to the orbit. Dandy would popularize the transfrontal approach to the orbit after a fortuitous case in 1921 in which he tracked the intraorbital extension of an intracranial tumor following the optic canal. During the approach the orbital roof was removed exposing the intraorbital contents "perfectly." He suggested that "in safe hands the intracranial approach involves very little risk and offers the maximum hope of cure, unless the frontal bone is involved, and is without cosmetic defects." (8) True, the transfrontal approach with removal of the orbital roof offered an excellent view of the orbital apical contents; however, limitations remained. To adequately visualize orbital contents, the frontal lobes had to be retracted above the superior orbital rim that remained after removal of the frontal flap. In addition, the burr hole at the anterior medial aspect of the flap often left a noticeable depression on the forehead. To improve exposure and advance cosmesis, a bicoronal incision could be substituted for the original frontal incision and hidden behind the hairline, and the frontal craniotomy could be extended to include the orbital rim. As early as 1913 Frazier (9) described this extension of the craniotomy inferiorly in an attempt to reach the pituitary fossa. Later this extension was adapted to improve exposure of the orbit by incorporating the orbital rim and zygomatic process of the frontal bone with the frontal bone in one fragment (10).

TAILORING A SURGICAL APPROACH

Problems in designing the appropriate operations for the tumor before the advent of imaging studies continued to plague us until the very recent past. This young patient presented at the University of Virginia in 1977 with proptosis of the left eye (Fig. 1A). The patient was prepared for surgery in the usual transcranial fashion but before beginning intervention, palpation around the globe with the subject asleep revealed a mass inframporal to the globe. Incision through the conjunctiva revealed a mass extending posteriorly. Dissection of an encapsulated tumor (Fig. 1B) resulted in complete removal obviating the planned craniotomy (Fig. 1C).

Imaging studies that provide a far more accurate method to preoperatively tailor a surgical approach could have prevented this error. In the 1970s, computerized tomography (CT) scanning provided critical orbital anatomical information for the first time (2). In particular, CT precisely located the lesion with respect to the cone and optic nerve and separated those lesions solely within the orbit from those with in-

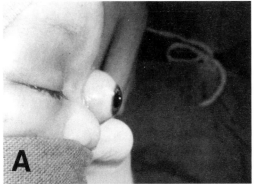

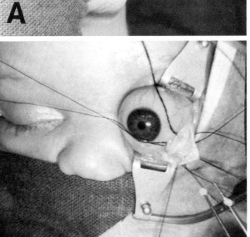

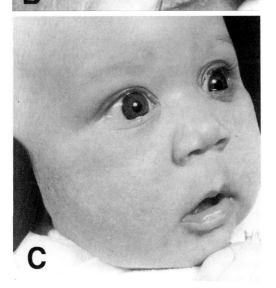

FIG. 1 Orbital surgery prior to modern imaging. (**A**) Without the aid of modern preoperative imaging, the patient is seen in the operating room prepped for a frontal craniotomy. Marked proptosis is evident. (**B**) An intraoperative photograph showing tumor in the inferolateral part of the globe. (**C**) Postoperative photograph showing resolved proptosis. The shaven head in anticipation of craniotomy is also seen.

tracranial extension. Subsequently magnetic resonance (MR) imaging has added additional soft tissue information about orbital pathology (1). Today, more objective decisions can be made regarding the most appropriate surgical approach to lesions affecting the orbit. Those lesions that remain inferior and medial to the optic nerve may be best approached anteriorly (16). Cosmesis may be respected although imperfectly by placing the incision in the lid crease (17). Conversely, pathology that primarily affects the optic nerve, particularly those extending through the canal, and tumors that extend beyond the boundaries of the orbit are most appropriately approached transcranially (13).

SUPRAORBITAL RIM APPROACH

Case Report

CLINICAL HISTORY

The 18-year-old woman in Figure 2 presented to the neuro-ophthalmology service at the University of Virginia in October 1987 complaining of prominence of her left globe (Fig. 2A). In covering her right eye she had noticed that vision was limited on the left. Visual acuity was 20/15 and 20/300, and she had 6 mm of proptosis on the left. An MR image revealed an optic nerve glioma extending back to, but not through, the optic canal (Fig. 2B). Follow-up imaging over the next 1.5 years demonstrated no change in the size of the tumor. Automated static perimetry, however, showed progressive visual loss paralleling acuity reduction from 20/400+ to 6/200 (Fig. 2C).

TREATMENT

A supraorbital rim approach (Fig. 2D) with extradural unroofing of the optic canal and sectioning of the optic nerve at the posterior aspect of the optic canal permitted the optic nerve glioma to be removed up to the back of the globe (Fig. 2E). The annulus of Zinn was opened between

---

FIG. 2 Supraorbital rim approach. (A) Preoperative photograph showing mild prominence of the left globe. (B) An MR image revealing a mass consistent with optic glioma that extends back to, but not through, the optic canal. (C) Preoperative automated static perimetry showing progressive visual field loss. (D) Artist's rendering of the supraorbital rim approach. Through a keyhole site, the craniotomy flap is extended with the craniotome, including a reverse cut at the medial supraorbital rim. The frontal process of the zygoma is cut back to the keyhole with the craniotome or sagittal saw. Subsequently, the bone flap is cracked forward and removed. Additional bone is removed from the orbital apex. (E) A drawing demonstrating the sectioning of the nerve and removal of the tumor. (F) Postoperative photographs in the nine cardinal positions of gaze demonstrate good cosmetic effect with a IV nerve palsy in the blind eye.

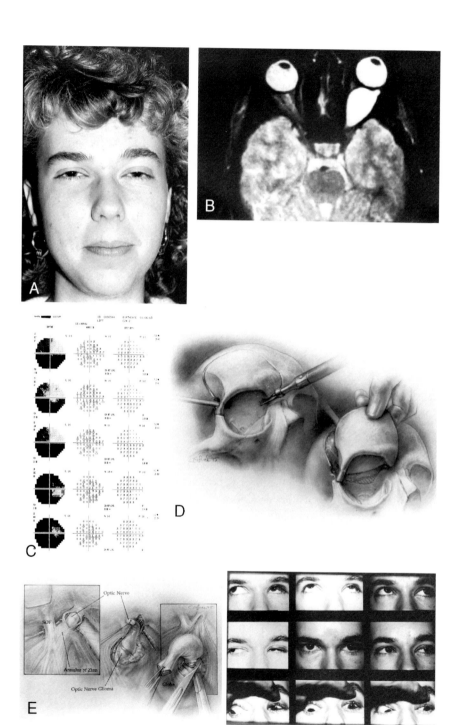

FIG. 2 Legend on page 56.

the levator/superior rectus complex and the superior oblique muscle. The trochlear nerve extending over the optic nerve was sectioned as its preservation was not necessary for excellent cosmetic results. Meticulous attention was paid to preservation of the rectus muscles and their innervation. The patient's postoperative motility and the cosmetic effect of her supraorbital bone flap demonstrated the success of this approach (Fig. 2**E**).

Cosmetic Modifications: The Frontal Sinus Approach

Continued research in the cosmetic aspects of the supraorbital approach suggested that the anterior table of the frontal sinus could be preserved by an osteoplastic approach to the frontal sinus with placement of the anterior burr hole through the posterior wall of the frontal sinus (Fig. 3**A**). This method offers improvements in the postoperative appearance of the bone flap. In addition, the frontal sinus may provide an extracranial approach to lesions of the anterior medial orbit or to pathology affecting the anterior ethmoids and the nose (6). If the sinuses are large enough, an osteoplastic approach may allow access to the orbit and anterior nasal cavity as well as the anterior ethmoids without entering the cranium. Even if not large enough for complete access, the frontal sinus can often be incorporated into the frontal bone flap.

Variations of this method have proven to be a major advance in access to tumors involving the anterior cranial fossa (Fig. 3**B**) when neurosurgeons and head and neck surgeons can employ a team approach to *en bloc* resection (4). The lateral margin can be positioned depending on the extent of tumor involvement within the orbit. If the medial wall of the orbit is entirely spared, dissection can be carried down through the lateral aspect of the ethmoid block. If the lamina papyracea has been violated, the superior cut can be made directly through the medial aspect of the orbital roof with dissection along the periorbita. If the tumor has extended to involve the periorbita, this area can be entered just below the superior oblique muscle margin. While retracting the orbital contents laterally, an inferior incision can be made through the periorbita again to the antrum thus allowing the entire medial wall of the orbit, including the periorbita, to be removed *en bloc* with the ethmoids presumably involved by the tumor. It is even possible to extend this incision to remove the involved trochlear and superior oblique muscle. This will, of necessity, create some degree of motility disturbance, but often these patients are amenable to subsequent extraocular muscle surgery preserving significant areas of binocular single vision. Further extension to within the cone or involving the

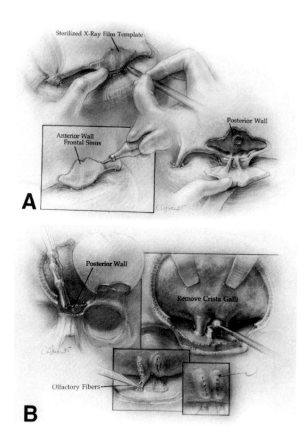

FIG. 3 The frontal sinus approach. **(A)** Frontal sinus approach: Whether used in conjunction with a formal craniotomy flap or alone in patients with large frontal sinuses, this approach affords excellent postoperative cosmesis. **(B)** The frontal sinus approach can be widened to approach the medial orbit and anterior cranial fossa. The posterior sinus wall is removed with rongeurs to improve extradural basal frontal fossa exposure. After the crista is removed, the olfactory fibers are dissected sharply and oversewn if necessary.

medial rectus muscle is usually an indication for exenteration if the pathology is malignant.

SURGICAL APPROACH TO TUMORS EXTENDING BEYOND THE CONFINES OF THE ORBIT

Benign tumors that secondarily affect the orbit can be removed even when the lesion extends intraconally. Probably the best example of this is an extension of meningioma from the lateral aspects of the greater wing of the sphenoid. Tumors arising in this location often extend to involve the temporal region as well as the orbit. This "three-compartment" meningioma requires attention to the details of its growth pattern if removal is to be complete (14).

Case Report

CLINICAL HISTORY

This 62-year-old man was referred to the University of Virginia in December 1993 with a 5-month history of increasing headaches, 5 weeks of increasing ocular prominence, and 1 week of double vision (Fig. 4A). His past history was remarkable for progressive decreased visual acuity that was originally attributed to "depression." He had undergone resection of a large sphenoid wing meningioma in 1988 elsewhere but the surgery had not extended to involve the orbit.

Examination demonstrated visual acuity of 20/25 on the right side and 20/400 on the left. He had diffuse depression in sensitivity on automated static perimetry. His external examination was remarkable for 11 mm

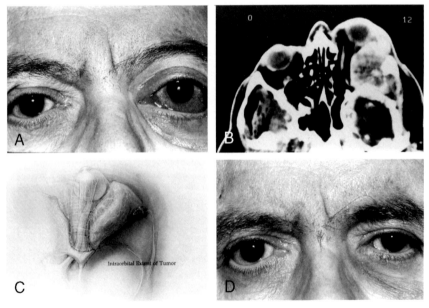

FIG. 4 Recurrent sphenoid wing meningioma. (**A**) Photograph showing presenting appearance with ocular prominence. (**B**) Preoperative CT scan showing an intracranial and intraorbital tumor after surgery elsewhere. (**C**) A drawing showing that after removal of the intracranial tumor components, the periorbita appeared intact. After opening the periorbita, a large tumor component was removed. (**D**) Postoperative photograph appearance showing reduction of proptosis. The patient's visual acuity and motility were preserved.

of proptosis on the left and 4 additional mm of inferior scleral show. He did have a mild left afferent pupillary defect and moderate restriction in motility in all directions. Computerized tomography scans demonstrated a significant recurrence of sphenoid wing meningioma involving the middle cranial and temporal fossae and orbital cavity (Fig. 4**B**).

TREATMENT

A preliminary pterional extradural approach was used, taking down all the bone of the lateral wall and roof of the orbit to the superior orbital fissure. The middle cranial fossa and temporal components could be removed easily. At that point the periorbita appeared to be intact (Fig. 4**C**). Dissection through the periorbita and the area of the superior rectus indicated the extent of meningioma involving the orbit with extension behind the globe. Two large nodules of tumor were removed with the periorbita representing almost the size of the globe itself. Postoperatively the patient had a 14-mm reduction in proptosis and preservation of his acuity and motility (Fig. 4**D**). Long-term improvement depends on aggressive removal of all involved tissues, including the periorbita and extension to within the orbital cavity; failure to recognize the orbital extent of these tumors often leads to residual proptosis and dystopia.

FIBROUS DYSPLASIA AS MODEL OF ORBITAL SURGERY

It is of significant historical interest that the first case discussed in Dandy's series (case 25) was a 28-year-old woman with severe headaches and exophthalmos originally seen at the Johns Hopkins Hospital in 1918 (Fig. 5**A**). She had previously been operated on by W. W. Keen in 1905 with exploration and removal of a portion of the orbital roof approaching the tumor within the orbit. Although described by Dandy as a "diffuse osteoma of the skull and orbit," the plain films and the description of the bone as "soft and spongy," suggest that this case represented fibrous dysplasia (Fig. 5**B**). Fibrous dysplasia may be isolated, as in the monostotic form, or, showing areas of multiple involvement (polyostic), may involve both the long bones and the bones of the skull base (15). This is particularly true of the sphenoid, frontal, and ethmoid complex bones. These tumors often affect the orbit, which produces globe displacement, proptosis, problems with motility, cosmetic surface deformities, and potential compromise of the optic nerve leading to decreased visual acuity. Because these lesions always extend beyond the confines of the orbit, a neurosurgical approach is usually warranted. Our experience at the University of Virginia demonstrates our increasing understanding of this disease process and ability to tailor the surgical approach to the problem.

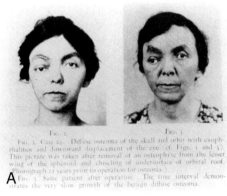

FIG. 2 Case 25. Diffuse osteoma of the skull and orbit with exophthalmos and downward displacement of the eye (cf. Figs. 1 and 3).
This picture was taken after removal of an osteophyte from the lesser
wing of the sphenoid and chiseling of undersurface of orbital roof.
Photograph 21 years prior to operation for osteoma.)
A FIG. 3 Same patient after operation. The time interval demonstrates the very slow growth of the benign diffuse osteoma.

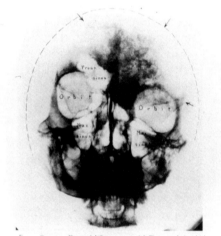

FIG. 1 Case 25. X-ray of diffuse osteoma (cf. Figs. 2 and 3), which
has obliterated right frontal sinus. Entire right orbit is placed lower
B than the left. The antrum is also lower, almost suggesting a congenital
displacement of these cavities.

FIG. 5 Fibrous dysplasia. (**A**) Two photographs of the patient described by W. E. Dandy
(8) showing a 21-year interval change. (**B**) An anterior-posterior skull radiograph of this
patient. Although Dandy described the mass as a "diffuse osteoma", the radiographic appearance and Dandy's description of the bone as "soft and spongy" suggest that the mass
represented what is now termed fibrous dysplasia.

Burring Procedure: A Case Report

CLINICAL HISTORY

The 39-year-old woman in Figure 6 was referred to the University of
Virginia in March 1994 with a 30-year history of progressive prominence of the globe. In 1967 she had undergone a surgical procedure for
thinning of the left cheek with some reduction in her proptosis. In the

2 years leading up to her admission at our institution, she had noted a progressive shift in her left globe as well as increasing prominence of her forehead (Fig. 6A). Visual acuity was correctable to 20/20 bilaterally with normal visual fields. The left globe was slightly lower than the right by about 3 mm, and she had a prominent forehead. Although her intermedial canthal distance was somewhat large, she wanted to do something to reduce the prominence of the forehead.

TREATMENT

A bicoronal incision and direct thinning of the bone with a shaping burr produced a cosmetic improvement (Fig. 6B). In this patient with a 30-year history, tailoring the operation to her wishes did not completely remove the abnormal growing tissue but did improve her overall acuity. Although the bone may continue to grow, developments are usually quite slow, allowing surgical remolding directly on the surface.

Acrylic Reconstruction

When the tumor is more extensive, often the bone cannot be left *in situ*. This young man (Fig. 7) had noted progressive displacement of the globe and gradually increasing prominence of his forehead. This had reached a point where simply tailoring the bone was inadequate. The surgical approach involved removal of the entire frontal complex with an acrylic reconstruction.

Management of the Downward Displaced Globe: A Case Report

Reconstituting the orbital roof and the forehead with methylmethacrylate often fails to allow adequate room for the globe to come up.

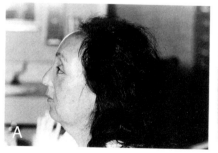 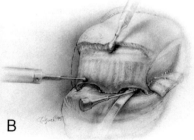

FIG. 6 Fibrous dysplasia: The burring procedure. (A) A preoperative photograph revealing a prominent forehead. (B) An artist's rendering of the operative procedure, including intraorbital burring and re-establishment of contours of forehead and orbital rims.

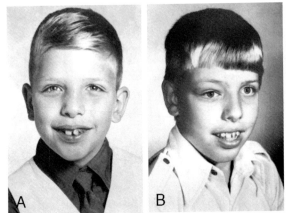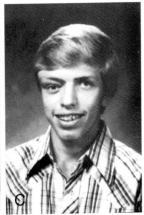

FIG. 7 Progressive fibrous dysplasia. Photograph of this child at 6 years of age (**A**), at 12 years of age (**B**), and at 19 years of age (**C**). At this point the child was referred to our institution. With this degree of involvement, a simple burring procedure would be inadequate.

Dandy's case was an early illustration of this, in which the globe dystopia persisted after surgery. While it may be necessary to literally lift the globe up, replacing autologous or alloplastic material within the orbital floor, may sometimes restore the globe to a more normal location simply by removing the offending downward compression of the thickened orbital roof.

CLINICAL HISTORY

This 46-year-old woman presented with a 5-year history of a prominent right globe being slowly displaced inferiorly. She attributed this to being "hit with a pillow" 20 years earlier. A CT scan done in 1988 had revealed fibrous dysplasia. On examination, visual acuity as well as ocular motility was entirely normal but the globe was displaced inferiorly by 3 to 4 mm with 2 mm of proptosis. Review of the MR image and CT scan (Fig. 8A) demonstrated that the superior portion of the orbital roof was in a normal position, while the inferior portion had displaced the globe inferiorly and forward.

TREATMENT

To allow approach to the inferior portion of the orbital roof, a bicoronal incision was made and the frontal supraorbital rim removed *in situ*. Although the frontal bone in this area involved by fibrous dysplasia was quite thick, the Gigli saw easily cut through it, permitting direct access to the inferior portion of the orbital roof (Fig. 8B). By hollowing

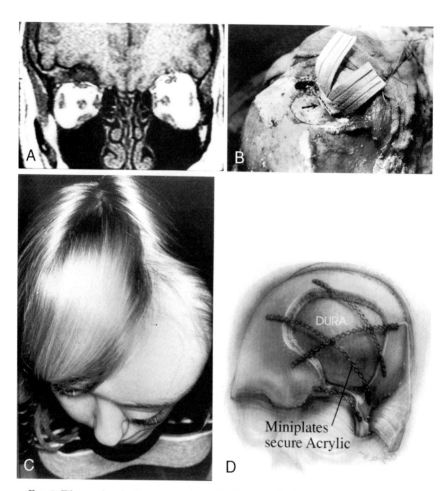

FIG. 8 Fibrous dysplasia compressing orbit downward. (**A**) A preoperative MR image. The superior edge of the superior orbital rim is in its normal position while its inferior edge is displacing the globe inferiorly and forward. (**B**) An intraoperative photograph shows the thickness of frontal bone and orbital roof that had been opened with the Gigli saw (*arrow*). The orbital roof was hollowed retaining the intracranial cortical table (*dotted line*). (**C**) A preoperative photograph of a different patient with more extensive globe dystopia requiring a more radical procedure. (**D**) An artist's rendering of this patient's operative procedure. The bone has been completely removed and will be replaced with cranioplastic material and held in position with microplates.

out the orbital cavity extending back to the edge of the sphenoid and then opening the restraining periorbita, the orbital contents were permitted to decompress posteriorly as well as superiorly. This maneuver resulted in resolution of both the dystopia and proptosis. Retention of the patient's own superior cortical table of the frontal bone had obvious advantages over placement of alloplastic material.

When involvement is more extensive, producing marked globe dystopia as well as external prominence, more radical procedures may be in order (Fig. 8C). The bone may be removed in its entirety and replaced by cranioplast or other alloplastic material. This may be positioned using wire or microplates (Fig. 8D).

Visual Loss in Fibrous Dysplasia: A Report of Three Cases

CLINICAL HISTORY

The chief concern in patients with fibrous dysplasia involves the potential for visual loss. Figure 9 depicts an 18-year-old woman who presented in June 1982 with a 4-week history of progessively decreasing visual acuity on the right side (Fig. 9A). She was 6 months pregnant and had noted an associated feeling of pressure; she also reported rapidly increasing proptosis and diplopia with attempt at up gaze. Examination revealed acuity of 20/50 on the right and 20/20 on the left; the globe was displaced by 7 mm, with 2 mm of ptosis and 9 mm of prop-

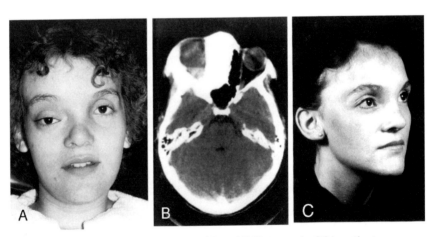

A   B   C

FIG. 9 Fibrous dysplasia causing visual loss. (A) Photograph of this patient upon presentation with dystopia and proptosis. Visual acuity was 20/50 OD 20/20 OS. (B) Preoperative CT revealing a large cystic cavity in the posterior orbit. (C) Postoperative photograph showing unchanged globe dystopia but marked reduction in proptosis.

tosis. In addition she had a right hypotropia increasing on up gaze. Funduscopic examination revealed mild disc edema and retinal and choroidal striae. A preoperative CT scan (Fig. 9B) revealed a large cystic cavity in the posterior orbit.

TREATMENT

The globe dropped back after a supraorbital approach allowed decompression of this cystic area and an additional soft, bony involvement of the apex. Postoperatively, the globe dystopia remained unchanged but the proptosis had decreased by 8.5 mm (Fig. 9C). Visual acuity returned to 20/20 on the right with resolution of her disc edema. This patient experienced rapid accumulation of a cystic component of fibrous dysplasia that produced acute compression of the globe and optic nerve which resulted in decreasing visual acuity. Although resembling mucoceles, these cysts are usually not mucosa-lined and represent enlargement of naturally occurring cysts within the fibrous dysplastic bone. By decompressing the cyst, acuity may be restored.

CLINICAL HISTORY

One of the more difficult aspects of dealing with fibrous dysplasia involves compromise of the optic canal. Figure 10 shows a 9-year-old girl who was evaluated at the University of Virginia in September 1994 and who had originally been seen 3 years earlier. Although visual acuity was 20/20 bilaterally, there was evidence of bilateral optic atrophy (Figs. 10, A and B) that was more worse on the right than on the left with a 1.2 log unit right afferent pupillary defect. Visual fields confirmed severe constriction with superior and inferior arcuate defects worse on the right than the left (Figs. 10, C and D). Follow-up CT and MR imaging revealed extensive compromise in both optic canals. She returned in September 1994 with reported progressive visual loss on the right side. Although she was somewhat hyperopic, acuity had dropped less than two lines. Visual fields, however, continued to demonstrate a central scotoma denser on the right than on the left.

TREATMENT

A transcranial orbitotomy was performed, with unroofing of the right optic canal. The canal was extensively involved with thick bone, with marked compromise to the optic nerve. Although the approach was done meticulously with the bone drilled down around the canal, postoperative visual acuity dropped to 2/200.

The mechanism of visual loss following unroofing the optic canal in cases of fibrous dysplasia remains unclear. The risk is not insubstantial

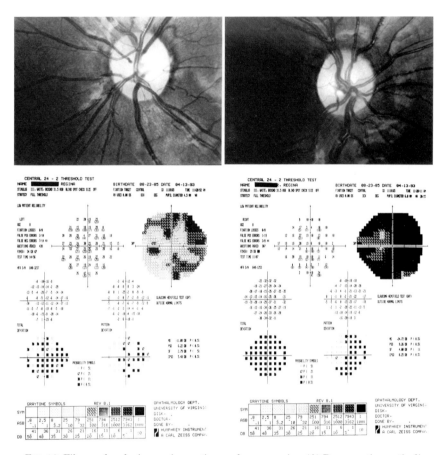

FIG. 10 Fibrous dysplasia causing optic canal compromise. (**A**) Preoperative optic disc photograph OS revealing optic atrophy. (**B**) Preoperative optic disc photograph OD revealing optic atrophy. (**C**) Preoperative automated static perimetry OS revealing severe constriction and superior and inferior arcuate defects. (**D**) Preoperative automated static perimetry OD revealing the same findings, only more severe.

FIG. 11 Fibrous dysplasia causing optic canal compromise. (**A**) A preoperative photograph from the front showing the cosmetic defect. Patient was blind OD. (**B**) A preoperative photograph in profile. (**C**) The preoperative CT scan reveals optic canal compromise bilaterally. Nevertheless, her visual acuity remains stable after 6 years' follow-up. (**D**) An intraoperative photograph in which correction of the cosmetic deformity was accomplished using wire across the orbital rim and acrylic. No attempt was made to decompress the left optic canal. (**E**) A postoperative photograph from the front revealing the improvement in the cosmetic deformity. (**F**) A postoperative photograph in profile again showing the results of the surgical correction. (**G**) An automated static perimetry at six years' follow-up revealing unchanged visual fields.

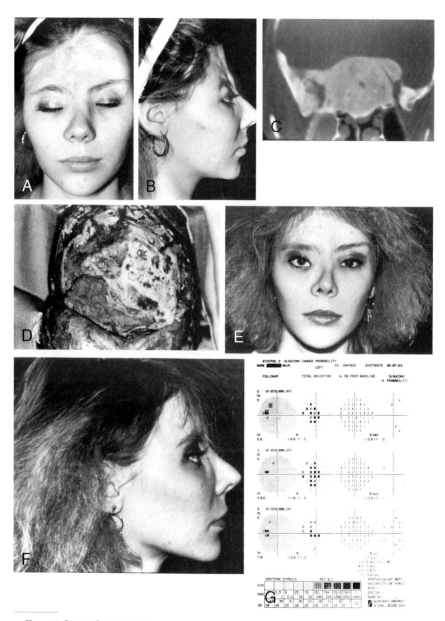

FIG. 11 Legend on page 68.

and the indications for intervention remain questionable. Although authors have suggested early aggressive intervention to prevent visual loss, progressive loss of visual acuity associated with fibrous dysplasia tends to be the exception rather than the rule.

CLINICAL HISTORY

Figure 11 shows a 19-year-old woman who was originally evaluated at the University of Virginia in May 1989. At 6 years of age, she was diagnosed as having fibrous dysplasia, and in 1978, at another institution, she underwent an initial surgical approach to the right orbit involving the right optic canal. After the surgery she lost the vision in her right eye. Subsequent CT scans revealed marked canal compromise both on the right and on the left sides, with severe narrowing (Fig. 11C). During her original evaluation in May 1989, visual acuity was 20/20 and 3 points. Her visual fields did demonstrate a relative central scotoma with some temporal breakout and she had been left with substantial cosmetic defect involving her right forehead (Figs. 11, A and B).

TREATMENT

She subsequently underwent surgery for cosmetic improvement on the right side (Figs. 11, E and F), but no attempt was made to decompress the left optic canal (Fig. 11D). Because of her loss of vision in one eye, her ophthalmic status was monitored closely. Follow-up MR imaging and CT scans continued to demonstrate marked canal compromise, but after 6 years of follow-up, visual acuity remains correctable to 20/20 on the left with normal color vision and no substantial change in her automated static perimetry (Fig. 11G).

CONCLUSION

It may be argued that, at times, the best surgical approach is no surgery at all. Successful treatment does not depend on only the technique of surgical approach and the advances thereof, but rather requires our continued improvements in understanding both the natural history of disease processes and the importance of appropriately timed intervention. This is true for fibrous dysplasia and may be said for all inflammatory and neoplastic processes that affect the skull and orbit. Appropriate case selection, improved preoperative planning made possible by the advent of imaging studies, and increasing attention to the cosmetic aspects of surgical approach will continue to improve the outcomes for our patients.

REFERENCES

1. Alper MG, Zimmerman LE, Sherman JL: Clinicopathologic correlation of orbital magnetic resonance imaging. **Trans Am Ophthalmol Soc** 84:192–220, 1986.
2. Ambrose J: Computerized transverse axial scanning (tomography), Part 2, clinical applications. **Br J Radiol** 46:1023–1047, 1973.
3. Berke RN: A modified Krönlein operation. **Trans Am Ophthalmol Soc** 51:193–227, 1953.
4. Biller, HF, Slotnick DB, Lawson W, et al.: Superior rhinotomy for en bloc resection of bilateral ethmoid tumors. **Arch Otolaryngol Head Neck Surg** 115:1463–1466, 1989.
5. Birch-Hirschfeld A: Operative Eingriffe im Bereich der Augenhohle, in Elschnig A (ed): *Qugenarztliche Operationslehre.* Berlin, Julius Springer, 1922.
6. Colohan AR, Jane JA, Newman SA, et al.: Frontal sinus approach to the orbit. Technical note. **J Neurosurg** 63:811–813, 1985.
7. Cushing H, Eisenhardt L: *Meningiomas. Their Classification, Regional Behavior, Life History, and Surgical End Results.* Springfield, Illinois, Charles C Thomas, 1938, p. 283.
8. Dandy WE: *Orbital Tumors. Results Following the Transcranial Operative Attack.* New York, Oskar Piest, 1941, p. 3-7.
9. Frazier CH: An approach to the hypophysis through the anterior cranial fossa. **Ann Surg** 57:145–152, 1913.
10. Jane JA, Park TS, Pobereskin LH, et al.: The supraorbital approach. Technical note. **Neurosurgery** 11:537–542, 1982.
11. Krönlein RU: Zur Pathologie und operativen Behandlung der Dermoidcysten der Orbita. **Beitr Klin Chir** 4:149–163, 1888.
12. Leone CR Jr.: Surgical approaches to the orbit. **Ophthalmology** 86:930–941, 1979.
13. Maroon JC, Kennerdell JS: Surgical approaches to the orbit. Indications and techniques. **J Neurosurg** 60:1226–1236, 1984.
14. Maroon JC, Kennerdell JS, Vidovich DV, et al.: Recurrent spheno-orbital meningioma. **J Neurosurg** 80:202–208, 1994.
15. Moore RT: Fibrous dysplasia. **Survey Ophthalmol** 13:321–334, 1969.
16. Smith B: The anterior surgical approach to orbital tumors. **Trans Am Acad Ophthalmol Otolaryngol** 70:607–611, 1966.
17. Wolfley DE: The lid crease approach to the superomedial orbit. **Ophthalmic Surg** 16:652–656, 1985.
18. Woods AC: Preface, in Dandy WE (ed): *Orbital Tumors. Results Following the Transcranial Operative Attack.* New York, Oskar Piest, 1941, vii–viii.
19. Wright JE, Stewart WB: Orbital surgery. **Int Ophthalmol Clin** 18:149–167, 1978.

5

Innovations in Surgical Approach: Lateral Cranial Base Approaches

J. DIAZ DAY, M.D., TAKANORI FUKUSHIMA, M.D., D.M.SC., AND STEVEN L. GIANNOTTA, M.D.

The discipline of cranial base surgery relies on a number of principles which, when adhered to, make individual approaches efficient, effective, and safe. Cranial base strategies always seek the *shortest trajectory* to the lesion. *Bone removal* is maximized in lieu of brain retraction. *Extradural exposure* is exaggerated to reduce brain retraction and preserve venous drainage. Surgical techniques are used that emphasize *cranial nerve preservation. Skeletonization-decompression* of neural and vascular foramina with sophisticated drilling techniques facilitates the attainment of the aforementioned goals. *Dural openings* are meticulously reconstituted.

The following two surgical approaches to the central cranial base are adaptations of previously applied strategies. By conscientiously adhering to the above principles, both have been expanded to serve as comprehensive techniques for complex pathologies, including giant aneurysms and large benign and malignant neoplasms.

THE EXTRADURAL ANTEROLATERAL TEMPOROPOLAR APPROACH

Development

Customarily, either the intradural pterional or subtemporal approaches have been used to access lesions of the central cranial base, including the upper clival, parasellar, and interpeduncular fossa regions. These standard approaches have proven versatile and adequate in most cases of upper basilar artery aneurysms, sella region tumors, and intracavernous pathologies. This is particularly true when the lesion is confined to one cistern or strongly lateralized. However, lesions such as giant basilar aneurysms or extensive tumors of the sellar region may not be adequately exposed using these approaches. Under such circumstances the more traditional approaches provide an unsatisfactorily narrow operative corridor. This results in a higher degree of brain retraction, hampered instrument and microscope maneuverability, and restricted access.

The extradural temporopolar approach takes advantage of extensive cranial base bone removal to affect an increased operative corridor with a reduction in brain retraction (5). Conceptually, it relies on definable corridors around the cavernous sinus to allow radical posterior temporal lobe retraction without sacrifice of the temporal tip-bridging veins. Such retraction results in a dramatically widened angle of attack, allowing radical angulation of the microscope through an arc of roughly 90° (Fig. 1). This is in comparison to the approximately 45° provided by the standard pterional approach. The widened angle of attack is advantageous in terms of viewing pathologic structures that extend medially or superiorly.

The extradural temporopolar approach is derived from the standard pterional schema first popularized by Yasargil for the treatment of anterior circulation aneurysms. Yasargil and Fox validated the versatility of this technique in his 1975 series of 28 aneurysms of the basilar tip (28). They advocated sacrifice of the posterior communicating artery as a means of widening the exposure of the basilar bifurcation. Drake combined the standard subtemporal approach to basilar aneurysms with the pterional approach to introduce the so-called "half-and-half" method for aneurysms located above the dorsum sellae (10). This strategy resulted in a more anterior trajectory. Sano's "temporopolar" approach capitalized on intradural posterior temporal pole retraction

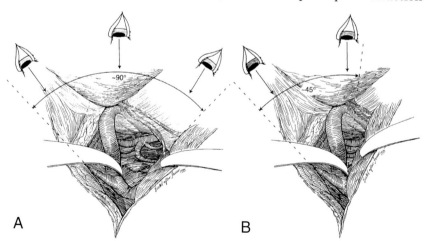

A **B**

FIG.1 (**A**) Wide viewing angle provided by the extradural temporopolar aproach. (**B**) Comparison view of the approach trajectory afforded by a standard pterional approach.

to affect a wider approach angle (27). Obligatory sacrifice of the temporal tip-bridging veins may result in compromised temporal lobe venous drainage.

The "transcavernous-transsellar" technique of Dolenc *et al.* further expanded the extradural temporopolar approach (8). Their approach utilizes extradural removal of the anterior clinoid process to expose the anteromedial cavernous triangle. The dura is opened in an inverted "T," and the frontal and temporal lobes are retracted intradurally. The posterior clinoid process is removed with the high-speed drill. Modest dissection of the medial cavernous triangle improves exposure to a high-positioned basilar bifurcation or large tumor.

Indications

Due to the extensive skull base and cavernous sinus dissection, the indications for this approach must be limited to complex pathologies. We have reserved its use for giant and high-positioned aneurysms of the upper basilar artery. Similarly, exposure of a particularly low positioned basilar tip aneurysm may benefit from the widened angle of attack afforded by this strategy. Tumors of the sellar region with large superior or posterior extensions, such as meningiomas or craniopharyngiomas, will be well exposed via this technique. It has also been used successfully for neurinomas of the abducens or trigeminal nerves (5).

Surgical Anatomy

Knowledge of the microsurgical anatomy of the cavernous sinus and its adjacent regions is a prerequisite for performing the extradural dissection of this approach. Particularly important is an intimate knowledge of the membranous coverings of the cavernous sinus. This anatomic construct is the basis for the defining maneuvers of the surgical approach. Also important for any approach to the cavernous sinus is familiarity with the triangle-shaped entry corridors, as described by various authors (4, 6, 8, 12–14, 26).

The cavernous venous plexus is bounded on all sides by the outer cavernous membrane. At the cranial base the periosteal layer of dura forms the outer cavernous membrane. The superior portion of the outer cavernous membrane is formed by a layer of connective tissue that incorporates the connective tissue sheaths of the third, fourth, and fifth cranial nerves. This sheath of connective tissue is contiguous with periosteum, meeting at the cranial base and enclosing the cavernous venous plexus. The outer cavernous membrane contains two condensations that surround the carotid artery at the foramen lacerum and as it passes into the epidural space inferior to the anterior clinoid process.

These condensations form the posterolateral and anteromedial fibrous rings.

The superior portion of the outer cavernous membrane forms the roof, or the outer portion of the lateral wall. The dura propria, which covers the inferior temporal lobe pole, is adjacent to this layer and is separable from the outer cavernous membrane, without disrupting its integrity. The dura propria may be separated from the outer cavernous membrane in the posterior and medial directions to the incisural edge and anterior petroclinoidal ligament. At these points, the dura folds over that of the posterior petrous bone coming from below, forming a reflection. This line of reflection, then, forms the limit of the extradural cavernous sinus dissection.

The full description of the triangular entry corridors into the cavernous sinus has been detailed elsewhere (4, 13, 14). The cavernous sinus triangles pertinent to the extradural temporopolar approach are the anteromedial, medial, superior, anterolateral, and far lateral (Fig. 2). The anteromedial triangle, originally described by Dolenc, outlines the epidural space that contains the subclinoidal segment of the carotid artery (8). The

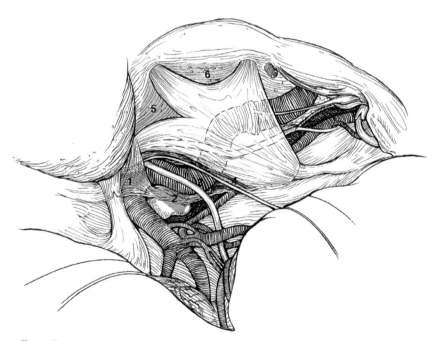

FIG.2 The triangular entry corridors into the cavernous sinus germane to the temporopolar approach. *1*, anteromedial; *2*, medial; *3*, superior; *4*, lateral; *5*, anterolateral; *6*, far lateral.

area is bounded by the optic nerve sheath dura, the medial wall of the superior orbital fissure, and the fibrous dural ring surrounding the carotid artery. The anterior clinoid process covers this triangle and is removed to expose the carotid artery below. The medial triangle provides the primary corridor to access the intracavernous carotid artery. The posterior clinoid process, the porus oculomotorius (the point of entrance of the oculomotor nerve into the wall of the cavernous sinus), and the angle of the subclinoidal carotid artery define the boundaries of this space. The superior triangle may be opened to expose the meningohypophyseal trunk. It is bounded by the third and fourth cranial nerves in the lateral wall of the cavernous sinus. It's posterior limit is the tentorial edge. The anterolateral triangle was first described by Sean Mullan as a means to exposing the superior orbital vein in the therapy of carotid-cavernous sinus fistulas (25). This space is delimited by the first and second divisions of the trigeminal nerve. Its anterior boundary is a line connecting the lateral edge of the superior orbital fissure and the medial lip of the foramen rotundum. The far lateral triangle is that located between the second and third divisions of the trigeminal nerve. These spaces will be exposed by the extradural temporopolar approach.

Surgical Technique

The patient is positioned supine with the head in rigid three-point pin fixation. The head is rotated 45° away from the side of approach with the vertex oriented approximately 15° downward. A routine "pterional" type scalp incision is made from the level of the zygomatic process to the midline. The scalp is elevated in two layers, and the temporalis muscle is elevated and retracted inferior and posterior (Fig. 3). This is done to clear muscle from the frontozygomatic recess and thus maximize the removal of bone over the temporal pole, providing a flat viewing trajectory across the temporal base. A frontotemporal craniotomy is typically made, removing the temporal squama to the cranial base. In approaching pathologies that extend considerably above the dorsum sellae, a more inferior-to-superior viewing trajectory may be desirable. In such cases, a transzygomatic or an orbitozygomatic craniotomy will result in a more extensive exposure (Fig. 4) (1, 11, 18). Removing the zygomatic arch allows more inferior retraction of the temporalis muscle, resulting in the ability to deviate the microscope for a superiorly directed view more radically. Further removal of the supraorbital bar results in expanding this increased angle of view frontally.

The dura is elevated from the anterolateral middle fossa to expose the foramen rotundum, superior orbital fissure, and the foramen ovale. Dura is elevated in the medial aspect from the floor of the anterior

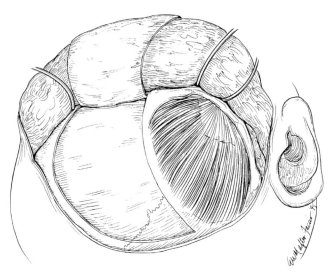

FIG.3 The scalp is reflected in two layers, preserving a vascularized pericranial flap medial to the superior temporal line. The lateral orbital rim and zygoma are exposed in preparation for a transzygomatic or an orbitozygomatic craniotomy.

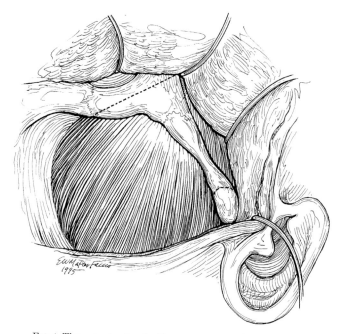

FIG.4 The osteotomies for the transzygomatic approach.

fossa. The sphenoid ridge is then reduced to result in a smooth contour from the anterior to the middle fossa across the superolateral orbit. To achieve a modest degree of mobility of the cranial nerve structures, the various neural foramina are unroofed using the high-speed drill under magnification. A length of approximately 5 to 8 mm of the second and third divisions of the trigeminal nerve is exposed by unroofing the foramen rotundum and foramen ovale, respectively. In similar fashion, the superior orbital fissure is skeletonized (Fig. 5).

The optic canal and anterior clinoid process are next addressed. The optic canal is unroofed in a 180° fashion to expose the optic nerve sheath. The anterior clinoid process is next removed extradurally, beginning by "coring out" the base of the process with a small diamond burr. The process is best removed as if debulking a mass, working in the soft center of the process and then thinning the outer cortex to a depressible shell of bone. Removal of the anterior clinoid is followed by reduction of the optic strut to complete the extradural bone removal.

At the apex of the superior orbital fissure, the meningo-orbital vessels are coagulated and divided. The cleavage plane between the periorbital fascia and the dura propria is then developed sharply, separat-

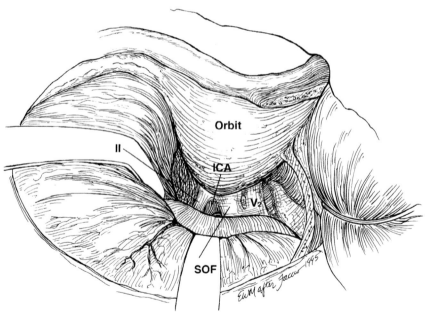

FIG.5 Illustrative view after extradural bone removal at the cranial base. *SOF,* superior orbital fissure; *ICA,* internal carotid artery.

ing dura propria from the outer cavernous membrane. Separation of these layers continues in the posterior and medial directions. The lateral limit of dural elevation is the foramen ovale. Posterior and medial, the limits of reflection are the incisura and petrous ridge. During this maneuver, a self-retaining retractor blade is placed on the temporal pole extradurally, and continuous posteriorly directed pressure is gently applied. As the dura propria is separated from the outer cavernous membrane, the temporal lobe is retracted posteriorly under protection of the overlying dura propria (Fig. 6).

A limited dural opening is then made in the shape of an "L." The incision begins over the sylvian fissure and extends to the optic nerve sheath, which is opened. The incision is then directed medially across the dura over the junction of the tuberculum and planum sphenoidale (Fig. 7). The fibrous dural ring surrounding the carotid artery entrance into the subarachnoid space is then incised to free the vessel of dural attachment. Beginning at the fibrous dural ring around the carotid artery, the fold of dura comprising the anterior petroclinoidal ligament is split. This dural split is continued lateral and posterior toward the porus oculomotorius. This maneuver will open the medial cavernous triangle. Cavernous sinus bleeding is controlled by judicious packing of oxidized cellulose. The superior border of the porus oculomotorius is opened and joined to the opening in the anterior petroclinoidal ligament. The oculomotor nerve may be mobilized at this point by releasing it from its connective tissue sheath. It may then be mobilized laterally and protected

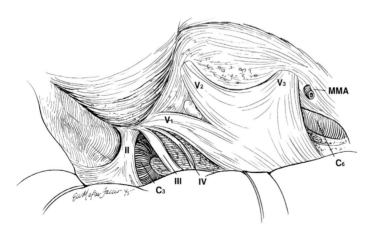

FIG.6 Elevation of the temporal dura propria from the outer cavernous membrane exposes the third through fifth cranial nerves in the lateral wall of the cavernous sinus. *MMA*, middle meningeal artery.

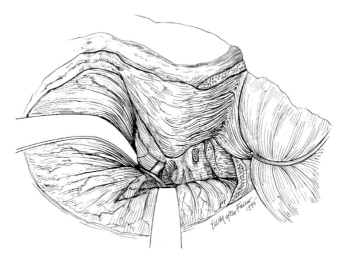

FIG.7 The dura is opened in an "L" directed along the sylvian fissure to the optic sheath, then extending across the tuberculum sellae.

by a soft cottonoid, opening the corridor to the interpeduncular fossa (Fig. 8). The membrane of Liliequist is opened sharply to open into the posterior fossa. To widen the exposure to the basilar artery, the posterior clinoidal process may be removed with the high-speed drill and a diamond burr (Fig. 9). The carotid artery may be mobilized to widen the exposure into the posterior fossa further, because it is not tethered by the fibrous dural ring (Fig. 10).

At the conclusion of the procedure, the dural opening is closed in a watertight fashion, using dural patch grafts as necessary. Superior cosmetic results are obtained by securing the bone flap with any of the titanium plating systems. The authors reapproximated the temporalis muscle along the superior temporal line, utilizing obliquely drilled bone channels to prevent sagging of the temporalis muscle postoperatively (7).

Summary

Several of the central tenets of contemporary cranial base surgery are satisfied by the extradural temporopolar approach. This technique reduces brain retraction by taking advantage of extradural cranial base bone resection. Release of neural and vascular structures traversing the cranial base by this removal of bone pays the added dividend of modest mobility of these substrates. The end result is a widened exposure without the added stress of overaggressive retraction. The approach further takes advantage of the construction of the

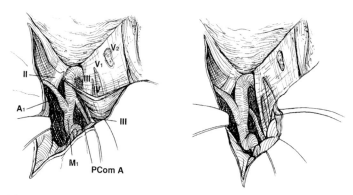

FIG. 8 A key maneuver is liberation of the carotid from the fibrous dural ring and opening the porus oculomotorius to gain mobility of the oculomotor nerve. *II*, optic nerve; *III*, oculomotor nerve; *IV*, trochlear nerve; V_1, ophthalmic division; V_2, mandibular division; A_1, anterior cerebral a.; M_1, middle cerebral a.; *PComA*, posterior communicating artery.

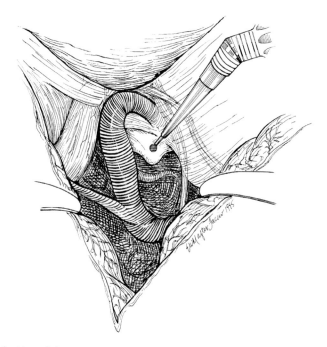

FIG. 9 Reduction of the posterior clinoid process enhances exposure to the posterior fossa.

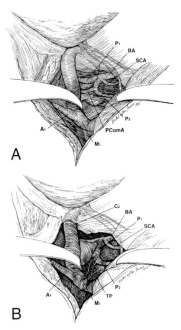

FIG.10 (**A**) Final exposure of the basilar caput. A_1, anterior cerebral artery; M_1, middle cerebral artery; P_1, P_2, posterior cerebral artery segments; *PComA*, posterior communicating artery; *BA*, basilar artery; *SCA*, superior cerebellar artery; (**B**) Same view with large basilar tip aneurysm. *TP*, thalamoperforating arteries; C_2, internal carotid artery.

lateral wall of the cavernous sinus to result in extradural retraction of the brain. This not only protects the brain by providing a natural barrier between the nervous tissue and retractor blade, but normal venous outflow routes are preserved. Taken as a whole, this strategy provides clear benefits by offering wide exposure for complex pathologic processes. The potential morbidity incurred by manipulation of cranial nerves and the carotid artery is not insignificant. Thus, the indications outlined should be satisfied to prevent placing the patient at an unnecessary risk for limited benefits.

THE EXTRADURAL ANTERIOR TRANSPETROSAL APPROACH (RHOMBOID APPROACH)

Development

In 1961, House described the extradural approach to the internal auditory canal via the middle fossa, aptly named the "middle fossa approach"

(20). This approach has been used mainly for the resection of intra-canalicular acoustic neurinomas, facial nerve decompression, and vestibular nerve section. Modifications of this basic approach followed, with the goal of expanding the exposure to the posterior fossa and, specifically, the petroclival region. Several authors incorporated removal of the bony labyrinth to expand the exposure to the lateral portion of the cerebello-pontine angle (2, 22). While advantageous in terms of exposing tumor in the cerebellopontine angle, hearing loss was a necessary by-product.

In 1985 Kawase et al. utilized an expanded middle fossa approach for aneurysms of the midbasilar trunk (24). Later, he described his experience with petroclival meningiomas (23). Working concurrently, House published a similar modification that extended the exposure to the petroclival region while preserving hearing (19, 21). These modifications involve extradural removal of apical petrous bone between the internal auditory canal and the petrosal sulcus. The boundaries of bone removal, as described by Kawase, et al., were the internal auditory canal, the trigeminal impression, and the posterior fossa dura. The inferior limit was the intrapetrous carotid artery. The approach as performed by House removed bone to the level of the petrosal sulcus, reaching the clivus bone as its inferior limit. This same idea was described by Hakuba et al. as a part of his combined retroauricular and preauricular transpetrosal-transtentorial approach (16, 17).

Indications

This approach, used alone, is indicated for apical petrous processes with or without extensions above the level of the incisura. Such lesions include meningiomas, trigeminal neurinomas, chordomas, and epidermoids. This approach is not well-suited to large lesions that extend beyond the boundaries of the petroclival region. It is best used in combination with another tactic if a significant component of tumor extends into the lower posterior fossa or anterior cavernous sinus. Vascular lesions that are accessible via this approach include midbasilar trunk aneurysms, especially at the origin of the anterior inferior cerebellar artery (AICA). Cavernous malformations, or other lesions, located laterally in the pons are also well exposed via the window created that leads into the posterior fossa.

As can be inferred from the discussion regarding the development of this technique, it lends itself well to combination with other approaches. Extradural petrous apex removal expands the exposure of the combined petrosal, subtemporal transcavernous, frontotemporal transcavernous, infratemporal fossa, translabyrinthine, transcochlear, and other approaches.

Surgical Anatomy

The anatomy pertinent to performance of the extradural bone removal in this approach has been described by several geometric constructs (3, 15, 24). For our version of the extended middle fossa approach, the authors view the middle fossa floor in terms of three triangular constructs and a rhomboid-shaped area that determines the volume of bone removal. Glasscock's posterolateral triangle (15) remains an important part of the construct, with the addition of two triangles. The premeatal triangle is defined by the intrapetrous carotid artery genu, the medial lip of the porus acusticus, and the geniculate ganglion. The postmeatal triangle describes the volume of bone on the posterolateral side of the internal auditory canal. It is defined by the geniculate ganglion, the lateral lip of the porus acusticus, and the petrous ridge (3, 13). The rhomboid construct is described by four points: (a) the greater superficial petrosal nerve (GSPN) junction with V3, (b) the porus trigeminus, (c) the petrous ridge at the posterior limit of the arcuate eminence (AE), and (d) the intersection of the axes of the GSPN and the AE (3) (Fig. 11).

Surgical Technique

The head is positioned in a 90° lateral position, with the vertex oriented approximately 15° toward the floor. The scalp is incised in the shape of a question mark that begins in front of the tragus of the ear. The height of the incision is just below the level of the superior temporal line. Scalp elevation is performed in two layers, splitting the temporal fat pad to protect the frontal branches of the facial nerve (29). The temporalis muscle and fascia are incised at the posterior aspect of the exposure and elevated subperiosteally, retracting the muscle forward. A key element to exposure is elevating periosteum and muscle from the root of the zy-

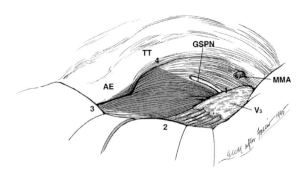

FIG.11 Left middle fossa floor with landmarks of the rhomboid complex highlighted. *AE*, arcuate eminence; *GSPN*, greater superficial petrosal nerve; *MMA*, middle meningeal artery, *TT*, tegmen tympani; V_3, mandibular division.

gomatic process. The muscle must be cleared from the zygoma root and pulled anteriorly. This provides a flat viewing trajectory across the middle fossa floor without requiring mobilization of the zygomatic arch, as suggested by others (3). With the temporal squama exposed, a 4-cm-square cranial flap is cut and is centered two-thirds anterior, one-third posterior to the external auditory meatus. After the flap has been removed, any remaining bone that overhangs the floor of the middle fossa must be removed with rongeurs or the high-speed drill (Fig. 12).

Dural elevation is begun posteriorly over the petrous ridge. The dura is elevated in the medial direction until the arcuate eminence is identified. The dura is then elevated in the anterior direction, identifying the greater superficial petrosal nerve running across the floor in the major petrosal groove. The middle meningeal artery will be seen emerging from the foramen spinosum, where it is coagulated and divided, which further increases the surface area of the middle fossa floor that is exposed. The medial limit of elevation is the trigeminal complex, lying in the trigeminal impression.

A key maneuver to increasing exposure is based on the anatomic construction of the cavernous sinus, as outlined for the temporopolar approach. The dura propria over the inferior temporal lobe may be separated from the connective tissue sheath of the trigeminal nerve. For this

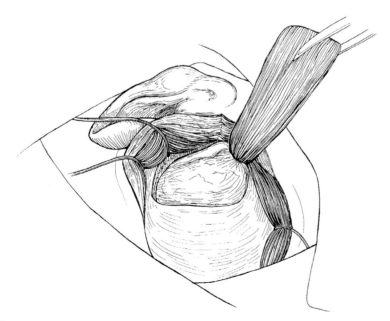

FIG.12 Left-sided approach showing temporal craniotomy and temporalis muscle flap to be used for closure of the middle fossa fenestration into the posterior fossa.

approach, separating the dura propria and outer cavernous membrane over V_3 and the lateral portion of the gasserian ganglion greatly facilitates the exposure of the middle fossa floor, which is illustrated in Figure 11.

With the middle fossa floor exposed, the critical landmarks necessary for guiding the extradural bone removal are identifiable. In obtaining maximal exposure and avoiding the internal structures of the hearing apparatus, it is important to proceed in a stepwise fashion. The drilling begins near the petrous ridge, along the bisection axis of the angle formed by the axes of the greater superficial petrosal nerve and the arcuate eminence. Removal of 3 to 4 mm of bone will expose the dura of the internal auditory canal and porus acusticus. After this dura is identified, it is best next to expose the intrapetrous carotid artery in the posterolateral triangle. The greater superficial petrosal nerve is divided, if necessary, as it passes deep to V_3. The bone over the posterolateral triangle is then removed to expose the carotid artery. The lateral limit of exposure is where the tensor tympani muscle is seen to cross over the artery. This marks the genu of the vessel, as it passes from the vertical to horizontal intrapetrous segment.

At this stage, the three points necessary to define the premeatal triangle have been identified: the carotid genu, the medial lip of the porus acusticus, and the intersection of the axes of the greater superficial petrosal nerve and the arcuate eminence. Within the basal one half of this construct is the cochlea. The bone between the internal auditory canal and carotid artery may then be safely removed (Fig. 13). Bone removal proceeds in a medial and inferior direction, inferior to the trigeminal

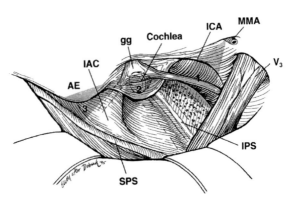

FIG.13 After petrous apex removal the extradural structures are seen, prior to dural incision. *AE,* arcuate eminence; *gg,* geniculate ganglion; *IAC,* internal auditory canal; *ICA,* internal carotid artery, *IPS,* inferior petrosal sinus; *MMA,* middle meningeal artery; *SPS,* superior petrosal sinus.

complex and cavernous sinus, out the petrous apex. The posterior fossa dura is exposed to the level of the inferior petrosal sinus.

To maximize the bone removal there are several key elements. First, bone must be removed from under the trigeminal complex to result in total resection of the petrous apex. This requires radical angulation of the microscope, as well as some "blind" drilling inferior to the nerve complex. Second, the carotid artery and the bone housing the cochlea must be undercut. This results in a wider window of bone opened and a larger posterior fossa dural surface to open. Thirdly, inferior bone removal should proceed beyond the level of the inferior petrosal sinus into the clivus. These maneuvers will result in a maximized window into the posterior fossa.

With drilling completed, the dura is opened. The initial step is to incise the dura parallel to the superior petrosal sinus on both the supra- and infratentorial sides. The incisions should extend from the region of the arcuate eminence to the fifth nerve entrance into Meckel's cave (the porus trigeminus). The superior petrosal sinus is then ligated near the trigeminal nerve. From this point, a parasagittal incision is made in the tentorium, approximately 8 to 10 mm in length. A suture is placed in the edge of the tentorium and retracted posteriorly. The dural ring around the trigeminal nerve root as it enters the porus trigeminus is opened to allow mobilization of the nerve. Next, the posterior fossa dura is incised and resected, opening the window into the posterior fossa. Laterally, the dura of the internal auditory canal is opened, exposing the seventh and eighth cranial nerves (Fig. 14).

Opening the dura exposes the pontine surface and medial cerebellopontine angle. In the depth of the exposure, the sixth nerve is viewed

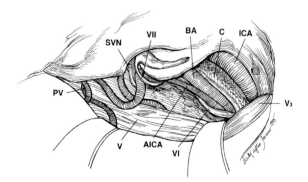

FIG. 14 Normal view of a left-sided approach to the posterior fossa. *AICA*, anterior inferior cerebellar artery; *BA*, basilar artery; *C*, clivus; *ICA*, internal carotid artery; *PV*, petrosal vein; *SVN*, superior vestibular nerve; *V*, trigeminal nerve; *VI*, abducens nerve; *VII*, facial nerve.

as it crosses behind the AICA. The trunk of the basilar artery is the deepest structure exposed, with the origin of the AICA typically framed in the depth of the exposure (Fig. 15). Deviation of the microscope through various angles is necessary to take full advantage of the operative corridor that has been created.

Summary

The extradural anterior transpetrosal approach possesses several advantages. First, the majority of the dissection is extradural, providing protection to the overlying neural structures. Second, only limited retraction of the temporal lobe is necessary, protecting venous outflow via the vein of Labbe'. Third, transposition of cranial nerves or vascular structures is unnecessary. Fourth, it enjoys natural compatibility with other surgical approaches to enhance exposure of the posterior cavernous sinus and petroclival region. The disadvantages are mostly related to the unfamiliar anatomy. Most surgeons are not accustomed to visualizing petrous apical anatomy from the middle fossa orientation. Therefore, practice of this technique in the cadaver laboratory is a mandatory prerequisite to its performance in the operating room. The cochlea, carotid artery, labyrinth, and cranial nerves five through eight are all at risk during drilling and dissection. When performed properly, this technique provides a solid adjunct to treating complex lesions of the central cranial base.

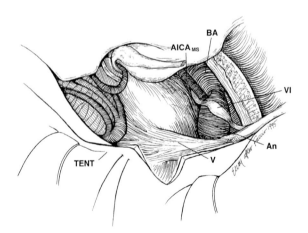

FIG.15 View of a left AICA aneurysm as seen through the approach. *AICAms*, meatal segment of anterior inferior cerebellar artery; *TENT*, tentorium; *An*, aneurysm; *BA*, basilar artery; *V*, trigeminal nerve; *VI*, abducens nerve.

REFERENCES

1. Al-Mefty O, Anand VK: Zygomatic approach to skull-base lesions. **J Neurosurg** 73:668–673, 1990.

2. Bochenek Z, Kukwa A: An extended approach through the middle cranial fossa to the internal auditory meatus and cerebellopontine angle. **Acta Otolaryngol (Stockh)** 80:410–414, 1975.

3. Day JD, Fukushima T, Giannotta SL: Microanatomical study of the extradural middle fossa approach to the petroclival and posterior cavernous sinus region: Description of the rhomboid construct. **Neurosurgery** 34:1009–1016, 1994.

4. Day JD, Fukushima T: Cavernous sinus neoplasms, in Youmans JR (ed): *Neurological Surgery: A Comprehensive Reference Guide to the Diagnosis and Management of Neurosurgical Problems*. Philadelphia, W.B. Saunders, 1996, ed 4, pp 2862–2881.

5. Day JD, Giannotta SL, Fukushima T: Extradural temporopolar approach to lesions of the infrachiasmatic and upper clival regions. **J Neurosurg** 81:230–235, 1994.

6. Day JD, Giannotta SL: Posterior circulation aneurysms, in Youmans JR (ed): *Neurological Surgery: A Comprehensive Reference Guide to the Diagnosis and Management of Neurosurgical Problems*. Philadelphia, W.B. Saunders, 1996, ed 4, pp 1335–1353.

7. Day JD, Levy ML, Fukushima T: Temporal muscle fixation. **J Neurosurg** 82:701, 1995.

8. Dolenc V: Direct microsurgical repair of intracavernous vascular lesions. **J Neurosurg** 58:824, 1983.

9 Dolenc V, Skrap M, Sustersic J, et al.: A transcavernous-transsellar approach to the basilar tip aneurysms. **Br J Neurosurg** 1:251–259, 1987.

10. Drake CG: The treatment of aneurysms of the posterior circulation. **Clin Neurosurg** 26:96, 1979.

11. Fujitsu K, Kuwabara T: Zygomatic approach for lesions in the interpeduncular cistern. **J Neurosurg** 62:340–343.

12. Fukushima T, Day JD, Tung H: Intracavernous carotid artery aneurysms, in Apuzzo MLJ (ed): Churchill Livingstone, *Brain surgery: Complication Avoidance and Management*. New York, 1992, vol 1, part 3, chap 30.

13. Fukushima T, Day JD: Surgical management of tumors involving the cavernous sinus, in Schmidek JJ, Sweet WH (eds): *Operative Neurosurgical Techniques: Indications, Methods, Results*. Philadelphia, W.B. Saunders, 1995, ed 3, pp 493–510.

14. Fukushima T: Techniques of carotid reconstruction. **Clin Neurosurg** 42:119–134, 1995.

15. Glasscock ME: Exposure of the intrapetrous portion of the carotid artery, in Hamberger CA, Wersall J (eds): *Disorders of the Skull Base Region: Proceedings of the Tenth Nobel Symposium, Stockholm, 1968.* Stockholm, Almqvist & Wicksell, 1969, p 135.

16. Hakuba A, Nishimura S, Inoue Y: Transpetrosal-transtentorial approach and its applications in the therapy of retrochiasmatic craniopharyngiomas. **Surg Neurol** 24:405–415, 1985.

17. Hakuba A, Nishimura S, Jang BJ: A combined retroauricular and preauricular transpetrosal-transtentorial approach to clivus meningiomas. **Surg Neurol** 30:108–116, 1988.

18. Hakuba A, Tanaka K, Suzuki T, *et al.*: A combined orbitozygomatic infratemporal epidural and subdural approach for lesions involving the entire cavernous sinus. **J Neurosurg** 71:699–704, 1989.

19. Hitselberger WE, Horn KL, Hankinson H, *et al.*: The middle fossa transpetrous approach for petroclival meningiomas. **Skull Base Surg** 3(3):130–135, 1993.
20. House WF: Surgical exposure of the internal auditory canal and its contents through the middle cranial fossa. **Laryngoscope** 71:1363–1385, 1961.
21. House WF, Hitselberger WE, Horn KL: The middle fossa transpetrous approach to the anterior-superior cerebellopontine angle. **Am J Otol** 7:1–4, 1986.
22. Kanzaki J, Kawase T, Sano K, *et al.*: A modified extended middle cranial fossa approach for acoustic tumors. **Arch Oto-Rhino-Laryngol** 217:119–121, 1977.
23. Kawase T, Shiobara R, Toya S: Anterior transpetrosal-transtentorial approach for sphenopetroclival meningiomas: Surgical method and results in 10 patients. **Neurosurgery** 28:869–876, 1991.
24. Kawase T, Toya S, Shiobara R, *et al.*: Transpetrosal approach for aneurysms of the lower basilar artery. **J Neurosurg** 63:857–861, 1985.
25. Mullan S: Treatment of carotid-cavernous fistulas by cavernous sinus occlusion. **J Neurosurg** 50:131, 1979.
26. Parkinson D: A surgical approach to the cavernous portion of the carotid artery: Anatomical studies and case report. **J Neurosurg** 23:474, 1965.
27. Sano K: Temporo-polar approach to aneurysms of the basilar artery at and around the distal bifurcation: Technical note. **Neurol Res** 2:361–367, 1980.
28. Yasargil MG, Fox JL: The microsurgical approach to intracranial aneurysms. **Surg Neurol** 3:7–14, 1975.
29. Yasargil MG, Reichmann MV, Kubik S: Preservation of the frontotemporal branch of the facial nerve using the interfascial temporalis flap for pterional craniotomy. **J Neurosurg** 67:463–466, 1987.

CHAPTER

6

Transpetrosal and Combination Approaches to Skull Base Lesions

MICHAEL T. LAWTON, M.D., C. PHILLIP DASPIT, M.D.,
AND ROBERT F. SPETZLER, M.D.

A decade ago skull base surgery became a major neurosurgical sub-specialty for dealing with complex lesions located at the anatomic border zones among the specialties of neurosurgery, otolaryngology, and plastic-craniofacial surgery. This collaborative effort assembled otologists' knowledge of temporal bone anatomy and facility with temporal bone removal, plastic surgeons' knowledge of maxillofacial anatomy and facility with facial disassembly and reconstruction, and neurosurgeons' knowledge of neuroanatomy and facility with microsurgical techniques. Intense interest and research spawned new techniques and their widespread application.

A critical component of many skull base approaches is the safe removal of the petrous bone (1, 2, 4–6, 11–14, 16, 19, 20, 24, 25, 28). Petrosectomy opens a corridor of exposure to the center of the skull base. The transpetrosal approaches are familiar to most neurosurgeons and include the retrolabyrinthine (28), translabyrinthine (4, 12, 19), transcochlear (13), and middle fossa approaches (5, 14). Still, exposure gained from these approaches can be limited at the region of interest medially or inadequate for larger lesions. Therefore, transpetrosal approaches have been used in combination with other approaches to gain even more exposure. For example, the combined supra- and infratentorial approach joins the subtemporal and transpetrosal exposures (6, 11, 24, 25), and the far lateral combined supra- and infratentorial approach adds to them the far lateral exposure (2, 3, 10, 21, 22, 27).

We have continued to experiment with combination approaches, and one that has proven useful is the orbitozygomatic-combined supra- and infratentorial approach. However, time and experience have tempered our enthusiasm for radical petrosectomy, and we have sought combination approaches that reduce the extent of temporal bone removal and corresponding morbidity, yet still provide adequate exposure.

This chapter reviews the surgical anatomy and techniques involved with the transpetrosal approaches, discusses the various combination approaches that use petrosectomy as their foundation, and identifies the current indications for these techniques. The discussion will focus on these technical issues, rather than on the results of our surgical series.

TRANSPETROSAL APPROACHES

We categorize the temporal bone dissection into three variations: retrolabyrinthine, translabyrinthine, and transcochlear (Table 1). The retrolabyrinthine approach removes temporal bone between the semicircular canals anteriorly and the posterior fossa dura on the posterior aspect of the temporal bone. The semicircular canals are skeletonized, but not violated, to maximize this working space. The translabyrinthine approach removes the semicircular canals, which causes loss of hearing (4, 12). Their removal increases the exposure anteriorly to the internal auditory canal. The transcochlear approach requires the facial nerve to be dissected from its bony canal and transposed to gain access to the cochlea for its removal (13). This approach enables almost complete removal of the petrous bone, with maximum exposure of the brainstem and clivus. The three types of temporal bone dissection represent a graduated increase in the amount of petrous bone resected with a corresponding increase in anterior exposure. The price of this increased exposure is progressively greater sacrifice of function in the seventh and eighth cranial nerves.

Extended Retrolabyrinthine Approach

The patient is positioned supine with the head turned away from the lesion, bringing the midline parallel to the floor and inclined slightly downward. The mastoid bone becomes uppermost in the operative field. A shoulder roll under the ipsilateral shoulder minimizes neck rotation. The skin is incised at the zygoma 1 cm anterior to the tragus and curves gently around the ear to the mastoid tip. The scalp flap is retracted inferiorly with fishhooks and a Leyla bar (23).

TABLE 1
Preservation of Cranial Nerve Function

Approach	Hearing	Facial Nerve
Retrolabyrinthine	Preserved	Preserved
Translabyrinthine	Sacrificed	Preserved
Transcochlear	Sacrificed	Transient paralysis or paresis

The neurotologist begins with a basic mastoidectomy. We prefer the MedNext (MedNext Co., Riviera Beach, FL) high-speed drill over the Osteon (Zimmer Assoc., Santa Barbara, CA) drill used previously, because it is more powerful, weighs less, and has less torque. The operating microscope and suction-irrigation are essential. An initial cut is made along the temporal line, the ridge that continues from the superior border of the zygomatic arch posteriorly to the mastoid cortex, marking both the inferior limit of temporalis muscle insertion and the floor of the middle fossa (tegmen of the temporal bone). A second cut is made perpendicularly, running inferiorly to the mastoid tip immediately behind the posterior canal wall. Mastoid cortex is then removed widely and rapidly with a large burr. It is important that the neurotologist remove superficial bone extensively, because residual bone along the posterior canal wall or mastoid tip constricts operating space, limits viewing angles, and obscures anatomic landmarks. Bone in the sinodural angle and covering the sigmoid sinus is removed completely to allow retraction of the sinus posteriorly.

The sigmoid sinus, middle fossa dura, and sinodural angle between them are the first important landmarks. The superior petrosal sinus lies deep to the sinodural angle and represents the posterior-superior margin of the temporal bone. Dissection into the mastoid antrum reveals the horizontal semicircular canal, which leads the surgeon to other anatomy, including the external genu of the facial nerve medially and inferiorly, the posterior semicircular canal posteriorly, and the epitympanum and superior semicircular canal anteriorly. The posterior and superior semicircular canals are skeletonized, when drilling is done as far anteriorly as possible (Fig. 1). Resection of temporal bone above and below the optic capsule exposes medial middle fossa dura, the superior petrosal sinus, and the jugular bulb. A large dural surface is thereby exposed which, when opened, accesses the cerebellopontine angle. The retrolabyrinthine approach provides excellent exposure of the angle but does not provide exposure of the anterior brain stem.

Translabyrinthine Approach

The translabyrinthine approach is used when greater exposure is needed. The initial part of this approach is the same as the retrolabyrinthine approach. The neurotologist proceeds by removing all three semicircular canals and skeletonizing the posterior half to two thirds of the internal auditory canal (IAC) (Fig. 2). The medial walls of the vestibule and superior semicircular canal ampulla represent the lateral wall of the IAC fundus, so minimal bone removal at this location exposes IAC. The superior vestibular nerve lies posterosuperiorly

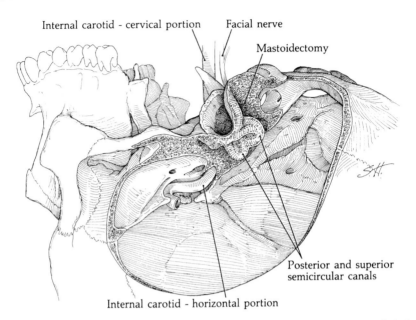

FIG.1 The extended retrolabyrinthine approach consists of mastoidectomy and skeletonization of the semicircular canals. (Reproduced with permission from Barrow Neurological Institute.)

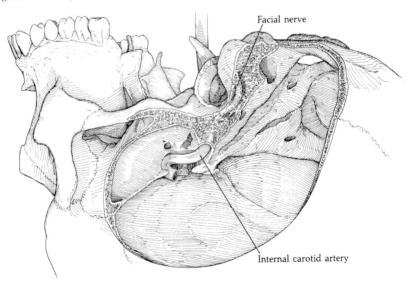

FIG.2 The translabyrinthine approach removes the semicircular canals and skeletonizes the descending segment of the facial nerve and internal auditory canal. (Reproduced with permission from Barrow Neurological Institute.)

in the canal and is encountered first. This nerve is separated from the facial nerve anterosuperiorly by a shelf of bone, Bill's bar. Therefore, the superior vestibular nerve is an important landmark in identifying the facial nerve as it exits the IAC and runs forward to the geniculate ganglion. The facial nerve is guarded carefully throughout the drilling with the aid of facial nerve monitoring. It is skeletonized with a diamond bit along its horizontal (tympanic) segment, external or second genu, and descending (mastoid) segment. The nerve is left in its thinned bony canal to minimize risk of injury. Additional exposure is gained by removing bone anteriorly and medially above the IAC in Kawase's triangle. Typically, the sigmoid sinus is unroofed to the jugular bulb to maximize inferior exposure beneath the IAC.

After this extensive bone removal, the exposure is more anterior than that of the retrolabyrinthine approach. The cerebellopontine angle, anterolateral brainstem, and inferior clivus are visualized. However, the exposure is obtained at the expense of ipsilateral hearing and has an increased risk of CSF leakage.

Transcochlear Approach

The transcochlear approach is a forward extension of the translabyrinthine approach that mobilizes the facial nerve, removes the cochlea, and opens into the cerebellopontine angle to expose anterolateral brainstem and clivus (13). This approach provides the maximum exposure that can be achieved by a transpetrosal approach by essentially resecting the entire petrous bone (Fig. 3).

The initial procedure is the same as for the translabyrinthine approach, except the external auditory canal is transected and oversewn in two layers. The facial nerve is skeletonized along its course from its entrance into the internal auditory canal to its exit from the stylomastoid foramen. An extended facial recess opening is performed. The facial recess is a tract of air cells bounded medially by the descending segment of the facial nerve, laterally by the chorda tympani, and superiorly by the fossa incudis. Opening the facial recess exposes the middle ear space, the stapes and incus, the promontory of the cochlea, Jacobson's nerve, and the horizontal segment of the facial nerve. The facial recess is opened into the epitympanum, and the ossicles are removed. The chorda tympani is sectioned inferiorly at its origin from the descending portion of the facial nerve, allowing the facial recess to be extended inferiorly to the hypotympanum and retrofacial area. The greater superficial petrosal nerve is sectioned anteriorly at its origin from the geniculate ganglion. These maneuvers free the facial nerve, which is transposed posteriorly after dissection from its bony canal.

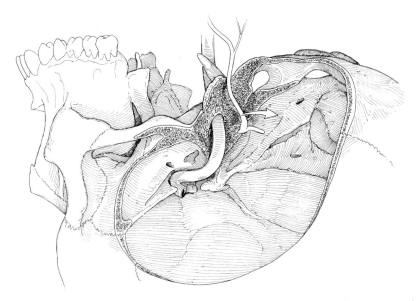

FIG.3 The transcochlear approach requires transposition of the facial nerve posteriorly and removal of the cochlea. (Reproduced with permission from Barrow Neurological Institute.)

The cochlea is then drilled out completely, beginning with the promontory that houses the basal turn. Bone removal is carried forward to the septum between the basal turn and the internal carotid artery. The internal carotid artery and internal jugular vein leave the carotid sheath and enter the skull base in proximity to each other. The jugulocarotid septum, a ridge of bone that separates the carotid artery as it turns anteriorly from the jugular vein as it turns posteriorly, is removed to expose the jugular bulb completely. The close relationship of the ninth, tenth, and eleventh cranial nerves must be remembered to avoid injuring them. During the extensive drilling of the temporal bone, the dura of the internal auditory canal is kept intact to protect this part of the facial nerve.

When the drilling is completed, the entire tympanic portion of the temporal bone is removed. Superiorly, the superior petrosal sinus is exposed from the sinodural angle laterally to Meckel's cave medially. Inferiorly, the inferior petrosal sinus and jugular bulb are exposed. Bone removal extends medially to the clivus and anteriorly to the internal carotid artery and periosteum of the temporomandibular joint. The bone surrounding the carotid artery can be removed superiorly to the middle fossa floor and medially to the siphon, thereby creating the exposure needed for a saphenous vein bypass graft from the petrous segment to supraclinoid segment of the carotid artery, if necessary (26).

The transcochlear approach yields the greatest exposure of the transpetrosal approaches. A wide triangular corridor is opened, leading directly to the clivus. The approach sacrifices hearing and increases the risk of CSF leakage. Mobilization of the facial nerve increases the risk of facial paresis or paralysis (25, 28).

COMBINATION APPROACHES

Combined Supra- and Infratentorial Approach

There are three essential components of the combined approach (6, 11, 24, 25, 28). First, one of the temporal bone dissections described above is performed. Second, a supra- and infratentorial craniotomy is made that causes the transverse sinus. Third, the tentorium is divided to connect the supra- and infratentorial compartments. Extensive exposure of the medial petrous and clival regions and associated neurovascular structures is obtained with minimal brain retraction.

When the neurotologist has completed the temporal bone drilling, an edge of middle fossa dura is exposed above the petrosectomy defect, and an edge of posterior fossa dura is exposed behind the sigmoid sinus (Fig. 4). These epidural locations serve as burrholes for a subtemporal-suboccipital craniotomy that crosses the transverse sinus. A large dural surface is exposed with visualization of the transverse, sigmoid, and superior petrosal sinuses. Before the dura is opened, the brain is relaxed with hyperventilation, mannitol, and removal of CSF through a lumbar drain. The dura is incised anteriorly over the temporal lobe and curves posteriorly and inferiorly to the superior petrosal sinus below, where it enters the sigmoid sinus. A second dural incision is made inferiorly in front of the sigmoid sinus, curving up to the superior petrosal sinus. The superior petrosal sinus is cauterized or clipped and divided. The surgeon should beware of a low-lying vein of Labbé that could be injured during the dural opening.

The sigmoid sinus may be sacrificed if the contralateral transverse and sigmoid sinuses are patent angiographically and communicate with the ipsilateral transverse and sagittal sinuses through a patent torcular herophili. As an added assurance, sigmoid sinus pressures are measured before and after test occlusion of the sigmoid sinus. We have observed no elevations of more than 7 mm Hg when angiographic patency of the sinuses has been confirmed (25). If the pressure were to rise by more than 10 mm Hg with test conclusion, the sinus should be kept intact. These measurements are made after the superior petrosal sinus has been divided. The sigmoid sinus can be sacrificed safely when

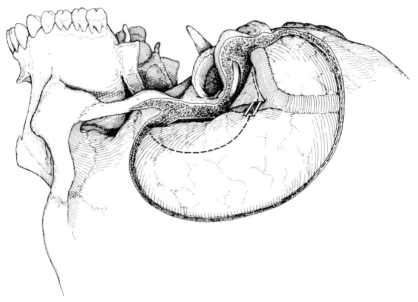

FIG.4   The dural incision of the combined supra- and infratentorial approach crosses superior petrosal sinus below where it enters the sigmoid sinus, thereby preserving sigmoid sinus. (Reproduced with permission from Barrow Neurological Institute.)

these angiographic and hemodynamic criteria are met. It is divided below its confluence with the superior petrosal sinus. The vein of Labbé consistently and reliably enters the transverse sinus above this junction and will therefore drain contralaterally. Notwithstanding these safety concerns, division of the sigmoid sinus is only necessary when additional exposure is needed, and the authors have not sacrificed the sigmoid sinus in more than 3 years.

When the dural incisions are completed and the superior petrosal sinus has been divided, the tentorium is incised medially to the tentorial hiatus, posterior to the fourth cranial nerve (Fig. 5). This crucial maneuver connects the supra- and infratentorial compartments and relaxes neural structures. The posterior temporal lobe is elevated, while the surgeon is careful to preserve the vein of Labbé, which is tethered to the transverse sinus. The petrous region, clivus, brainstem, cranial nerves, and vessels of the posterior circulation are well visualized. The lesion is accessed by working between adjacent cranial nerve bundles. The approach gives wide exposure along the skull base from the foramen magnum to above the dorsum sella with minimal brain retraction.

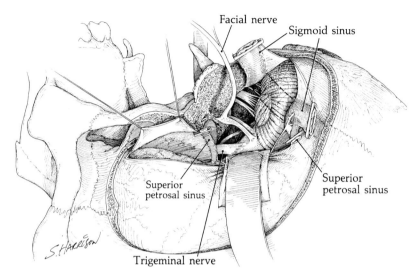

Facial nerve

Sigmoid sinus

Superior
petrosal sinus

Superior
petrosal sinus

Trigeminal nerve

FIG.5 Incising the tentorium medially to the tentorial incisura exposes the cranial nerves, brainstem, vasculature, and clivus. Note that the sigmoid sinus has been divided. (Reproduced with permission from Barrow Neurological Institute.)

Far Lateral-Combined Supra- and Infratentorial (Combined-Combined) Approach

Occasionally, petroclival lesions span the entire length of the posterior fossa from above the petrous apex to below the foramen magnum. For these lesions, a combination approach joining the transpetrosal, subtemporal, and far lateral approaches overcomes the limitations of just a transpetrosal approach (2, 3). This approach is the most extensive of the combination approaches and is referred to as the "combined-combined" approach. The far lateral approach has been well described elsewhere (10, 21, 22, 27, 28) but is simply a lateral extension of a unilateral suboccipital approach that removes additional lateral occipital bone, the inferior foramen magnum, the posterior half of the condyle, and the arch of the first cervical vertebra. Bone removal gives a more anterior angle to the inferior clivus and upper cervical region, enabling access to the anterolateral brainstem, lower cranial nerves, and the vertebrobasilar junction. When used with the combined supra- and infratentorial approach, the entire petroclival region is exposed.

An important modification to the far lateral approach is the patient's position (27, 28). The authors use a modified park bench position with the patient on his or her side, lesion side upward. The operating table is extended by placing a 3/4-inch plastic board under the mattress and pulling both the mattress and board 20 cm beyond the edge of the table. The patient is positioned so that the dependent arm hangs over the extended end of the table, cradled in a paddled sling in the gap between the Mayfield head holder and its attachment to the table. This position improves venous return, minimizes brachial plexus compression, and enables better positioning of the head.

Unlike other transpetrosal approaches, the head is not placed in the straight lateral position. Three maneuvers position the head optimally: (a) flexion in the anteroposterior plane until the chin is one finger's breadth from the sternum, (b) rotation 45° away from the side of the lesion (down), and (c) lateral flexion 30° down toward the opposite shoulder. The clivus is then perpendicular to the floor, allowing the surgeon to look down the axis of the basilar artery and work between horizontally arrayed cranial nerves. The ipsilateral mastoid process becomes the highest point in the operative field, and the posterior cervical-suboccipital angle is opened maximally to increase the surgeon's operating space.

The hockey stick incision used for the far lateral approach is enlarged, beginning anteriorly at the zygoma, coursing superiorly around the pinna and toward the inion, and ending inferiorly in the midline at C4. A myocutaneous flap is elevated to expose the lateral temporal bone, mastoid, posterior cranium, and laminae of C1 and C2. A cuff of nuchal fascia is left to reattach the cervical muscles at the end of the procedure.

Bone removal consists of four parts: petrosectomy, C1 laminotomy, craniotomy, and condylar expansion. The neurotologist first drills the temporal bone. Rotation of head can be adjusted during the petrosectomy to bring the head parallel to the floor to facilitate drilling. The arch and lateral mass of C1 are exposed, and the vertebral artery is dissected along its course from the transverse foramen to its dural entry point. The arch of C1 is removed with the Midas Rex (Midas Rex, Inc. Fort Worth, TX) drill. The lateral cut is made at the sulcus arteriosus, and additional atlantal bone is removed until the transverse foramen is reached. The foramen can be opened dorsally and the artery mobilized, if necessary. The craniotomy cut then connects the foramen magnum with the anterior margin of the petrosectomy overlying the inferior temporal lobe, crossing the transverse sinus. A second cut connects the lateral foramen magnum with the posteroinferior margin of the petrosectomy, immediately behind the sigmoid sinus. The underlying dural sinuses are dissected carefully from the bone flap, which is then removed. Finally, the lateral aspect of the foramen magnum, jugular tubercle, and posteromedial two thirds of the occipital condyle are removed. The extreme lateral removal of bone minimizes retraction and maximizes exposure of the anterior brainstem along this route.

The dura can be opened either in two flaps in front of and behind the sigmoid sinus to preserve this structure or in a single flap that sacrifices the sigmoid sinus. The two dural flaps are simply the standard openings for the combined approach plus the standard opening for the far lateral approach. The latter opens the dura in the midline at the C1 level and extends laterally in an L shape below the dural entry point of the vertebral artery and extends superiorly to the sinodural angle. The lateral cuts enable the dura and vertebral artery to be pulled laterally against the margin of the craniotomy. When the presigmoid dural opening of the combined approach is completed, two windows of exposure are opened on either side of the preserved sigmoid sinus. In contrast, sacrificing the sigmoid sinus and crossing it below the sinodural angle joins these two incisions to create a single flap extending from the anterior margin of the craniotomy over the temporal lobe, across the sigmoid sinus, and down to the C1 level (Fig. 6). When the tentorium is incised to the hiatus, a large unobstructed opening is created that exposes the anterolateral brainstem from the midbrain to the upper cervical spinal cord (Fig. 7).

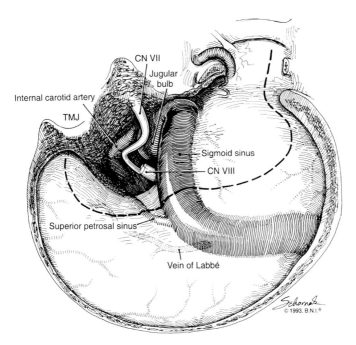

FIG.6 The dural opening for the far lateral-combined supra- and infratentorial ("combined-combined") approach. Alternately, the dura can be opened in two flaps in front of and behind the sigmoid sinus to preserve this structure. (Reproduced with permission from Barrow Neurological Institute.)

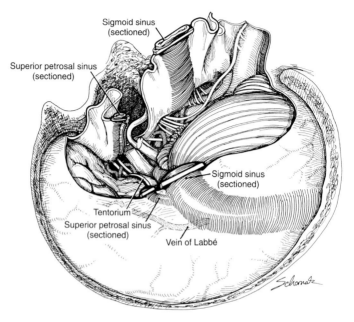

FIG.7   An overview of the exposure provided by the far lateral-combined supra- and infratentorial ("combined-combined") approach. (Reproduced with permission from Barrow Neurological Institute.)

Arachnoid dissection reveals the second through twelfth cranial nerves, both vertebral arteries, posteroinferior cerebellar arteries, anterior spinal artery, vertebrobasilar junction, basilar artery, and the entire length of the clivus (Fig. 8) (7). Division of the dentate ligaments facilitates surgical manipulation of neural structures.

Extended Middle Fossa Approach

The middle fossa approach is different from the other transpetrosal approaches. Instead of approaching petroclival lesions laterally by drilling out the petrous pyramid, the middle fossa approach accesses these lesions from anterior and above, leaving the lateral temporal bone intact and removing just its medial portion (5, 14). The advantage of this approach is that it provides a direct route to small lesions in and around the IAC but keeps the hearing apparatus intact. The middle fossa approach is used extensively in acoustic neuroma surgery to remove small, intracanalicular tumors with less than 5-mm extension into the cerebellopontine angle. The chances of preserving hearing are good in patients with useful preoperative hearing, usually defined as

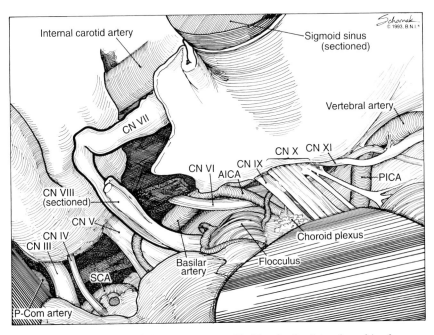

FIG.8   A close-up view of the exposure provided by the far lateral-combined supra-
and infratentorial ("combined-combined") approach. *CN*, cranial nerve; *AICA*, anterior
inferior cerebellar artery; *PICA*, posterior inferior cerebellar artery; *SCA*, superior cerebellar artery; *P-Com*, posterior communicating. (Reproduced with permission from Barrow Neurological Institute.)

speech reception thresholds less than 50 dB and speech discrimination
scores greater than 50% (5, 14).

A complete understanding of the surgical anatomy is essential when
performing the middle fossa approach. The dissection is demarcated
anteriorly by the middle meningeal artery where it leaves the foramen
spinosum. Medial to this initial landmark is the greater superficial petrosal nerve originating from the geniculate ganglion of the facial nerve
and running superficially along the middle fossa floor in an anteroposterior direction. The greater superficial petrosal nerve is the lateral
limit of the dissection. The posterior limit of the dissection is the arcuate eminence, a bony prominence along the middle fossa floor that
marks the underlying superior semicircular canal. Perpendicular to
the arcuate eminence is the petrous ridge, which defines the medial
limit of the dissection.

The crux of this approach is identifying the IAC, which can be done
in two ways. The first technique follows the greater superficial petrosal

nerve posteriorly to the geniculate ganglion of the facial nerve, then drills out the facial nerve retrograde to expose the IAC. The second technique, which the authors prefer, approximates the location of the IAC by bisecting the approximately 120° angle formed between the greater superficial petrosal nerve and arcuate eminence. Petrous bone is then removed over the IAC medially where there are no adjacent neurovascular structures, and drilling is relatively safe. The dura of the canal is exposed working from medial to lateral. Remembering that the IAC runs along the same axis as the external auditory canal can help orient the surgeon to the surgical field.

The patient is positioned supine with the head turned away from the lesion and inclined slightly downward. The skin and temporalis muscle are incised and reflected anteriorly. A 5 × 5-cm craniotomy is made in the squamous portion of the temporal bone two thirds anterior and one third posterior to the external auditory canal, with the flap extending inferiorly to the middle fossa floor. The dura is elevated from the middle fossa floor medially to the petrous ridge, and a House-Urban or another self-retaining middle fossa retractor is placed with its tip over the lip of the petrous ridge. The middle meningeal artery is followed along the dura to the foramen spinosum, and the greater superficial petrosal nerve is identified approximately 1 cm medially. The greater superficial petrosal nerve and geniculate ganglion are often dehiscent and vulnerable to injury during the dissection. The arcuate eminence and the greater superficial petrosal nerve are identified, and the IAC is drilled out beginning medially. Bone is removed around the porus acusticus and around the IAC until its upper three quarters of dura are exposed. The lateral IAC (fundus) is surrounded by important anatomy. The cochlea is immediately anterior. Its basal turn is particularly vulnerable to entry when drilling in the angle between the greater superficial petrosal nerve and the IAC, and perforation of the cochlea results in hearing loss. The vestibule and ampulla of the superior semicircular canal are immediately posterior to the fundus. As drilling proceeds laterally, the exposure is narrowed to avoid the cochlea and superior semicircular canal. Dura of the IAC is exposed laterally to Bill's bar, the vertical shelf of bone that separates the facial nerve anteriorly from the superior vestibular nerve posteriorly. Dura is opened along the axis of the IAC to expose the tumor. The preservation of hearing depends on preserving the IAC artery and on dissecting the tumor from medial to lateral to avoid traction on the cochlear nerve that might avulse these fragile nerve fibers (5).

The extended middle fossa approach removes more of the medial petrous bone in Kawase's triangle (16) and anterior petrous bone up to the horizontal portion of the petrous internal carotid artery. The tentorium is cut to enter the posterior fossa and expose the anatomy. Labyrinthectomy also can be added when hearing preservation is not attempted. The middle fossa approach is technically difficult due to limited exposure and limited anatomical landmarks. Drawbacks include the fact that the facial nerve lies between the surgeon and the tumor during the resection, forcing the surgeon to work over the facial nerve. The nerve is vulnerable in this position and must be protected from injury and excessive manipulation. Bleeding in the posterior fossa is at the depth of the operative field and can be difficult to control.

RECENT TRENDS IN TRANSPETROSAL SURGERY

Orbitozygomatic-Combined Supra- and Infratentorial Approach

We have continued to experiment with new combination approaches to provide the exposure needed for complex skull base lesions. An approach that we have used extensively in recent years is the orbitozygomatic approach (8, 9, 15, 17, 18). The technique removes the superior orbital rim and roof, lateral orbital rim and wall, and zygomatic arch in a single piece to allow downward retraction of the globe and an upward viewing angle to the anterior brainstem. It is ideal for gaining added exposure of the basilar artery terminus for high-riding aneurysms. We began using this approach mainly for these lesions and have had good results. The orbitozygomatic approach also provides a route to cavernous malformations that surface on the anterior midbrain. In addition, removing the zygoma gives the surgeon wide exposure of the middle fossa and an upward angle to medial lesions. When the orbitozygomatic craniotomy is combined with the combined supra- and infratentorial approach, the anterior, middle, and posterior fossae are widely exposed. A lesion at the center of the skull base encasing important arteries and cranial nerves can be accessed from various angles to optimize the dissection of these structures.

Combination Approaches with Conservative Petrosectomy

Radical petrosectomy is the foundation for most of the skull base approaches discussed above. A guiding principle in the management of complex skull base lesions has been to create maximum surgical exposure by removing bone rather than retracting brain. The transpetrosal approaches fulfill this important principle. However, the morbidity associated with radical petrosectomy is considerable. The evolution of surgical techniques and instruments has substantially reduced operative mortality associated with these procedures. For example, in our series of more than 120 combined supra- and infratentorial approaches, there has been no operative mortality. Nonetheless, facial nerve paralysis can be expected in a third of patients undergoing this procedure (28). Leakage of CSF can be expected in 15% (28) of patients despite meticulous dural closure, abdominal fat grafts, temporalis muscle flaps, occlusion of the eustachian tube, and prophylactic lumbar spinal drainage for 3 days. Deficits involving the lower cranial nerves are less common but debilitate patients and lead to tracheostomy, feeding tubes, other medical complications, and extended rehabilitation. Therefore, the complications associated with radical petrosectomy frequently necessitate prolonged hospitalization, additional procedures, and higher costs. In the current cost-conscious medical environment, surgical treatments with these associated side effects are being evaluated critically.

Experience with this level of morbidity has inspired greater caution in using radical petrosectomy in our skull base approaches. Instead, we have sought combination approaches that reduce the extent of temporal bone removal and correspondingly reduce morbidity but still provide adequate surgical exposure to deal with the lesion without undue brain retraction. By necessity, approaches with conservative petrosectomy provide a different angle of exposure than the radical approaches. Instead of a direct lateral route through the petrous corridor, alternative approaches must reach the anterolateral brainstem either from an anterosuperior or posteroinferior position. Two such approaches are the extended orbitozygomatic approach and the extended far lateral approach. The former extends the lateral exposure of the orbitozygomatic approach by removing the medial petrous bone in Kawase's triangle, and the latter extends the lateral exposure of the far lateral approach by removing retrolabyrinthine temporal bone and retracting the sigmoid sinus anteriorly. We have developed increasing facility with these approaches and increasing confidence that less extensive petrosectomy does not hinder the operation. Furthermore, the corresponding morbidity rate with these approaches has decreased.

Extended Orbitozygomatic Approach

The orbitozygomatic approach was introduced by Hakuba as a route for accessing lesions located high in the interpeduncular fossa and parasellar regions (8, 9). The authors have modified the orbitozygomatic approach by removing the medial petrous bone in Kawase's triangle to gain added exposure inferiorly and laterally. The approach essentially combines the orbitozygomatic exposure with that of the middle fossa approach, and little has been written about this modification for midbasilar lesions.

Kawase's triangle is not a true triangle but rather a quadrangle (16). It is formed by the IAC posteriorly, the greater superficial petrosal nerve laterally, the trigeminal ganglion anteriorly, and the medial edge of the petrous bone medially. The quadrangle extends inferiorly to the inferior petrosal sinus. Between these important neurovascular boundaries are simply temporal bone and air cells. Resection of Kawase's quadrangle opens a large space through which the basilar artery is exposed down to the vertebrobasilar junction. The extended orbitozygomatic approach therefore accesses the anterior brainstem from the midbrain to the pontomedullary junction and provides lateral exposure to the midpoint of the petrous ridge. This approach is an excellent alternative to a radical transpetrosal approach in patients with facial nerve function and preservable hearing. The utility of this approach is demonstrated in case 1 (Fig. 9).

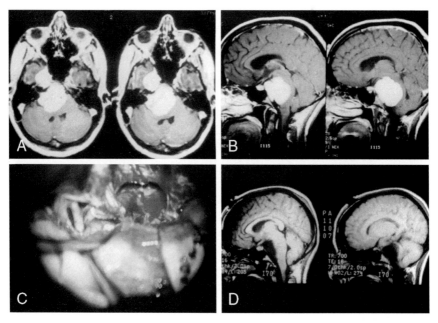

FIG.9   This 29-year-old female presented with right tinnitus and facial paresthesia. Neurologic examination revealed only decreased sensation in the V_1 and V_2 distributions of the trigeminal nerve. (**A**) Axial and (**B**) sagittal T1-weighted magnetic resonance (MR) images with gadolinium demonstrate an enhancing tumor centered about Meckel's cave and extending anteriorly into the right cavernous sinus. (**C**) An intraoperative photograph shows the right optic nerve and carotid artery (*upper left*), and a retractor elevating the temporal lobe (*lower left*). Tumor and bone in Kawase's triangle have been removed through an extended orbitozygomatic approach, providing inferior exposure into the posterior fossa (*upper right*). (**D**) Sagittal T1-weighted MR images with gadolinium demonstrate good resection of the trigeminal schwannoma with decompression of the brainstem.

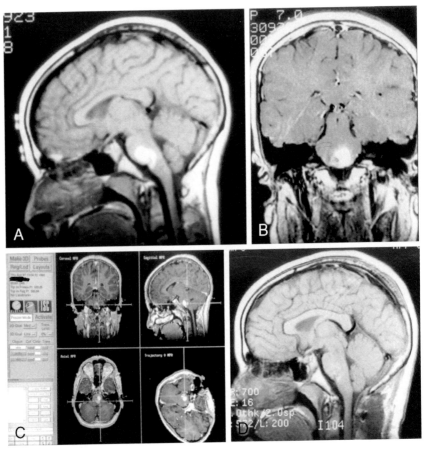

FIG.10 A 13-year-old patient with a severe headache, left abducens nerve palsy, and right hemiparesis. (A) Sagittal and (B) coronal T1-weighted magnetic resonance (MR) images demonstrate a pontine cavernous malformation that comes to the pial surface at the inferior belly of the pons in the midline. (C) The extended far lateral approach exposes this overhanging pial surface along the axis of the lesion, as shown in the intraoperative ISG wand display (*lower right*). (D) Postoperative sagittal T1-weighted MR image demonstrates complete resection of the cavernous malformation.

Extended Far Lateral Approach

The far lateral approach has already been discussed in relationship to the combined-combined approach. The extended far lateral approach is simply the standard far lateral craniotomy plus a retrolabyrinthine drilling. The mastoidectomy is extended inferiorly to skeletonize the sigmoid sinus completely from the sinodural angle to the jugular bulb. When this limited petrous bone removal is added to the far lateral craniotomy, the dura can be incised more laterally and superiorly, and the reflected dura can be pulled forward to retract the sigmoid sinus anteriorly. Thus, the exposure gained is more than that of the standard far lateral approach and less than that of the combined-combined approach. Still, this modified approach gives the exposure needed to accomplish the surgical goal while minimizing operative morbidity. The utility of the extended far lateral approach is demonstrated in case 2 (Fig. 10).

CURRENT INDICATIONS FOR TRANSPETROSAL APPROACHES

We have developed a plan for selecting the best approach or combination of approaches for dealing with petroclival lesions (Table 2). The critical factors are lesion location, size, pathology, and the patient's preoperative neurologic function. Classically, the clivus is divided into thirds, and lesions located in the upper third are treated with a pterional or subtemporal approach. This orbitozygomatic approach has largely supplanted the pterional-subtemporal approach at this institution, but the authors routinely drill down lateral temporal bone as part of the orbitozygomatic craniotomy to provide subtemporal exposure if needed. Lesions confined to the middle third of the clivus are accessed through one of the transpetrosal approaches, and lesions of the lower third of the clivus are exposed through a far lateral craniotomy.

Usually, small lesions can be exposed adequately with one of these approaches. However, larger lesions are more likely to need one of

TABLE 2
Selection of Appropriate Approach

Approach	Lesion Location
Orbitozygomatic	Upper third of the clivus
Transpetrosal	Middle third of the clivus
Retrolabyrinthine	CP[a] angle
Translabyrinthine	CP angle and anterolateral brainstem
Transcochlear	CP angle and anterior brainstem
Far lateral	Lower third of the clivus
Combined	Upper two thirds of the clivus and middle cranial fossa
Combined-combined	Entire clivus and middle cranial fossa
Orbitozygomatic-combined	Upper two thirds of clivus, entire middle cranial fossa, and anterior cranial fossa

[a]CP, cerebellopontine.

the combination approaches. The extended orbitozygomatic approach gives more inferior exposure than the standard orbitozygomatic approach and can be considered for larger lesions of the upper clivus. Similarly, the extended far lateral approach gives more superior exposure than the standard approach and can be considered for larger lesions of the lower clivus. These extended approaches are associated with less morbidity than the extensive approaches and are therefore considered first. If this exposure is insufficient to deal with these larger lesions, then one of the transpetrosal approaches is recommended, usually the combined supra- and infratentorial approach. If the lesion involves the entire clivus and foramen magnum, the combined-combined approach may be required.

Once a decision has been made to drill the temporal bone, the surgeon must estimate the amount of temporal bone resection needed to obtain adequate exposure. This evaluation is balanced with an assessment of preoperative neurologic function, specifically the function of the seventh and eighth cranial nerves. When the patient has good preoperative hearing and the surgeon wants to preserve it, temporal bone removal is limited to a retrolabyrinthine drilling. This approach exposes only the cerebellopontine angle and not the anterolateral brainstem, but it preserves both hearing and facial nerve function. Patients with poor preoperative hearing are well suited to translabyrinthine drilling, which gives anterolateral exposure of the brainstem at the expense of hearing and an increased risk of CSF leakage. When large lesions compressing the brainstem produce preoperative hearing loss and facial nerve deficits, a trancochlear approach is ideal. The increased exposure of the anterior brainstem is often critical, and the preoperative deficits lessen the impact of the greater risk of facial paresis or paralysis.

Pathology is an important factor in selecting the approach. Vascular lesions typically require a more focused area of exposure. The pial surface of a cavernous malformation and the neck of an aneurysm must be visualized adequately (20). Such visualization can often be accomplished through more limited exposures that spare the patient extensive temporal bone drilling. In contrast, tumors typically require wide exposure, and extensive temporal bone resection is unavoidable. This is the case with meningiomas, chordomas, chondrosarcomas, glomus tumors, and skull base carcinomas. However, some tumors are soft and more easily removed, and less exposure is needed for their removal. Schwannomas, epidermoids, and dermoid tumors may be dealt with through a more conservative craniotomy (Fig. 9) (29).

CONCLUSIONS

Petrosectomy is the essential component of many of the important skull base approaches. The transpetrosal approaches enable safe surgical treatment of many petroclival lesions. The combination approaches further increase surgical exposure for more complex lesions. When appropriate, alternative approaches with conservative temporal bone removal provide adequate exposure and reduce the morbidity associated with radical temporal bone removal. Selecting the best surgical approach requires careful evaluation of lesion location, size, pathology, and the patient's preoperative neurologic function. Successful management of these difficult lesions requires a multidisciplinary team that is critically dependent on the neurotologist.

REFERENCES

1. Al-Mefty O, Fox JL, Smith RR: Petrosal approach for petroclival meningiomas. **Neurosurgery** 22:510–517, 1988.
2. Baldwin HZ, Miller CG, van Loveren HR, *et al.:* The far lateral/combined supra- and infratentorial approach: A human cadaveric prosection model for routes of access to the petroclival region and ventral brain stem. **J Neurosurg** 81:60–68, 1994.
3. Baldwin HZ, Spetzler RF, Wascher TM, *et al.:* The far lateral-combined supra- and infratentorial approach: Clinical experience. **Acta Neurochir (Wien)** 134:155–158, 1995.
4. Brackmann DE, Green JD: Translabyrinthine approach for acoustic tumor removal. **Otolaryngol Clin North Am** 25:311–329, 1992.
5. Brackmann DE, House JR III, Hitselberger WE: Technical modifications to the middle fossa craniotomy approach in removal of acoustic neuromas. **Am J Otol** 15:614–619, 1994.
6. Daspit CP, Spetzler RF, Pappas CTE: Combined approach for lesions involving the cerebellopontine angle and skull base: Experience with 20 cases—preliminary report. **Otolaryngol Head Neck Surg** 105:788–796, 1991.
7. De Oliveira E, Rhoton AL Jr, Peace D: Microsurgical anatomy of the region of the foramen magnum. **Surg Neurol** 24:293–352, 1985.
8. Hakuba A, Liu S, Nishimura S: The orbitozygomatic infratemporal approach: A new surgical technique. **Surg Neurol** 26:271–276, 1986.
9. Hakuba A, Tanaka K, Suzuki T, *et al.:* A combined orbitozygomatic infratemporal epidural and subdural approach for lesions involving the entire cavernous sinus. **J Neurosurg** 71:699–704, 1989.
10. Heros RC: Lateral suboccipital approach for vertebral and vertebrobasilar artery lesions. **J Neurosurg** 64:559–562, 1986.
11. Hitselberger WE, House WF: A combined approach to the cerebellopontine angle: A suboccipital-petrosal approach. **Arch Otolaryngol** 84:49–67, 1966.
12. House WF: Translabyrinthine approach, in House WF, Luetje CM (eds): **Acoustic Tumors, Vol. 2: Management:** Baltimore, University Park Press, 1979, p. 43.
13. House WF, Hitselberger WE: The transcochlear approach to the skull base. **Arch Otolaryngol** 102:334–342, 1976.

14. House WF, Shelton C: Middle fossa approach for acoustic tumor removal. **Otolaryngol Clin North Am** 25:347–359, 1992.

15. Ikeda K, Yamashita J, Hashimoto M, *et al.:* Orbitozygomatic temporopolar approach for a high basilar tip aneurysm associated with a short intracranial internal carotid artery: A new surgical approach. **Neurosurgery** 28:105–110, 1991.

16. Kawase T, Toya S, Shiobara R, *et al.:* Transpetrosal approach for aneurysms of the lower basilar artery. **J Neurosurg** 63:857–861, 1985.

17. Lee JP, Tsai MS, Chen YR: Orbitozygomatic infratemporal approach to lateral skull base tumors. **Acta Neurol Scand** 87:403–409, 1993.

18. McDermott MW, Durity FA, Rootman J, *et al.:* Combined frontotemporal-orbitozygomatic approach for tumors of the sphenoid wing and orbit. **Neurosurgery** 26:107–116, 1990.

19. Morrison AW, King TT: Experiences with a translabyrinthine-transtentorial approach to the cerebello-pontine angle. **J Neurosurg** 38:382–390, 1973.

20. Sekhar LN, Kalia KK, Yonas H, *et al.:* Cranial base approaches to intracranial aneurysms in the subarachnoid space. **Neurosurgery** 35:472–483, 1994.

21. Sen CN, Sekhar LN: An extreme lateral approach to the intradural lesions of the cervical spine and foramen magnum. **Neurosurgery** 27:197–204, 1990.

22. Sen CN, Sekhar LN: Surgical management of anteriorly placed lesions at the craniocervical junction—an alternative approach. **Acta Neurochir (Wien)** 108:70–77, 1991.

23. Spetzler RF: Two technical notes for microsurgery. **Barrow Neurological Institute** 4:38–39, 1988.

24. Spetzler RF, Daspit CP, Pappas CTE: Combined approach for lesions involving the cerebellopontine angle and skull base: Experience with 30 cases. **Skull Base Surg** 1:226–234, 1991.

25. Spetzler RF, Daspit CP, Pappas CTE: The combined supra- and infratentorial approach for lesions of the petrous and clival regions: Experience with 46 cases. **J Neurosurg** 76:588–599, 1992.

26. Spetzler RF, Fukushima T, Martin N, *et al.:* Petrous carotid-to-intradural carotid saphenous vein graft for intracavernous giant aneurysm, tumor, and occlusive cerebrovascular disease. **J Neurosurg** 73:496–501, 1990.

27. Spetzler RF, Grahm T: The far-lateral approach to the inferior clivus and the upper cervical region: Technical note. **Barrow Neurological Institute.** 6:35–38, 1990.

28 Spetzler RF, Hamilton MG, Daspit CP: Petroclival lesions. **Clin Neurosurg** 41:62–82, 1993.

29 Yasui T, Hakuba A, Kim SH, *et al.:* Trigeminal neurinomas: Operative approach in eight cases. **J Neurosurg** 71:506–511, 1989.

7

The Transcondylar Approach to the Lower Clivus, Foramen Magnum and C1-C2

CHANDRANATH SEN, M.D.

Tumors arising ventrally and ventrolaterally to the brainstem and cervicomedullary junction pose some special problems for the neurosurgeon. These include difficulty of access, and/or involvement of the vertebral artery (VA) and lower cranial nerves either by the tumor itself or the path of the surgical approach. Some of these tumors may also invade extradural tissues. The majority of the tumors, either benign (meningioma, schwannoma, glomus tumors, and others) or locally aggressive (chordoma and chondrosarcoma) are amenable to radical resection, which provides the best chance for long-term control or cure. Aneurysms arising from the VA and vertebrobasilar junction may share these difficulties.

A standard lateral suboccipital approach may not be adequate to achieve such a radical resection or safely clip the aneurysm with full visualization. A more lateral approach along with control and mobilization of the VA as it enters the dura allows better visibility anterior to the brainstem and favorably influences the safety and completeness of the operation.

ANATOMIC CONSIDERATIONS

The Bony Anatomy

The foramen magnum can be circular or oval in shape, making the surface in front of the brainstem shallow or deep. The occipital condyles are on the lateral boundaries of the foramen magnum. Each condyle is directed anteromedially and the articular surface faces laterally. The hypoglossal canal is in the medial third of the condyle while a large condylar emissary vein emerges from its posterior aspect. Thus the shape of the foramen magnum determines how much of an obstacle the occipital condyle poses. That is, the condyles are more of a hindrance in a deep and oval foramen magnum than in a round one. This in turn determines what trajectory of the surgical approach would be necessary to view its anterior surface and the extent of the condylar resection that may be needed, if any.

The Vertebral Artery

The third portion of the VA begins at the foramen transversarium of C2 and ends where it enters the dura. Within the foramen of C2 it turns laterally and posteriorly, exiting at a different plane above C2 than below C2. It then passes through the foramen transversarium of C1 directly above. The artery turns sharply posteriorly on the posterior arch of C1 after emerging from the foramen of C1 and curves around the occiput-C1 articulation to enter the dura on the lateral aspect of the thecal sac. Between C2 and C1 and above C1 the artery may be redundant to some extent, allowing for the mobility in these spinal segments. The artery is surrounded by a periosteal sheath and venous plexus all the way up to its dural entry. Between C2 and C1 the ventral ramus of the C2 nerve root crosses the artery from posterior to anterior. Above C1 the artery closely adheres to the joint capsule of occiput-C1 as it turns around it to enter the dura. The artery pierces the dura in an oblique fashion immediately posterior to the occipital condyle and lateral mass of C1.

The Cranial Nerves

The cranial nerves IX and XII are most often either related to the tumor or in the field of the surgical approach. Within the jugular foramen the ninth, tenth, and eleventh nerves lie medial to the jugular bulb. The inferior petrosal sinus may travel in between the nerves on its way to join the medial surface of the jugular bulb. All the nerves are surrounded by dense connective tissue in the jugular foramen. The twelfth nerve exits separately, inferiorly and medially to the jugular foramen. The hypoglossal canal occupies the medial part of the occipital condyle and is directed superiorly and laterally to a point of exit that is higher than the intracranial entrance. This produces a situation in which the nerves in the jugular foramen are directed inferiorly and laterally while the hypoglossal nerve is directed superiorly and laterally, which becomes an important issue in dealing with extradural tumors. The hypoglossal nerve is accompanied by an emissary vein and a branch of the ascending pharyngeal artery in the canal.

PRINCIPLES OF THE SURGICAL APPROACH

Mobilization of the VA is a key step in the approach to lesions at the anterior surface of the foramen magnum. To accomplish this the artery needs to be completely freed from the dura circumferentially at its entrance. This is facilitated by resection of bone from the posterior aspect of the occipital condyle, in front of the VA. Extradural tumors invading the occipital condyle and the bone around the hypoglossal and jugular foramen are also accessed in a similar manner. Preservation of the cranial nerves requires their dissection from a normal to an abnormal area in the region of their respective foramina.

THE SURGICAL APPROACH

Position

Positioning for the operation requires attention (11). Flexion and extension of the head on the spine leads to changes in the dimensions of the foramen magnum, which can cause further compromise of an already compressed cervicomedullary junction. Rotation of the head leads to distortion of the relation of the extradural VA. Therefore, for tumors in this region the patient is positioned in a full lateral decubitus with the head and neck in a neutral position. Intraoperative neurophysiologic monitoring is a useful adjunct during positioning, as well as during the surgical procedure.

Soft Tissue Dissection and Vertebral Artery Exposure

An inverted horseshoe incision is used if an occipitocervical fusion operation is anticipated, otherwise a gentle "C"-shaped incision can be used. The muscle dissection in the posterior cervical triangle is performed in anatomic layers, detaching each muscle from its lateral attachment and reflecting it medially. This method of dissection serves two purposes: it maintains the surgeon's orientation to the area throughout the approach and isolation of the VA; it clears away the muscle bulk from a wide arc so that the surgeon may view the area from far laterally, as well as medially, which is usually necessary for the anteriorly located lesion, both aneurysms and tumors.

The prominent transverse process of C1 and the muscles (superior and inferior oblique and levator scapulae) attached to it form an important landmark for the identification and mobilization of the third portion of the VA. When dissecting in the vicinity of the C1 transverse process, the course of the accessory nerve must be kept in mind. The nerve crosses from anterior to posterior, lateral to the internal jugular vein. A profusion of veins marks this area. The muscles are detached from the C1 transverse process and reflected medially. After all the muscles' dissection is completed, the posterior arch of C1, the mastoid process, and the lateral suboccipital region have been exposed. The VA is exposed below or above the C1 transverse process, as determined by the lesion. If better access to the lateral mass of C1 is required, the VA is displaced out of the transverse foramen of C1. For this, a subperiosteal plane is established between the venous sheath surrounding the VA and the transverse foramen of C1, and the transverse process is rongeured away, allowing the artery to be displaced posteriorly, providing a clear access to the lateral mass of C1.

Bony Opening

The extent of the bony opening is determined by the nature and extent of the lesion at hand. If the tumor has a large posterior fossa extent, then the craniotomy must be carried up to the transverse sinus and laterally; the sigmoid sinus is completely unroofed down to the jugular bulb (Fig. 1). For lower lesions, a C1 hemilaminectomy may be needed with a less extensive posterior fossa exposure. Since the occipital condyle is just anterior to the VA where it enters the dura, the extent of the condyle drilling is determined by the amount of room needed in front of the artery in the particular case. Typically, for purely intradural lesions like an aneurysm or a meningioma, only about the posterior one third is drilled away along with the jugular tubercle. However, for tumors like chordomas that invade the condyle, all the involved bone needs to be removed, and this may be the entire condyle (Fig. 2). The internal jugular vein and the internal carotid artery (ICA) are directly anterior to the lateral mass of C1. Drilling in the vicinity of the VA is performed under the microscope and with a diamond bur. Venous bleeding from the condylar emissary vein is controlled with Surgicel packing.

Tumor Removal

The posterior fossa dura is opened posterior and parallel to the sigmoid sinus and posterior to the VA dural penetration. The location of the eleventh nerve intradurally is ascertained, and the dural incision is then incrementally carried all around the artery to free it up from the dural tether (Fig. 3). Tumor resection proceeds using the standard microsurgical principles of progressive debulking and dissection from the brainstem and cranial nerves. The brainstem and tumor interface is best visualized from the lateral vantage point, while the anterior surface of the foramen magnum is visualized from more posteriorly. The VA is followed from a normal area to the tumor-involved one, looking for the posterior inferior cerebellar artery and the anterior spinal artery. Identification and preservation of these branches is greatly facilitated by completely mobilizing the extradural VA and untethering it at the dural entry.

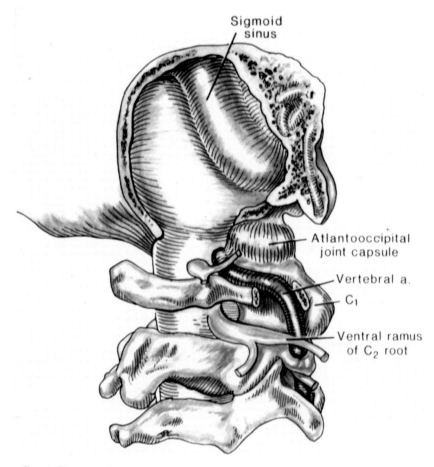

FIG. 1 Diagram showing the salient points of the exposure. This includes exposure of the sigmoid sinus down to the jugular bulb, exposure of the extradural VA all the way to its dural entry. The angle of the view is more from a lateral perspective than posteriorly. Also, note the relation of the occiput-C1 joint capsule to the artery.

In the case of chordomas and chondrosarcomas, after the soft portion of the tumor is removed, the involved bone is drilled away with a diamond bur. Drilling of the entire condyle exposes the twelfth nerve to injury, and this must be carefully approached. If the jugular foramen is involved, the sigmoid sinus and the jugular vein must be ligated, and the jugular foramen is opened to remove the tumor (Fig. 3). The cranial nerves are carefully dissected and preserved if possible and, subsequently, the surrounding bone is drilled. Watertight dural closure is

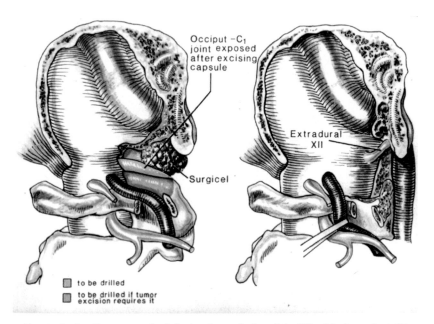

FIG. 2   In the diagram on the *left,* the close relation of the VA with the occiput-C1 articulation is seen. A portion of the occipital condyle needs to be drilled away to expose the dura in front of the artery. Drilling more of the condyle exposes the extradural portion of the twelfth nerve below the jugular bulb, as seen on the *right.* Also note that the artery has been displaced from the foramen transversarium of C1, clearing the access to the anterior part of C1.

usually not possible around the VA. All the mastoid air cells are thoroughly waxed, and an autologous piece of fat is laid over the dural defect. The muscles are then reapproximated in layers.

POSTOPERATIVE CARE

A cervical collar is not necessary; however, if the entire condyle has been resected, a stabilization procedure needs to be performed. A lumbar subarachnoid drain is inserted the next day and maintained for 5 days. This is used prophylactically to prevent a CSF collection in the subcutaneous tissues and also an external CSF fistula. If manipulation of the lower cranial nerves has occurred during surgery, the patient must be closely watched for dysfunction, which can lead to airway compromise or aspiration and dysphagia. A low threshold for performing a tracheostomy and/or a percutaneous gastrostomy is crucial in ensuring a steady and early recovery of the patient.

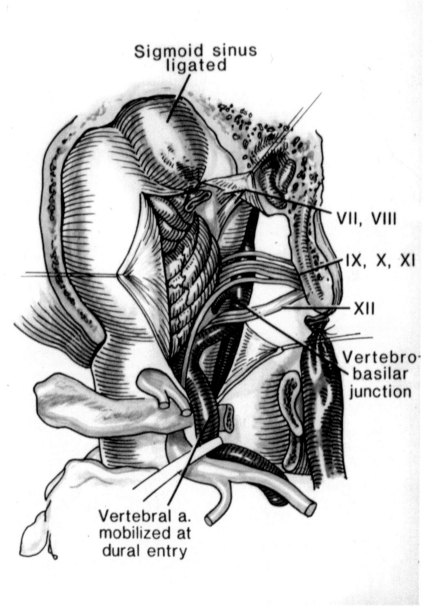

Sigmoid sinus ligated

VII, VIII

IX, X, XI

XII

Vertebro-
basilar
junction

**Vertebral a.
mobilized at
dural entry**

FIG. 3 In this diagram, the dura has been opened all around the entry point of the VA, freeing it up completely from this attachment. The jugular foramen has also been entered after ligating the sigmoid sinus and the internal jugular vein. From the lateral view, the vertebral artery can be followed up to the origin of the basilar artery.

ILLUSTRATIVE CASES

This 24-year-old woman had undergone a prior suboccipital craniectomy for a tumor that was subsequently diagnosed as a chordoma. Two
years later, progressive growth of the residual tumor was documented
by magnetic resonance (MR) and completed tomography (CT) scans.
The tumor was located entirely anterior to the spinomedullary junction
and involved the occipital condyle, lower clivus, and also extended into
the jugular foramen and behind the ICA (Fig. 4, **A** and **B**).

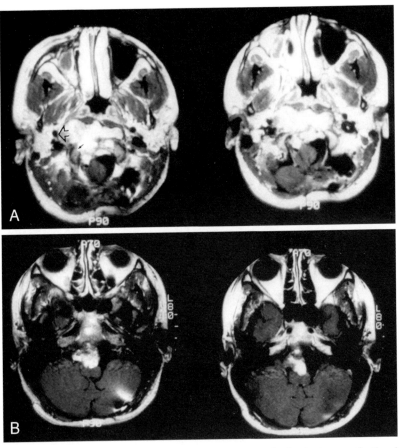

FIG. 4 (**A**) In case 1, the tumor is entirely anterior to the brainstem, projecting intradurally as well as involving the extradural tissues behind the retropharyngeal muscles medial to the internal carotid artery (*open arrow*). The medial portion of the occipital condyle is invaded by the tumor (*small arrow*). (**B**) In a higher axial section, the
tumor is seen extending further up the clivus and is almost midline in its location.

Tumor resection was performed in two stages. At the first operation the preauricular subtemporal and infratemporal approach was taken, and the ICA in the petrous bone was completely uncovered and mobilized laterally, allowing removal of tumor in this area and also drilling of the infiltrated petrous bone (8). At the second operation (1 week later) an extreme lateral transcondylar approach was taken. Since the tumor was in the jugular foramen, the bony opening was extended superiorly to the level of the transverse sinus. The VA was exposed at C2 and followed up into the dura. It was displaced from the transverse foramen of C1, because the tumor involved the occiput-C1 articulation. Complete tumor removal was achieved including the involved bone (Fig. 5). A unilateral fusion with titanium plate and screws was performed but failed. Subsequently, the patient underwent occipitocervical fusion with a contoured stainless steel pin, wire, and bone.

She suffered unilateral lower cranial nerve palsies, which she compensated for in the course of a few months. The hardware was removed 4 years later to allow proper imaging, and she remains free of disease (Fig. 6). In view of the apparently complete tumor resection, radiation therapy has been witheld.

A 45-year-old man was evaluated for neck and occipital pain. The MRI revealed a foramen magnum tumor suggestive of a meningioma (Fig. 7, **A** and **B**). The important features in the preoperative imaging

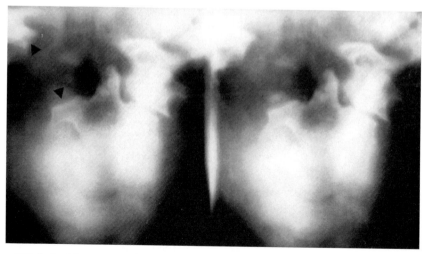

FIG. 5 In this postoperative coronal polytomography, complete removal of the lateral mass of C1 and the occipital condyle (*arrows*) is noted, compared to the normal side. This is an unstable situation that will result in a painful torticollis if not stabilized.

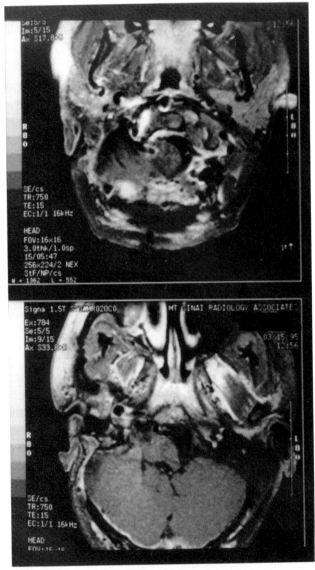

FIG. 6 The postoperative MR was obtained 4 years after the operation. The posterior instrumentation was removed after good fusion was documented. No evidence of tumor residue or recurrence is noted.

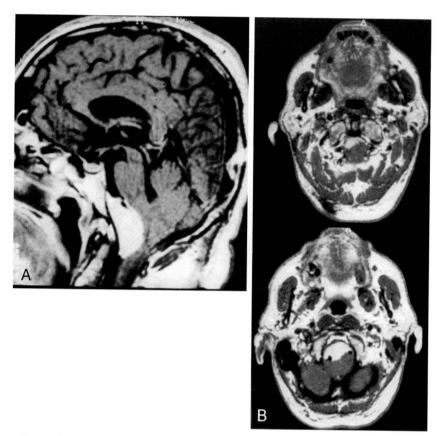

FIG. 7 Sagittal (**A**) and axial (**B**) MR images in case 2. The tumor is noted to be completely anterior to the brainstem. From the axial scan it can be seen that the opposite pole of the tumor will be difficult to reach from a standard posterolateral approach. Partial condyle resection and a more lateral view improved the access in this case.

indicated that this was entirely anterior to the brainstem, extending to the opposite hypoglossal foramen, and the ipsilateral VA was partially encased within the tumor (Fig. 8).

The operation was performed as described above. A "C"-shaped incision was used, and the bony exposure was taken down to C1. The vertebral artery was exposed above C1 and completely released at its dural entry and was mobilized posteriorly to allow tumor removal anterior to it. Only a small amount of bone was removed from the condyle, and no stabilization was necessary (Fig. 9). Because of subcutaneous CSF collection, a lumbar spinal drain was inserted for 5 days postoperatively. Postop imaging showed complete tumor removal.

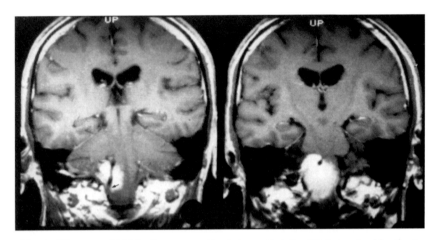

FIG. 8 The coronal MR in the same patient shows that the VA is involved by the tumor as soon as it enters the dura (*arrow*). In this case releasing the artery at its dural attachment greatly facilitates its dissection from the tumor. A short segment of the distal VA is surrounded by the tumor.

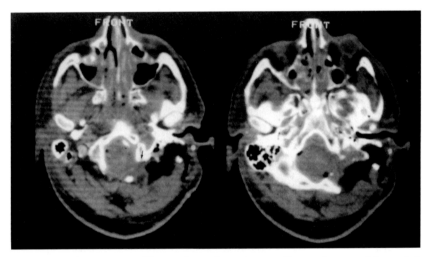

FIG. 9 The postoperative CT scan shows that only a small posterior part of the condyle has been drilled away from the access, allowing complete removal of the tumor (*arrow*).

DISCUSSION

The usual difficulties associated with these lesions are related to: access to the ventral surface of the lower clivus and the craniocervial junction, involvement of the VA at its entry into the dura, involvement of the lower cranial nerves and in certain tumors, and involvement of the extradural tissues. Although the standard lateral suboccipital approach may be sufficient in most instances, there is a 5 to 15% incidence of morbidity and mortality associated with surgery for purely ventral lesions (7, 13).

Heros described a lateral extension of the suboccipital craniectomy that proved helpful in providing a more lateral view in front of the brainstem and successfully used it in the management of VA aneurysms (6). George *et al.* carried the craniectomy further laterally and used this approach for anterior tumors at the foramen magnum (4). The benefits of the lateral perspective were evident in their superior results. Despite the lateral extension of the exposure, the dural entry point of the VA still seems to be a hindrance, because the artery remained fixed at this point.

As is readily apparent on studying the anatomy of the artery above C1, the vessel closely skirts the atlanto-occipital joint capsule and enters the dura immediately posteromedially to this joint (3). Thus, to release the VA at its dural entry, the dura must be opened circumferentially around the artery. The occipital condyle may obstruct opening the dura in front of the artery. Therefore, drilling this portion of the condyle creates enough room anterior to the VA to allow the dura to be opened around the artery to free it up from the dural attachment. The artery can now be mobilized posteriorly and dissected from the tumor, at the same time facilitating access to the ventral foramen magnum (2, 9, 10, 12). Another step that is helpful in this lateral approach is a laterally placed skin incision and layer-by-layer dissection of the posterior triangle muscles. These muscles are subsequently detached from their lateral attachment and displaced medially and inferiorly. This maneuver removes the muscle bulk from the lateral portion of the exposure, providing an unimpeded view from the lateral perspective (9, 10).

For purely intradural tumors, condylar resection is not always necessary to release and mobilize the VA. If needed, resection of only a small portion of the posterior end of the condyle will suffice. The need for and the amount of resection is determined by the exact location of the tumor (ventral or ventrolateral), the shape of the bony foramen magnum, and the exact relation of the VA to the tumor or the aneurysm (whether the pathology involves the artery close to the point where it enters the dura). When dealing with extradural tumors that invade the condyle and extradural tissues, radical resection of the tumor requires drilling of the entire condyle and also, frequently, entry into the jugular bulb and foramen with the attendant risks to the lower cranial nerves. Chordomas and chondrosarcomas and some large glomus jugular tumors are the ones most frequently encountered in this area requiring this approach. Aggressive resection is usually warranted in these situations due to their high propensity for local recurrence.

Partial condyle resection does not produce any instability, but removal of the entire condyle on one side produces painful torticollis and should be stabilized posteriorly with occipitocervial fusion. The published results indicate that the approach itself does not increase the morbidity, except for the risk of CSF leakage due to inadequate dural closure (1, 2, 5, 10, 12). The most significant morbidity is related to the lower cranial nerve dysfunction, and this is related to their dissection from the tumor or their manipulation but not to the surgical approach itself. The distinct advantage of the approach is the better access and control of the VA, as well as a shortened operating distance.

REFERENCES

1. Babu RP, Sekhar LN, Wright DC: Extreme lateral transcondylar approach: Technical improvements and lessons learned. **J Neurosurg** 81:49–59, 1994.
2. Bertalanffy H, Seeger W: The dorsolateral, suboccipital, transcondylar approach to the lower clivus and anterior portion of the craniocervical junction. **Neurosurgery** 29:815–821, 1991.
3. de Oliveira E, Rhoton AL Jr, Peace D: Microsurgical anatomy of the region of the foramen magnum. **Surg Neurol** 24:293–352, 1985.
4. George B, Dematons C, Cophignon J: Lateral approach to the anterior portion of the foramen magnum. **Surg Neurol** 29:484–490, 1988.
5. George B, Lot G, Velut S, et al.: Tumors of the foramen magnum. **Neurochirurgie** 39(suppl 1):1993.
6. Heros RC: Lateral suboccipital approach for vertebral and vertebrobasilar artery lesions. **J Neurosurg** 64:559–562, 1986.
7. Meyer FB, Ebersold MJ, Reese DF: Benign tumors of the foramen magnum. **J Neurosurg** 61:136–142, 1984.
8. Sen C, Sekhar LN: The subtemporal and preauricular infratemporal approach to intradural structures ventral to the brain stem. **J Neurosurg** 73:345–354, 1990.
9. Sen CN, Sekhar LN: An extreme lateral approach to intradural lesions of the cervical spine and foramen magnum. **Neurosurgery** 27:197–204, 1990.
10. Sen C, Sekhar LN: Surgical management of anteriorly placed lesions of the craniocervical junction—An alternative approach. **Acta Neurochir** 108:70–77, 1991.
11. Sen C, Sekhar LN: An extreme lateral transcondylar approach to the foramen magnum and cervical spine, in Rengachary S, Wilkins RH (eds): *Neurosurgical Operative Atlas (AANS)*. Baltimore, Williams & Wilkins, 1992, vol 2, pp 323–329.
12. Spetzler RF, Grahm TW: The far-lateral approach to the inferior clivus and the upper cervical region: Technical note. **Barrow Neurological Institute** 6:35–38, 1990.
13. Stein BM, Leeds NE, Taveras JM, et al.: Meningiomas of the foramen magnum. **J Neurosurg** 20:740–751, 1963.

8

Surgical Approaches to Aneurysms of the Upper Basilar Artery

JOEL D. MacDONALD M.D., AND ARTHUR L. DAY, M.D.

Aneurysms of the upper basilar artery represent a unique surgical challenge to the neurosurgeon. Because of the variability of size, location, and orientation of these lesions, no single approach is suitable for every situation. With the evolution of skull base surgical techniques, wide access can now be gained to all levels of the upper basilar region via one of four basic approaches: (a) transsylvian plus-or-minus orbitozygomatic osteotomy, (b) temporopolar, (c) anterior subtemporal plus-or-minus medial petrosectomy, and (d) lateral petrosectomy (presigmoid). The determination of which approach to use is based on considerations of the level of the aneurysm, its laterality, the existence of other aneurysms, and the neurologic status of the patient. This chapter will briefly discuss each component of the decision process and present two examples of surgical management. Utilizing these approaches, many lesions that were once believed too treacherous for direct attack can now be treated safely.

SURGICAL APPROACHES

Transsylvian

The pterional transsylvian approach to the upper basilar artery was first advocated by Yasargil *et al.* who noticed that the apex of the basilar bifurcation usually lies 15 to 17 mm deep to the intracranial internal carotid artery (13) (Fig. 1). Extensive extradural sphenoid ridge removal, combined with an interfascial temporalis muscle dissection, allows wide separation of the sylvian fissure with minimal frontal and temporal lobe retraction (14). The carotid, anterior cerebral, and middle cerebral arteries can be extensively dissected to provide three avenues to the basilar apex and interpeduncular cistern (Fig. 2A). The first route passes between the optic nerve and carotid artery through the opticocarotid space. The second route passes lateral to the carotid artery and is dependent on an elongated and mobile carotid artery. The

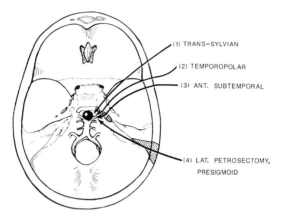

FIG. 1 Schematic representation of (1) transsylvian, (2) temporopolar, (3) anterior subtemporal, and (4) lateral petrosal surgical routes. *Hatched areas* indicate medial and lateral petrosal bone resection, respectively. Note the trajectory each approach provides relative to the basilar apex lesion and associated perforating vessels.

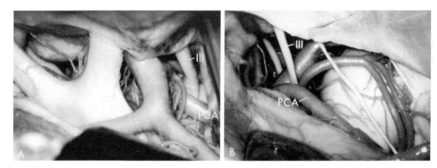

FIG. 2 Anatomic dissection illustrating the exposure gained by (**A**) trans-sylvian approach and (**B**) anterior subtemporal approach. The posterior cerebral artery (*PCA*) and
cranial nerve III (*III*) are labeled for orientation.

final route proceeds above the carotid bifurcation between the anterior
and middle cerebral arteries.

Removal of the orbital roof and zygoma have been described as methods of increasing the superior extent of surgical access (1, 8). The periorbita and globe can be retracted inferiorly, resulting in a flatter angle
of approach for clip application to high-riding apex lesions. Removal of
the anterior clinoid process and mobilization of the internal carotid
artery at the dural ring will also enhance exposure by increasing the
ability to displace the carotid artery.

Temporopolar

Like the transsylvian approach, the temporopolar approach begins with a pterional craniotomy but includes more inferior and anterior temporal bone removal. After the bridging veins to the sphenoparietal sinus are coagulated and sectioned, the temporal tip is gently elevated and retracted posteriorly to provide a view of the incisura. The basis for this maneuver is that the temporal lobe can seemingly tolerate retraction along its long axis better than in the medial-to-lateral direction. As originally described, little dissection of the sylvian fissure is required, and adequate exposure to lesions lying above the posterior clinoid can be achieved (11, 12). Visualization of lesions lying at or just below the level of the posterior clinoid process, however, may be obscured by this bony process. Broad sylvian fissure splitting will greatly reduce temporal lobe morbidity and improve incisural exposure (14). When combined with sacrifice of the anterior temporal lobe venous drainage, however, a large area of the cortical surface is instrumented and thus may be damaged.

Anterior Subtemporal

The lateral subtemporal approach devised by Drake once represented the mainstay of surgical management of basilar apex aneurysms but was accompanied by a high incidence of intratemporal contusion or hematoma formation (5, 6). Subsequent modification to an anterior subtemporal approach now permits the temporal lobe to be gently elevated without damage to the temporal lobe or its venous structures in most instances (7). This approach is used extensively at our institution for most typical basilar bifurcation aneurysms. A muscle-splitting temporalis incision mobilizes the bulk of the muscle anteriorly. The primarily temporal craniotomy exposes the lower edge of the inferior frontal lobe and the lateral sphenoid ridge and is extended toward the anterior temporal region until flush with the floor of the middle fossa. The superior edge of the zygomatic arch is drilled off to further enhance the subtemporal view to the incisura while minimizing temporal lobe retraction. Two retractor blades are used to elevate the temporal lobe gently and distribute the force, thereby avoiding any focal angular distortion of the cortical surface like that encountered when a single retractor is used. The surgical route is obliquely oriented across the anterior floor of the middle fossa. The tentorial edge is incised posterior to the entry point of the fourth cranial nerve and tacked laterally. The resultant space allows visualization of a 2.0-cm interval centered at the level of the posterior clinoid process (Fig. 2**B**).

The anterior subtemporal approach can be modified to include extradural resection of the medial petrous apex (3, 9). A rhomboidal segment of bone medial to the greater superficial petrosal nerve and between the trigeminal groove and arcuate eminence is resected. The tentorial incision is directed more laterally to the edge of the fifth cranial nerve. The nerve and dura then prolapse into the petrosectomy defect. The resultant exposure is particularly useful to access low-lying lesions below the posterior clinoid base.

Lateral Petrosectomy (Presigmoid)

The lateral petrosal approach combines a retrosigmoid and posterior temporal craniotomy with additional mastoid and lateral petrosal bone resection to expose the dura anterior to the sigmoid sinus (2, 10). The sigmoid sinus is unroofed, and the vestibular labyrinth is skeletonized to attain a trajectory that is flat against the petrous bone. After the superior petrosal sinus is sacrificed, the dura is incised anteriorly to the sigmoid sinus. The tentorium is then divided to the incisura. Although the presigmoid view may be quite limited, this approach may be useful for lesions of the midbasilar artery that approximate the midclival level.

ANEURYSM CHARACTERISTICS

Laterality

For most solitary basilar apex aneurysms, a right-sided approach is favored. Brain retraction can be confined to the nondominant frontal and/or temporal lobes, thereby limiting the potential for speech deficits, should retraction injury occur. A left-sided approach is preferable in several circumstances: (a) with patients presenting with a left cranial nerve III palsy or right hemiparesis, where a right-sided approach would jeopardize the intact cranial nerve or hemisphere; (b) coexistent basilar and left-sided anterior circulation aneurysm (both can sometimes be treated with a single left-sided craniotomy); and (c) lateral orientation of the basilar aneurysm toward the left side. Any laterality (as seen in a superior cerebellar/posterior cerebral junction lesion) places the aneurysm neck closer to the ipsilateral incisura, thereby facilitating visualization and clip application. The contralateral posterior thalamoperforating arteries arising from the contralateral P1 segment are farther away, well seen, and more easily preserved (Fig. 3C).

Level

The level of a basilar bifurcation relative to the posterior clinoid process is the chief determinant for the type of approach to be used (Fig. 4). This relationship can best be assessed from a lateral an-

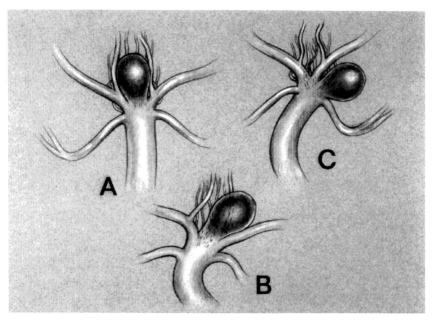

FIG. 3 Schematic representation of the relationship of the basilar apex aneurysm to perforating vessels. (**A**) A midline lesion. (**B**) An apex lesion eccentric to the left. (**C**) A left superior cerebellar/posterior cerebral aneurysm.

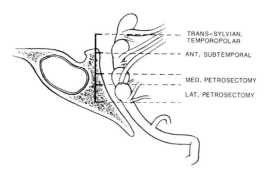

FIG. 4 Schematic representation of surgical approach based on level of the basilar apex aneurysm relative to the posterior clinoid process and clivus.

giogram. A lesion lying at or above the posterior clinoid can be adequately reached by either a transsylvian, temporopolar, or anterior subtemporal approach. For a high-riding bifurcation lesion, a pterional transsylvian approach, perhaps combined with fronto-orbital basal bone removal, provides excellent visualization. The requisite detachment of the oculomotor nerve from the uncus and more extensive temporal lobe retraction make the anterior subtemporal route less attractive in this situation unless the zygoma is also removed. A low-lying aneurysm behind or below the posterior clinoid process can be exposed well by combining the anterior subtemporal approach with a medial petrosectomy. Finally, for a lesion at the middle third of the clivus, a lateral petrosal presigmoid approach is considered.

NEUROLOGIC STATUS

Timing

The timing of surgical intervention is dependent on the clinical status of the patient. At our institution, early surgery (within 72 hours) is undertaken in all patients of Hunt-Hess grade III or better. Poorer grade patients frequently have a component of acute hydrocephalus contributing to their neurologic state. A brief interval of ventricular drainage often results in rapid improvement of clinical grade. By clipping the aneurysm early, prophylactic or therapeutic medical therapy for vasospasm can be maximized.

Vasospasm

For late-presenting patients in florid clinical vasospasm, surgical therapy is generally delayed, as spastic arteries and injured brain do not tolerate mechanical manipulation well. This is especially true in the region of the basilar apex.

Size

The size of the aneurysm does not usually affect the timing of surgery, except in cases of giant lesions. When the already tight confines of the interpeduncular cistern are further embarrassed by hemorrhage and the mass of a giant aneurysm, exposure can be quite difficult. It may be wise to allow the brain and vessels to recover to some degree before a planned procedure, particularly if the aneurysm is partially calcified or has significant intraluminal thrombus. Circulatory arrest may facilitate exposure to larger or giant lesions when the neck is bulbous and there is little chronic intra-aneurysmal thrombus.

Intraventricular Hemorrhage

Retraction of the temporal lobe against an intraventricular cast of blood can limit exposure and increase the incidence of temporal lobe retraction injury. For optimal brain relaxation, extensive cerebrospinal fluid drainage is mandatory, and an intraventricular clot prevents complete fluid evacuation. Delayed surgery allows the clot to liquefy and improves the chances of benign brain retraction.

CASE 1

A 54-year-old female presented with subarachnoid hemorrhage. Neurologic exam showed lethargy but no focal deficits (Hunt-Hess grade III). CT scan showed thick subarachnoid clot in the perimesencephalic cisterns. Cerebral angiography demonstrated a right-sided middle cerebral artery aneurysm measuring 1.0 cm (Fig. 5A) and a 1.0-cm basilar apex aneurysm eccentric to the left at the junction of the superior cerebellar and posterior cerebral arteries (Fig. 5, **B** and **C**).

The dilemma in this case is whether to attempt a single approach for both lesions or to utilize two separate approaches. Both a right transsylvian or temporopolar approach with wide fissure dissection are

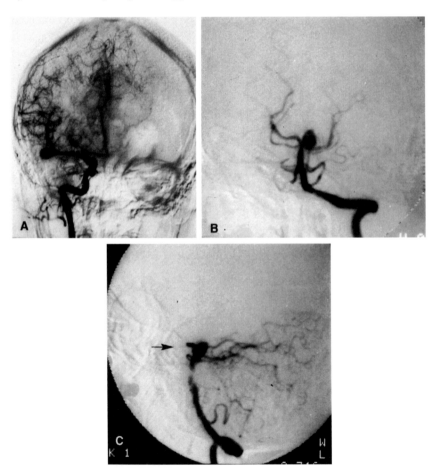

FIG. 5 (**A**) Right carotid angiogram showing 1.0-cm right middle cerebral aneurysm. (**B**) AP and (**C**) lateral left vertebral angiogram showing 1.0 cm eccentric posterior cerebral/superior cerebellar aneurysm. *Arrow* indicates the posterior clinoid process.

attractive options. These strategies however, provide a limited view of the neck of the left eccentric basilar aneurysm, which is clearly the lesion that has bled. The ability to define and protect associated perforating arteries from this approach is limited by the contralateral eccentricity, by the increased distance of reach, and by the trajectory angle of exposure.

A left anterior subtemporal approach, however, affords a more direct path to the aneurysm neck. Perforating vessels can be freed from the fundus and swept posteriorly. The clip can then be applied from a lateral perspective, with the perforators directly visualized during clip application. Considering that the basilar aneurysm is the lesion of greatest difficulty and greatest risk (to the patient and during surgery), the authors chose to proceed with clipping of the basilar aneurysm from a left anterior subtemporal approach. The right middle cerebral aneurysm was clipped via a right trans-sylvian approach at a separate sitting. The patient made an uneventful recovery.

CASE 2

A 37-year-old female presented with subarachnoid hemorrhage. She was awake and alert with no focal deficits and was assigned a Hunt-Hess grade I. A CT scan showed thick subarachnoid clot in the perimesencephalic cistern. An angiogram demonstrated an aneurysm of the basilar apex with the neck lying 1.5 cm below the posterior clinoid process (Fig. 6, **A** and **B**).

This case illustrates the difficulties posed by a low-lying bifurcation aneurysm with the neck well below the posterior clinoid process. The upward slope of the medial petrous apex obstructs the visualization of the neck and proximal basilar artery. The posterior cerebral artery, which must ascend to reach the tentorial edge, also lies in the way (Fig. 6A). Even with extensive temporal retraction, the exposure achieved through a standard anterior subtemporal approach is inadequate for safe clip application. The addition of an extradural medial petrosectomy, however, yields an avenue for attack that is flush with the floor of the temporal fossa (Fig. 7, **A** and **B**). The neck and perforating vessels can be easily dissected along with a short segment of the proximal basilar artery for potential temporary occlusion. This aneurysm was managed in this way, and the patient recovered without incident.

CONCLUSION

Four basic approaches can be used to access aneurysms of the upper basilar region including trans-sylvian, temporopolar, anterior subtemporal, and lateral petrosal, presigmoid. Selection of the best approach

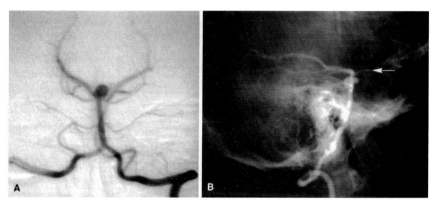

FIG. 6 **(A)** AP and **(B)** lateral angiogram showing low-lying basilar bifurcation aneurysm. *Arrow* indicates posterior clinoid process.

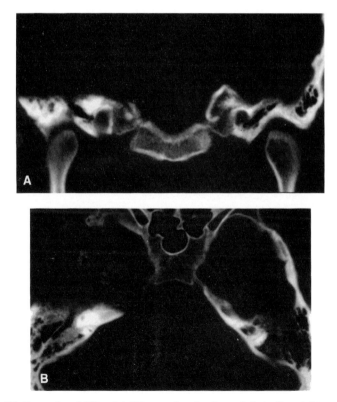

FIG. 7 **(A)** Coronal and **(B)** axial CT scan showing bone defect after right medial petrosectomy. Note bone removal flush with floor of temporal fossa.

varies according to the level and laterality of the lesion as well as the clinical status of the patient. We prefer the anterior subtemporal approach in most situations because of the wide exposure, lateral perspective for clip application, and the anterior oblique visualization of the associated perforating vessels it provides.

ACKNOWLEDGMENTS

The authors thank David A. Peace for his help and advice in the preparation of illustrations and figures.

REFERENCES

1. Al-Mefty O: Supraorbital-pterional approach to skull base lesions. **Neurosurgery** 21:474–477, 1987.
2. Al-Mefty O, Fox JL, Smith RR: Petrosal approach for petroclival meningiomas. **Neurosurgery** 22:510–517, 1988.
3. Day JD, Fukushima T, Giannotta SL: Microanatomical study of the extradural middle fossa approach to the petroclival and posterior cavernous sinus region: Description of the rhomboid construct. **Neurosurgery** 34:1009–1016, 1994.
4. Oliviera ED, Tedeschi H, Siqueira M, *et al.*: Surgical approaches for aneurysms of the basilar artery bifurcation, in Matsushima T (ed): *Surgical Anatomy for Microsurgery VI: Cerebral Aneurysms and Skull Base Lesions*. Fukuoka City, Japan, Scimed Publications, 1993, pp 34–42.
5. Drake C: Bleeding aneurysms of the basilar artery: Direct surgical management in four cases. **J Neurosurg** 18:230–238, 1961.
6. Drake CG: Gordon Murray lecture: Evolution of intracranial aneurysm surgery. **Can J Surg** 27:549–555, 1984.
7. Heros RC, Lee SH: The combined pterional/anterior temporal approach for aneurysms of the upper basilar complex: Technical report. **Neurosurgery** 33:244–250, 1993.
8. Jane JA, Park TS, Poberskin LH, *et al.*: The supraorbital approach: Technical note. **Neurosurgery** 11:537–542, 1982.
9. Kawase T, Shiobara R, Toya S: Middle fossa transpetrosal-transtentorial approaches for. **Acta Neurochir (Wien)** 129:113–120, 1994.
10. Malis L: The petrosal approach. **Clin Neurosurg** 37:528–540, 1990.
11. Sano K, Shiokawa Y: The temporo-polar approach to basilar artery aneurysms with or without zygomatic arch translocation. **Acta Neurochir (Wien)** 130:14–19, 1994.
12. Sundt TM: *Surgical Techniques for Saccular and Giant Intracranial Aneurysms.* Baltimore, Williams & Wilkins, 1990, pp 213–223.
13. Yasargil MG, Antic J, Laciga R, *et al.*: Microsurgical pterional approach to aneurysms of the basilar bifurcation. **Surg Neurol** 6:83–91, 1976.
14. Yasargil MG, Reichman MV, Kubik S: Preservation of the frontotemporal branch of the facial nerve using the interfascial temporalis flap for pterional craniotomy: Technical article. **J Neurosurg** 67:463–466, 1987.

II

General Scientific Session II—Innovations in the Treatment of Craniofacial Disorders and Spinal Dysraphisms

9

Treatment of Craniosynostosis

JOHN A. JANE, SR., M.D., PH.D., AND JOHN A. JANE, JR., M.D.

In this chapter the authors' techniques for the treatment of craniosynostosis are discussed. No attempt is made to present alternate methods; rather, these treatment modalities represent the methods in use at the University of Virginia. They have been developed in collaboration with the Department of Plastic Surgery at the University of Virginia, most notably, Milton Edgerton, John Persing, and Kant Lin; resident staff members throughout the years have also made major contributions.

The topics that will be discussed are (a) sagittal synostosis; (b) unilateral coronal synostosis; (c) metopic synostosis; (d) lambdoid synostosis; (e) bicoronal synostosis; (f) multiple suture synostosis; and (g) the late correction of synostosis.

Figure 1 shows a 5-month gestational skull in which the sutures are widely open. The biologic significance of this is well known: open sutures permit head deformation during passage through the birth canal and subsequently allow the brain to grow. Skull growth takes place in response to growth of the brain and occurs perpendicular to each suture. Thus, when a suture closes, growth perpendicular to that suture ceases. For example, the premature closure of the sagittal suture, the head is narrow. The subsequent compensations, which result in stereotypic deformities, follow other well-defined, albeit unusual, rules.

SKULL GROWTH AFTER SINGLE SUTURE CLOSURE

Figures 2**A**–**C** demonstrate the changes that occur in sagittal, coronal, and metopic synostosis. Figure 2 emphasizes that a single suture closure results in deformity throughout the entire skull; the deformity is not just limited to the area of the closed suture. It also demonstrates an interesting puzzle: if skull growth is dependent on the growth of the brain and our skulls are generally round because our brains are generally round, then why does a single-suture closure result in any

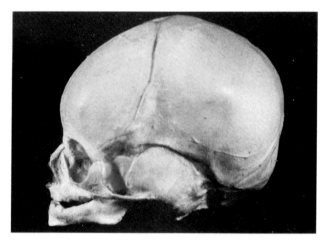

FIG. 1 Normal fetal skull. A photograph of a normal 5-month gestational skull showing widely patent sutures that permit brain growth and easy passage through the birth
canal.

deformity at all? In other words, why don't other sutures compensate
for the lack of growth at a single site and reconstitute a round skull?
For example, with sagittal synostosis, if the growing round brain is
the prime mover, why doesn't growth take place at the squamosal suture (Fig. 2**A**) to compensate and return the skull to a normal shape?
Why does the growth instead take place unilaterally at the lambdoid
and coronal sutures and bilaterally at the metopic suture?

  In fact, we do not know the mechanisms that cause the compensations seen in craniosynostosis. Nevertheless, the compensations are
not random, and the application of certain rules does predict the
growth of the skull after single suture closure. These rules are as follows: (a) Compensation takes place at sutures that are immediately
adjacent to the closed suture, not at distant unconnected sutures. (b)
Those sutures that are perpendicular to the closed suture compensate

FIG. 2 Single suture closure. (**A**) Sagittal synostosis. An artist's depiction of sagittal synostosis, offering sites at which growth could compensate for the suture closure if the skull
truly grew only in response to brain growth. In fact, other sutures do not compensate by
returning the skull to its normal contour, and while the mechanism is unknown, predictable pathologic compensations occur. The closure of the sagittal suture causes deformities throughout the skull, including frontal bossing and temporal narrowing. (**B**) Coronal synostosis. Notice that growth at sutures adjacent and perpendicular to the closed
suture occurs away from the closed suture. (**C**) Metopic synostosis. Notice that growth at
sutures adjacent to but not perpendicular to the closed suture occurs bilaterally.

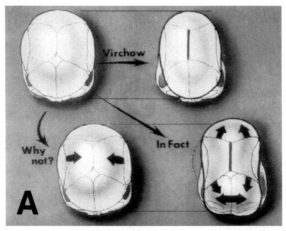

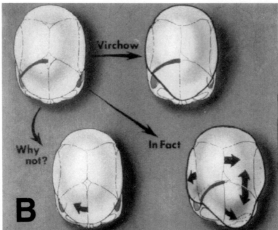

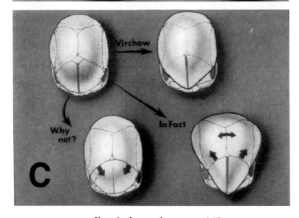

FIG. 2 Legend on page 140

by growing unilaterally and away from the closed suture. (c) Those sutures that are in line and not perpendicular to the closed suture compensate by growing bilaterally. These rules are depicted in Figure 2**B** and **C** and predict all of the well-known characteristics of each type of premature closure. The practical point that arises from these considerations is that surgery should be directed primarily toward the compensations that have occurred rather than the primary suture closure. The benefit of early correction is that surgery can be directed at preventing these compensations and correcting those that are found.

SAGITTAL SYNOSTOSIS

The Anterior "Π" Procedure

The frontal bossing and temporal narrowing are clearly seen in Figure 3. Surgery that simply addresses the sagittal suture does not correct the frontal bossing and, therefore, does not resolve what may be the most striking deformity. The correct procedure encompasses the length of the head, the bossing, and the narrowness of the skull. The aim must be to produce a pleasing round head at the time of surgery, to allow further normal growth, and not to leave bone defects of any size.

The procedure that accomplishes all of these desiderations is called the anterior "Π" procedure. Figure 3**B** shows the bone plates that are removed. The coronal suture is removed (Fig. 3**C**), the sagittal suture is elevated, and bone is removed from the temporal fossa. To make sure that the bone plates can slide toward one another, the dura is separated from the bone both frontally and underneath the sagittal suture (Fig. 3**D**). Figure 3 **E** shows the skull being shortened and held together and the bone plates being replaced. We believe that changing the relationship of the skull to the dura actually corrects the condition and allows normal skull growth to proceed. Before-and-after pictures are shown in Figure 3**F** and **G**. Note that this procedure has corrected the frontal bossing and the temporal depression.

FIG. 3   Sagittal synostosis: the anterior "Π" procedure. (**A**) An artist's rendering of sagittal synostosis, with arrows showing the direction of compensatory bone growth. Note the classic frontal bossing and temporal narrowing. (**B**) This drawing shows the bone plates removed perpendicular and lateral to the sagittal suture. (**C**) In this drawing the coronal suture is removed and the sagittal suture is elevated above the dura. Notice that the removed bone now resembles the Greek symbol "Π". (**D**) In this intraoperative photograph the coronal suture has been removed and the dura

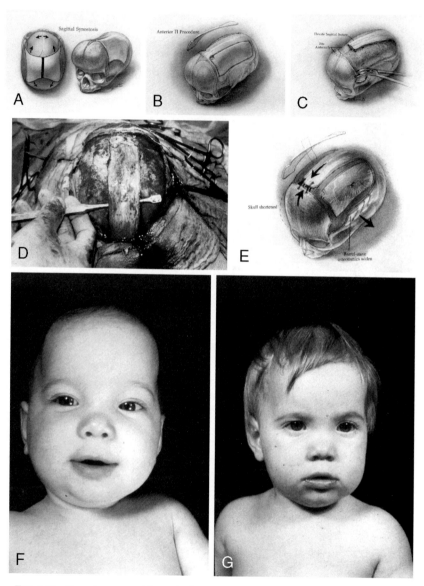

FIG. 3 *Continued* separated from the bone, allowing the bone plates to be squeezed together. (**E**) Drawing of the anterior "Π" procedure at completion; the skull is shortened and the bone plates have been replaced. (**F**) Preoperative photograph of patient with sagittal synostosis. Notice the frontal bossing and temporal narrowing. (**G**) Postoperative photograph of the same patient. Notice the correction of the frontal bossing and the lack of temporal narrowing.

Anterior Sagittal Synostosis

In children who primarily experience closure of their anterior sagittal suture, a depression will occur at the vertex with frontal bossing as the principal deformity. Figures 4**A** and **B** show front and side views of a child with closure of the anterior sagittal suture. Compensation has

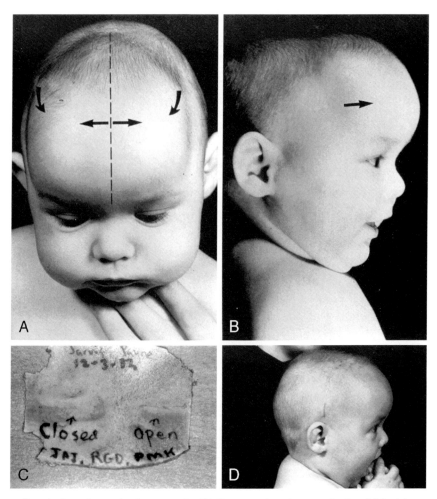

FIG. 4 Anterior sagittal synostosis. (**A**) Preoperative photograph of a child with an anterior closure of the sagittal suture. (**B**) Preoperative photograph in profile of the same child. Notice that the primary deformity is frontal bossing. (**C**) An intraoperative photograph of the bone fragment carrying the sagittal suture that is open posteriorly and closed anteriorly. (**D**) A postoperative photograph showing a marked reduction in the anterior-posterior dimensions of the skull.

occurred mainly at the coronal suture anteriorly, but the metopic suture has also contributed to the bulging forehead. In this situation, the sagittal suture has to be removed and the skull shortened, using a bifrontal craniotomy with dural plication and bone remolding. Figure 4**C** shows the bone opened posteriorly and closed anteriorly and the postoperative result (Fig. 4**D**).

Other Variations of Sagittal Synostosis

We estimate that approximately 10% of our sagittal synostosis patients have posterior compensation. This condition results in an occipital knob (Fig. 5**A**). Here, the so-called "reverse Π" is performed. As seen in Figure 5**B**, the bone plates are elevated, the bone is carefully removed across the posterior part of the sagittal sinus, and the skull is shortened by pulling the knob forward (Fig. 5**C**). If the knob is closer to the foramen magnum, we will go around the entire knob, using it as a piece that can be brought forward. Care must be taken to dissect the transverse sinus and torcula from the bone and to hold the knob forward by means of plates. Figure 5**D** shows an adequate postoperative result using the reverse "Π" procedure.

Other variations in sagittal synostosis also occur. In the so-called "golf-tee" deformity there is closure of the posterior part of the sagittal suture that is compensated by frontal bossing and widening of the skull surrounding the open anterior portion of the sagittal suture. Figure 6**A** illustrates the golf-tee deformity in lateral and superior views. In Fig. 6**B**, the bone has been removed, allowing the skull to be shortened anteriorly and the posterior part of the skull to expand. To hold the correction in place, plates are used, as seen in Figure 6**C** and **D**. Figures 6**E** and **F** show a good cosmetic result.

Another variation on posterior sagittal synostosis is so-called "bathrocephaly" (Fig. 7), in which there appears to be a podium at the posterior part of the skull. The correction for this condition requires a slightly different approach, in which the posterior part of the skull is remodeled with the patient in the prone position (Fig. 7**B**). The sagittal suture is re-formed with the use of miniplates to achieve an agreeable posterior projection. Sagittal synostosis is particularly interesting because its manifestations are so protean. The proper correction cannot be achieved by using a single procedure. In Greek legend, Procrustes' bed of a given length would not fit everyone. His solution was to either stretch the guest or cut off his legs, depending on his height. We recommend planning multiple alternatives, depending on the particular anatomy of the patient.

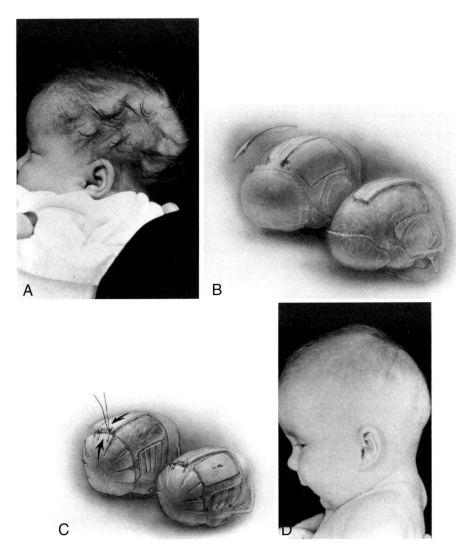

FIG. 5 Occipital knob: the reverse "Π" procedure. (A) A preoperative photograph of a child with sagittal synostosis and posterior compensation, resulting in an occipital knob. (B) In this setting, a reverse "Π" procedure is performed. Here the plates and lambdoid sutures have been removed. (C) In this drawing the knob is pulled forward and held with wire. (D) A postoperative photograph showing a more normal skull contour.

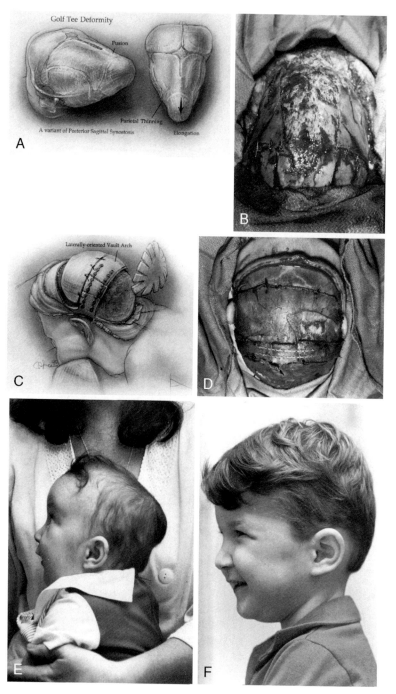

FIG. 6 Legend on page 148

FIG. 6 The "golf–tee" deformity. (**A**) A drawing depicting the fused posterior sagittal suture, the compensation of the lambdoid suture, and frontal bossing. (**B**) An intraoperative photograph showing the lateral expansion of the brain after bone removal. (**C**) A drawing showing the vaulting used to hold the lateral expansion in place. (**D**) An intraoperative photograph of the vaulting utilizing plates. (**E**) A preoperative photograph of a child with the "golf-tee" deformity. (**F**) The postoperative photograph of the same child.

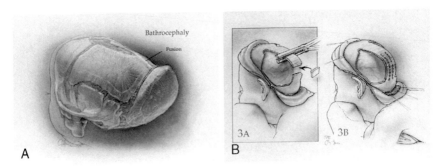

FIG. 7 Bathrocephaly (**A**) An artist's rendering of bathrocephaly. The posterior skull resembles a podium. (**B**) A drawing of the surgical procedure after correction with plates. This procedure is performed in the prone position.

UNILATERAL CORONAL SYNOSTOSIS

As seen in Figures 8**A** and **B**, unilateral coronal synostosis is characterized by ipsilateral flattening, contralateral frontal bossing, ipsilateral enlargement of the middle fossa, and a mild contralateral parietal bulge with the radix of the nose deviated toward the side of the synostosis. In the past, we routinely corrected this deviation, but we no longer consider it critical. A very severe example is seen illustrated in Figure 8**C**, showing the bony plate, consisting of the frontal and parietal bones, which has failed to grow, and the expected compensations at the squamosal, sagittal, coronal, and metopic sutures (Fig. 8**D**).

Figure 9 shows a technique, the tongue-and-groove procedure, for correcting the older patient with severe unilateral coronal synostosis. One of the most important considerations here is the necessity of rotating the temporalis muscle anteriorly. Figure 10**A** shows a less severe case of coronal synostosis; here, the orbital rim and temporalis have advanced bone chips that have been placed in the temporal fossa to make sure that there is no concavity (Fig. 10**B**). The result (Fig. 10**C**) is quite good, except that the contralateral left parietal area is still slightly more prominent. This has no cosmetic significance whatsoever.

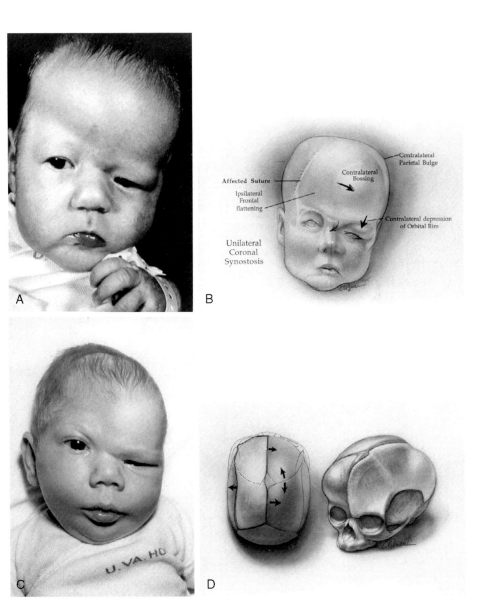

FIG. 8 Unilateral coronal synostosis. (**A**) A preoperative photograph of a child with unilateral coronal synostosis. (**B**) An artist's drawing of the child with arrows depicting the compensatory growth. (**C**) A preoperative photograph of a different child with a more severe form of coronal synostosis. (**D**) An artist's rendering of the expected compensations in unilateral coronal synostosis.

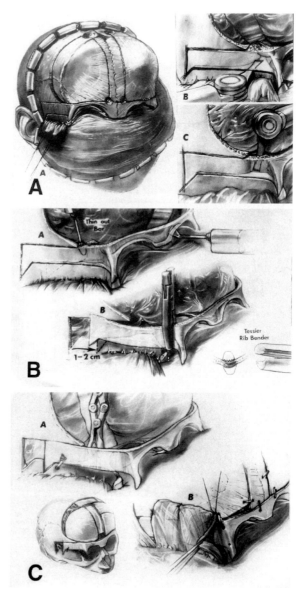

FIG. 9 Late correction of unilateral coronal synostosis. (**A**) A drawing of the tongue-and-groove procedure for late correction of unilateral coronal synostosis. (**B**) A drawing showing the advancement of the bone flap, including the superior orbital rim. (**C**) A drawing showing the fixation of the advanced bone and the necessary advancement of the temporalis muscle.

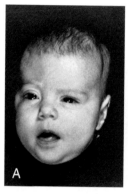 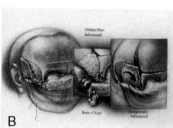 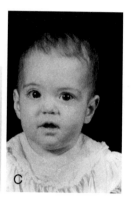

FIG. 10 Coronal synostosis (**A**) A preoperative photograph of a child with a mild form of coronal synostosis. (**B**) This drawing emphasizes the need to place bone chips in the temporal fossa and advance the temporalis muscle. (**C**) A postoperative photograph showing a good cosmetic result, except for some residual left parietal prominence.

METOPIC SYNOSTOSIS

Figure 11**A** shows a case of metopic synostosis with an anteriorly displaced coronal suture and a pear-shaped skull. The characteristics, as seen here, are midfrontal keel, biparietal widening, and hypotelorism.

The correction can take place in stages with very minor degrees of metopic synostosis; merely shaving down the keel may be adequate (Fig. 11**B**). As the disease progresses it is necessary to remove the thick glabellar bone (Fig. 11**C**). The dura is plicated over the frontal keel, and the orbital rim is advanced (Fig. 11**D**). Finally, the frontal bone is tailored in advance, as are the orbital rims (Fig. 11**E**). Figure 11**F** shows the very thick bone that is seen in this condition. Figure 12 shows a boy with typical metopic synostosis; his postoperative photographs show a good result.

LAMBDOID SYNOSTOSIS

The diagnosis of lambdoid synostosis presents an area in which there is some disagreement. The authors consider true lambdoid synostosis, in which there is actual fusion of the lambdoid suture, to be exceedingly rare. When this occurs, the skull grows in the predicted fashion: the ear on the same side is displaced downward. There is some slight anterior movement caused by growth at the squamosal suture (Fig. 13**A**) and a contralateral bulge because of growth at the sagittal and lambdoid sutures. Figures 13**B** and **C** show a case of true lambdoid synostosis.

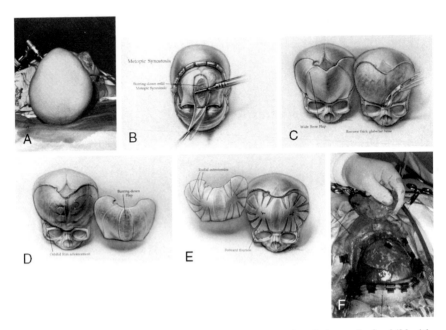

FIG. 11 Metopic synostosis (**A**) An immediate preoperative photograph of a child with metopic synostosis, showing a midfrontal keel, biparietal widening, and hypotelorism. (**B**) A drawing of the procedure used to correct this minor deformity, in which simple burring is adequate to correct the cosmetic defect. (**C**) A drawing of an alternative procedure that may be required for more severe cases in which the thick glabellar bone must be removed. (**D**) The dura is plicated and the orbital rim is advanced. (**E**) Finally, both the bone flap and the orbital rim are tailored and replaced. (**F**) An intraoperative photograph showing the thick bone characteristic of metopic synostosis.

What is more common than true lambdoid synostosis is posterior plagiocephaly. This has been described as positional molding, functional lambdoid, or lazy lambdoid. If the condition is unilateral, then a "parallelogram" skull results (Fig. 14**A**). With a bilateral press, the deformity is very marked but symmetrical.

Figure 14**B** illustrates bilateral molding with a dramatically deformed posterior portion of the skull. It is our opinion that helmet molding is relatively ineffective when such striking deformities occur. Figures 14**C** and **D** show how the sagittal bone has been expanded to give a corrected projection; plates are then used to correct it, and the bone flaps are replaced. The pre- and postoperative radiographs show the correction that was obtained (Fig. 14**E**).

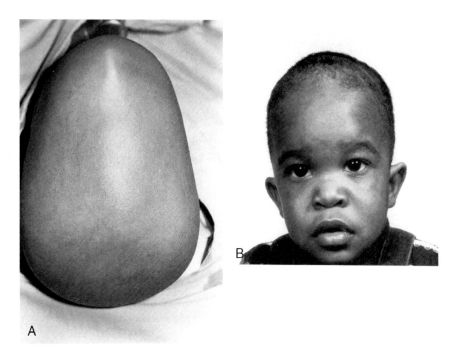

FIG. 12   Metopic Synostosis. (**A**) A preoperative photograph of a child with metopic synostosis. (**B**) A postoperative photograph showing a good cosmetic result.

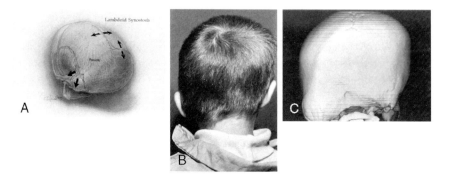

FIG. 13   Lambdoid Synostosis. (**A**) A drawing showing the compensatory bone growth in lambdoid synostosis. (**B**) A preoperative photograph of a child with true lambdoid synostosis. Notice that the ear on the effected side is displaced downward. (**C**) A preoperative three-dimensional reconstructed CT scan of the same child.

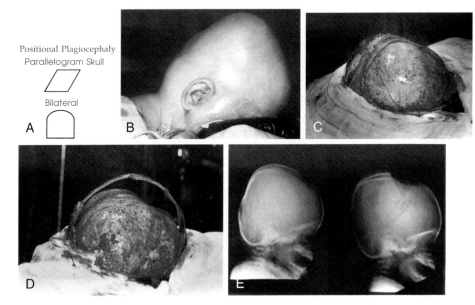

FIG. 14 Posterior plagiocephaly. (**A**) A schematic depicting the result of unilateral and bilateral positional plagiocephaly. (**B**) An immediate preoperative photograph of a child with bilateral plagiocephaly. (**C**) An intraoperative photograph of the same child with biparietal craniotomies. (**D**) An intraoperative photograph showing an expanded sagittal bone fixated with plates. (**E**) Preoperative (*left*) and postoperative (*right*) radiographs showing the correction.

BICORONAL SYNOSTOSIS

Bicoronal synostosis is characterized by a high vertex, brachiocephaly, and recessed superior orbital rims (Fig. 15). Figure 15**D** and **E** illustrate the repair with a cap being left on so that the overall height can be reduced. The orbital rims can be managed as seen above or just by advancing them. Figure 15**F** shows a remodeled frontal bone as well as an orbital rim. The pre- and postoperative computerized tomography (CT) scans (Figs. 15**G** and **H**) show adequate lengthening of the skull accompanied by diminishment of the bitemporal width. The pre- and postoperative plain films are seen here (Fig. 15**I**). Figure 15**J** reveals a good cosmetic result.

With single suture closure, excellent results can be regularly achieved. Bilateral coronal synostosis and multiple suture closure have presented as difficult technical problems that have prevented consistently superb results. Early in our approach, two-stage procedures were decided on with the forehead vertex and orbital rims done as the first step and brachycephaly corrected at a later time. While the orbital rim appearance was adequate, the vertex remained high, probably because of lack of room posteriorly. This, therefore, led into a more radical single-stage procedure utilizing the Park modification of a prone position.

MULTIPLE SUTURE SYNOSTOSIS

There are many problems associated with achieving truly good results when more than one suture is involved. The basic principle seems to be clear: the entire skull must be remodeled. This one-stage correction is best done with the patient in a modified prone position so that access from maxilla to foramen magnum is possible. The skull is narrowed

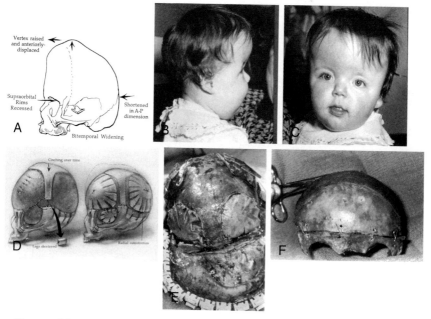

FIG. 15 Bilateral bicoronal synostosis. (**A**) A line-drawing of a patient with bicoronal synostosis. Note the high vertex, brachiocephaly, and recessed superior orbital rims. (**B**) A preoperative photograph of a patient with bicoronal synostosis. (**C**) Another preoperative photograph of the same child. (**D**) An artist's depiction of the operative procedure. An ample craniotomy is performed, leaving a "cap" that is used to reduce the overall height. Before replacing the bone flaps, the dura is plicated and the orbital rims are advanced. (**E**) An intraoperative photograph of the completed procedure. (**F**) An intraoperative view of the tailored frontal bone and orbital rim.

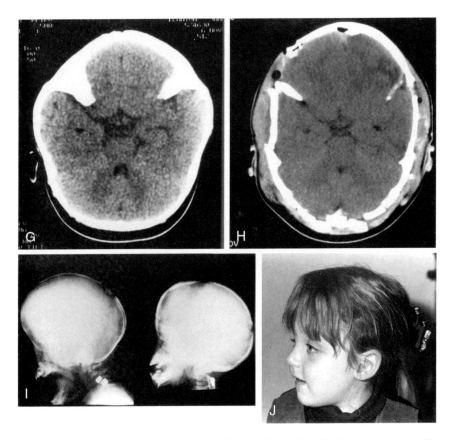

FIG. 15 *Continued* (**G**) A preoperative CT scan of this child. (**H**) The postoperative CT scan showing an overall lengthening of the skull and a reduction in the bitemporal diameter. (**I**) Preoperative (*left*) and postoperative (*right*) radiographs showing the operative results. (**J**) A postoperative photograph showing the good cosmetic result.

FIG. 16 Turricephaly. (**A**) An immediate preoperative photograph of a child with turricephaly. (**B**) A preoperative photograph of the same child. (**C**) Preoperative plain radiographs confirmed multiple suture closure. (**D**) A postoperative photograph of the same child with adequate cosmetic results. (**E**) The same child in adolescence revealing good social performance. (**F**) The child also exhibits normal intellectual development.

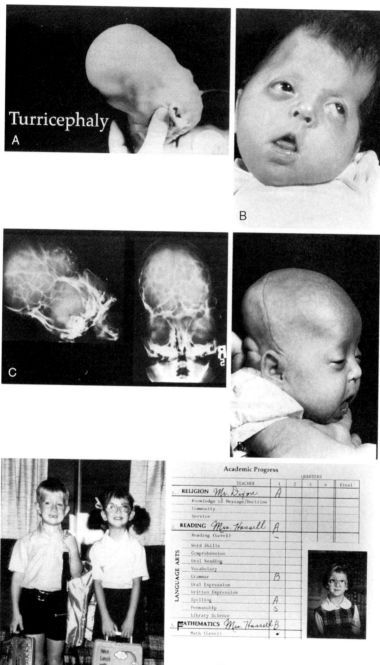

FIG. 16   Legend on page 156

in multiple fragments and, based upon the deformity, the appropriate reconstruction is carried out. Figure 16**A** and **B** show a child with multiple suture closure as confirmed by preoperative films (Fig. 16**C**). Total skull removal and remolding was performed with an adequate result (Fig. 16**D**). Her psychological status was important, and we found that she did well (Figs. 16**E** and **F**).

Another case of multiple suture closure is seen in Figure 17. The patient is placed in the face-up position so that access from the foramen to maxilla is possible. The skull has been exposed with each orbit seen as well (Fig. 17**B**). The skull is removed and remolded (Fig. 17**C**). The pre- and postoperative pictures show adequate correction (Fig. 17**D**).

LATE CORRECTION OF CRANIOSYNOSTOSIS

Late correction of untreated or poorly treated synostosis is a major procedure that becomes more difficult as times passes. Figure 18**A** and **B** shows anterior-posterior and lateral views of a 3-year-old girl whose parents decided that her untreated sagittal synostosis needed correction. This was done by removing her entire skull and remolding it, using a kerfing technique to mold the bone (Fig. 18**C**). Her postoperative appearance is good (Fig. 18**D**).

A boy (Fig. 19**A**) had an anterior sagittal synostosis; strip craniotomy was initially performed by the author. This was inadequate, as it did not address the frontal bossing, and at the age of 3½ he returned for further correction. Figure 19**B** shows the old skin incision and the persistent frontal bossing, and Figure 19**C** shows the technique that was used to correct his deformity, which was mainly frontal and did not require posterior attention. His postoperative appearance is good (Fig. 19**D**).

Late correction of coronal synostosis can often be accomplished in a simple extracranial fashion. A girl (Fig. 20**A**) had an asymmetrical brow that was repaired by a simple onlay acrylic technique (Fig. 20**B**).

CONCLUSIONS

(a) Fusion of a single suture results in deformities throughout the entire skull. (b) These deformities are predictable, based on the site of fusion. (c) Often, correction of these compensatory deformities must be the principal goal of the surgeon. An effort should be made at the time of the initial surgery to achieve an immediate pleasing aesthetic response; however, early surgery will allow the growing brain to aid in the correction.

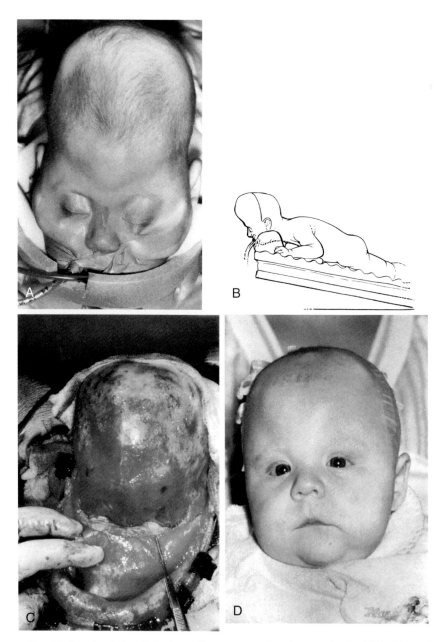

FIG. 17 Turricephaly. (**A**) An immediate preoperative photograph of a child with turricephaly. Note the prone, head-up position. (**B**) A line-drawing of the prone, head-up positioning used for this case. (**D**) An intraoperative photograph with the skull and superior orbital rims exposed. (**D**) A postoperative photograph of this child with good cosmetic result.

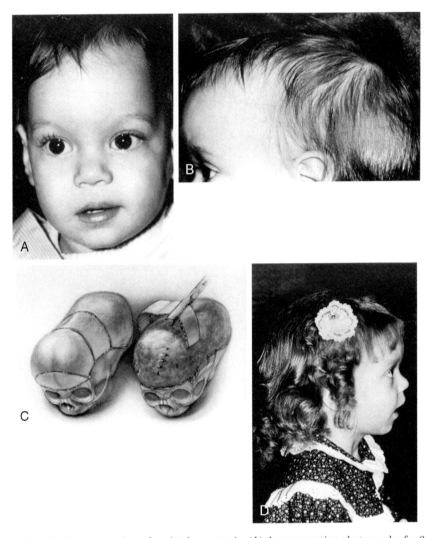

FIG. 18 Late correction of sagittal synostosis. (**A**) A preoperative photograph of a 3-year-old girl with previously uncorrected sagittal synostosis. (**B**) A preoperative photograph of the same child, showing the dramatic anterior-posterior length of her skull. (**C**) A drawing of the procedure performed requiring complete removal of the skull and substantial tailoring before replacing the bone flaps. (**D**) A postoperative photograph revealing a good postoperative appearance.

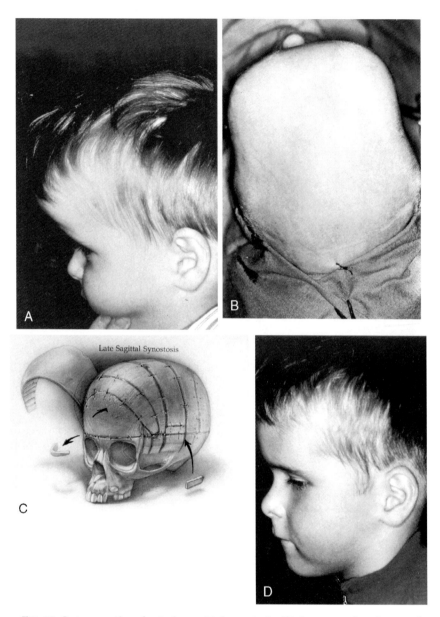

FIG. 19 Late correction of anterior sagittal synostosis. (**A**) A preoperative photograph of a boy with anterior sagittal synostosis. A simple strip craniectomy had been unsuccessful. (**B**) An immediate preoperative photograph revealing the frontal bossing as well as the previous surgical scar. (**C**) An artist's depiction of the surgical procedure showing the radical craniotomy that must be performed in late corrections. (**D**) A postoperative photograph showing a good correction of the frontal bossing and restoration of the normal skull dimensions.

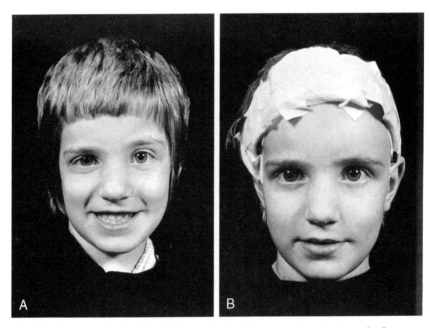

FIG. 20   Late correction of coronal synostosis. (**A**) preoperative photograph of a young girl with uncorrected coronal synostosis revealing an asymmetric brow. (**B**) A postoperative photograph of the same girl after surgical correction using a simple onlay acrylic technique.

10

Electrophysiologic Monitoring during Tethered Spinal Cord Release

LAWRENCE H. PHILLIPS II, M.D., AND JOHN A. JANE, M.D., PH.D.

Surgery on the cauda equina always carries some risk of nerve injury. Release of a tethered spinal cord is one of the procedures that carries an especially high risk for injury. There are several indications and types of procedures that could be done for release of a tethered spinal cord. This condition exists when some developmental or acquired abnormality, usually in the lumbosacral region, exists that prevents the normal rostral-caudal elongation of the spinal cord during growth. The tension on the neural elements that this abnormality produces eventually results in a progressive neurologic deficit. It is believed that neurologic deterioration can be prevented or relieved by releasing the restraint on the spinal cord or nerve roots.

The dysraphic conditions, such as myelomeningocele, are the major cause for spinal cord tethering, but at times the only abnormality is a so-called "tight filum," or failure of elongation of the filum terminale. In the case of the dysraphic anomaly, inadvertent nerve injury can occur when distorted anatomy prevents precise identification of viable nerve tissue. Additionally, the cause of tethering in such cases is often scarring from previous surgical procedures in the same area. Nerve tissue can become embedded in scar and be very difficult to identify.

The anatomy of the tight filum is usually more easily identified; however, nerve roots can often be closely associated with the filum, particularly the sacral nerve roots that innervate the bowel and bladder (3, 5). These fibers are often difficult to visualize, even with the use of the operating microscope. Blindly sectioning the filum in these circumstances can lead to potentially devastating injury to bowel and bladder function.

Intraoperative monitoring (IOM) of various peripheral and central nervous system functions has been adopted in many centers to reduce the risk for injury to neural elements. Monitoring strategies have included somatosensory evoked potential (SSEP) recording (4, 13), bladder and rectal manometry (6, 11, 13), ultrasound (10), blood flow measurement (12), and various types of muscle recording, including recording of ongoing spontaneous electromyography (EMG) activity (4), as well as the response to electrical stimulation of nerve roots within the operative field (3–5, 13). In some centers, combinations of these techniques are used (4, 13).

The utility of many of these techniques has yet to be established. The goal for IOM in most surgical procedures is to detect injury to nerve at a sufficiently early stage that the procedure can be modified to prevent the damage from becoming more extensive or permanent. Arguably, some IOM techniques, by their nature, are either too insensitive or not sufficiently timely to meet this goal. For example, the generation time for an SSEP may be so long that any nerve injury detected is so far after the fact that nothing can be done about it. (13).

Motor readings, either of ongoing electrical activity in muscle or of evoked compound muscle action potentials, provide the most immediate and extensive type of information. Recordings from multiple lower extremity muscles and either the external urethral sphincter or anal sphincter can be made simultaneously using modern multichannel recording equipment. We have developed a technique for IOM that involves recording from four to six lower extremity muscles and the external and sphincter while electrical stimulation is applied within the surgical field. This technique has converted IOM from a passive procedure that waits for injury to occur to one that is actively involved in guiding the surgical dissection.

METHODS OF MONITORING

All patients who are to undergo IOM for tethered cord release undergo preoperative examination in the diagnostic EMG laboratory. This preoperative examination will precisely define the amount of innervation present before surgery. One can then decide which muscles to select for monitoring and also defined realistic goals for the surgery.

The recordings methods the authors use are evolved from those originally developed for IOM during selective dorsal rhizotomy (7). When this series was begun, a 5-channel recording instrument (TECA Mystro) was used, but the later cases were done on an 8-channel instrument (Nicolet Viking II). In the 5-channel recordings, intramuscular monopolar needle electrodes were placed in the anterior tibial and medical gastrocnemius muscles bilaterally with subcutaneous reference electrodes, and the fifth channel was used for recordings from the anal sphincter (see below). The extra channels of the Nicolet instrument are also used to record bilaterally from the vastus lateralis muscles.

Recordings from the anal sphincter are accomplished by inserting a commercially available bipolar plug electrode into the sphincter. When the case involves a newborn infant, the plug electrodes are too large to insert, and subcutaneous electroencephalogram needle electrodes are used instead. One electrode is inserted into each side of the sphincter.

This recording arrangement is planned to provide coverage of each spinal and root segment from L2 to S2 (9). If preoperative studies revealed complete denervation in specific muscles, others were substituted in the recording array, but most cases have been done using the montage described above.

The intramuscular recordings are displayed at a gain setting of 1 m V per vertical deflection. The anal sphincter recordings, which are technically surface recordings, are displayed at a gait setting of 100 m V per vertical deflection. The recordings are made with a 10-Hz low-frequency filter and a 1.0-kHz high-frequency filter.

Two recording methods are used. The first involves continuous recording of ongoing muscle activity. The recording machine is left in a free-running mode with a display speed of 5-seconds full sweep, and the volume of the audio output is increased to allow the operating team to hear it. When peripheral nerve undergoes traction or compression, it will spontaneously discharge. This produces trains of neurotonic discharges in muscles supplied by the nerve (1, 2). These bursts of discharges are recognized by the operating team, who notify the surgeon that nerve is at risk for permanent damage.

The second recording method involves electrical stimulation within the operating field. The stimulator is a modified commercial device designed for intraoperative use. Bipolar platinum stimulating wigs are mounted on a surgical forceps to facilitate manipulation within tight spaces (8).The stimulator is connected to the stimulus output of the monitoring machine and led onto the surgical drapes by gas-sterilized cables. The stimulator output is set to deliver a 0.05 msec stimulus, and the current is adjusted in a range from 0 to 100 mA. Recordings are made with a display window of 100 msec full sweep.

Stimulation is performed when there is any question about the identification of tissue within the wound. The stimulator is applied to the tissue, and recordings are made from all seven recording sites simultaneously. A compound muscle action potential evoked in any recording site is considered a positive response and indicates the presence of active nerve. The stimulus intensity required is noted and a judgment is made about the proximity of active nerve to the stimulating electrode according to the criteria noted in Table 1.

Attention to technical details is important during stimulation. Care must be taken to keep the field dry, because blood, cerebrospinal fluid, or other fluids can "short out" or shunt current between the stimulator

TABLE 1

Interpretation of Stimulation Results in 37 Patients with Tethered Spinal Cord

Stimulus Intensity	Interpretation
1–10 mA	Stimulator directly on nerve
11–25 mA	Nerve near stimulator, but intervening tissue
>25 mA	Spread of stimulus to distant nerve tissue

poles. This would result in inadequate delivery of stimulating current to the tissue. The stimulator must also be maintained in firm contact with the underlying tissue during the entire period of stimulation to ensure full current delivery to the intended area.

No attempt was made to perform quantitative postoperative assessments; however, follow-up studies were performed during routine clinical visits. A global assessment of neurologic function was made from those visits.

RESULTS

This series was performed over a 2-year period. During that time we performed the IOM protocol on 37 patients with various lesions in the lumbosacral region; their diagnoses are listed in Table 2. Some patients had more than one diagnosis; thus the total number of diagnoses is 46. There were 18 females and 19 males, ranging in age from 4 days to 46 years (Fig. 1). In general the younger patients had some form of myelomeningocele, lipomyelomeningocele, or meningocele. Older patients had either a tight filum or some type of tumor with a question of cord tethering involving the tumor.

We often find that innervation that cannot be visually identified can be demonstrated by electrical stimulation. An example is shown in Figures 2 and 3. The patient was a 3-year-old girl who had myelomeningocele closure done in the newborn period. She was able to walk and run with some mild impairment but had not yet been toilet trained. At 3 years of age, increasing weakness in her legs was noted, and a magnetic resonance (MR) image revealed that the cord ended at the level of S2 with an overlying lipoma.

When the defect was exposed, stimulation of the lipoma with stimulus intensities up to 100 mA did not produce responses in leg muscles or the anal sphincter, thus indicating the absence of active nerve tissue. After resection of the lipoma, the neural placode (Fig. 2) was believed to be tethered caudally. Stimulation of the placode at the sites denoted from A to E in Figure 2 with stimulus intensities ranging from 2 to 8 mA produced clear compound muscle action potentials at each stimulation site. Stimulation site E is especially noteworthy, because

TABLE 2
Diagnoses Found in 37 Patients in Intraoperative Monitoring Series

Diagnosis	Number
Diastematomyelia	4
Myelomeningocele	21
Tumor	5
Lipomyelomeningocele	12
Tight filum	3
Other developmental anomaly	1

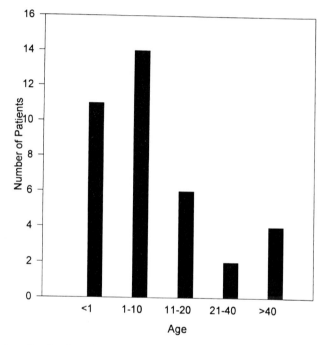

FIG. 1   Age distribution of the 37 patients monitored in this series. All individuals listed in the <1 year age group were operated on in the neonatal period for a closure of a myelomeningocele.

it appeared to have some adhesive scarring, and the authors had planned to section it. The response to stimulation clearly demonstrated the presence of active nerve; thus, it was concluded that some sacral nerve roots were present. Although this structure appeared to be at least partially responsible for the tethering, the authors elected to leave it intact. The patient was unchanged postoperatively, although follow-up MR images continued to indicate a low-lying cord.

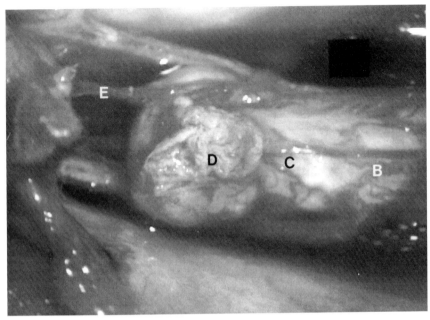

FIG. 2   Intraoperative photograph of the neural placode from the case described in the text. The rostral end of the placode is to the right, and the level of the lesion is at approximately S1-S2. The letters from *A* to *E* denote stimulation and correspond to the electrophysiologic recordings in Figure 3.

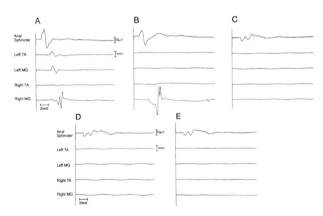

FIG. 3   Intraoperative recordings made in response to stimulation at the sites noted in Figure 2. The *letters* from *A* to *E* correspond to stimulation sites from rostral to caudal on the placode. Recording sites are respectively: anal sphincter (AS), left tibialis anterior (*Left TA*), left medial gastrocnemius (*Left MG*), right tibialis anterior (*Right TA*), and right medial gastrocnemius (*Right MG*). Traces A–C represent the response to stimulus strengths up to 100 mA. The responses in traces D–F were obtained with stimuli of less than 10 mA intensity.

This case illustrates how the IOM protocol is typically used to map innervation. When the possibility of active nerve being present arises during dissection, the authors stimulate the area in question. The initial stimulus intensity is 0 to 1 mA, and it is progessively increased until a response is seen in any of the channels. If no response is seen by the time a 100-mA stimulus is delivered, the authors conclude that there is not active nerve tissue in the vicinity of the stimulation site. As indicated in Table 1, responses evoked by a stimulus of less than 10 mA indicate that the stimulator is in direct contact with nerve. If a stimulus of between 10 and 25 mA produces a response, we know that active nerve is in the vicinity of the stimulator but that there is often intervening tissue. Careful dissection often reveals that stimulus intensity greater than 25 mA produces a response; the authors conclude that nerve is being excited at some distance from the stimulator by a spread of current through the tissue.

Overall, active nerve tissue present in close proximity to either the filum terminale or the tissue producing the tethering has been demonstrated in a surprisingly high percentage of cases. Twenty of the 37 patients (54%) demonstrated these findings. This is particularly noteworthy, because our initial plan in these cases was to resect the tissue in question. In the majority of cases, further dissection revealed nerve that would have been transected, had the initial plan been followed. Avoiding injury to these nerve fibers is at least partially responsible for the demonstrated outcomes (Table 3).

We have also used monitoring for those patients who develop increased spasticity in their lower extremities after neonatal repair of their myelomeningoceles. Although the lesions are complete neurologically, the increase in the spasticity has become exceedingly bothersome. Despite this deficit many such patients have retained anal and urethral sphincter tone, which facilitates toilet function, even though they do not have any volitional control. Often, as they grow, increasing spasticity in the legs makes wheelchair seating and toileting a problem. The neural placode appears to be tethered caudally in such cases, and the authors first attempt to untether it using the procedure described above. In some cases, however, the tethering structures appear to be nerve roots, especially sacral roots that supply innervation to the

TABLE 3
Postoperative Results in 37 Patients with Tethered Spinal Cord

Outcome	Number (%)
Improved	13 (35.1%)
No change	17 (46.0%)
Worse	2 (5.4%)
No follow-up	5 (13.5%)

sphincters. The authors believe that it would be disadvantageous to transect these roots to untether the placode.

In these patients the authors believe that more or less normal spinal reflex arcs are maintained up to some level, producing an "autonomous placode," which lacks normal suprasegmental input. The authors use electrical stimulation to map out the level at which the suprasegmental input is lost. The method we use is shown in Figures 4 and 5. Starting rostrally on the placode the authors stimulate at progressively more caudal levels until we find a level at which compound action muscle potentials can be recorded in the legs and/or the anal sphincter. Typically, there will be a reproducible distinct level below which stimulation will produce responses and above which no response can be seen. The authors consider this to be the level at which the autonomous placode begins; we then section through the placode, and, at this point, the ends retract dramatically. The relief of spasticity is usually immediate and gratifying.

The example shown in Figures 4 and 5 illustrates the procedure. The patient was a 10-year-old female with Arnold-Chiari malformation and

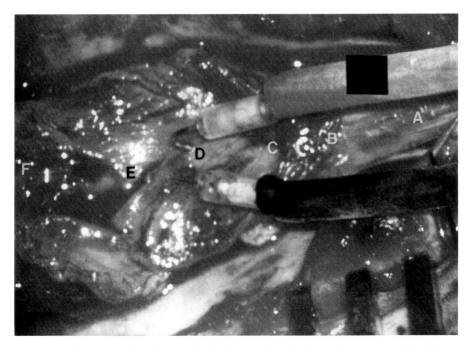

FIG. 4 Intraoperative photograph of what was found to be an "autonomous placode" be electrical stimulation. As in Figure 2, the letters indicate points of stimulation that correspond to the responses shown in Figure 5. The two poles of the stimulator are shown in contact with point *D*. See the text for a description of the case.

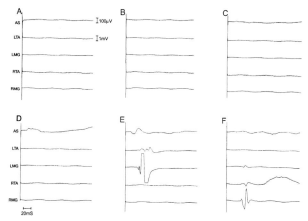

FIG. 5 Intraoperative recordings made in response to stimulation at the sites noted in Figure 4. The notations are the same as those in Figure 3. The pattern that denotes an "autonomous placode" is illustrated. No response is obtained with maximal (100 mA) stimulation at rostral sites (A–C). Stimulus strengths of 10 mA or less at sites D through F produce responses in various channels. The transition between points C and D probably corresponds to the point where the placode loses suprasegmental input.

myelomeningocele who was paraplegic and anesthetic from the waist down. She first sought attention for increasingly troublesome spasticity at age 5, when neuroimaging studies revealed that the spinal cord ended at the sacral level. An attempt at untethering was made. Electrical stimulation revealed evidence of an "autonomous placode" and preserved innervation to lower extremity muscles and the anal sphincter. Multiple adhesions, which were thought to be possibly tethering the cord, was lysed, but she continued to have problems with spasticity postoperatively. By age 10, her symptoms caused increasing difficulty, as the authors re-explored the region of the placode. Electrical mapping again revealed that responses could be obtained in the legs and anal sphincter with stimulation up to a point of transition from normal appearing cord to the placode (between points C and D in Figure 4, which correspond to the responses shown in Fig. 5). These findings were remarkably similar to those the authors had obtained with similar studies during the operation on the patient at age 5. The placode was sectioned between points C and D, and the cord immediately retracted rostrally at least 2 cm. Postoperatively muscle tone was markedly reduced.

Another example is seen in Figure 6. Stimulation is carried out above the level of the placode, and it is quite typical to find no response in the lower extremities (Fig. 6A). Over a very short area of transition between the cord and placode, a sudden response is obtained in the lower

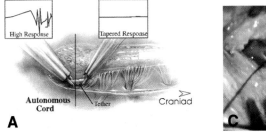

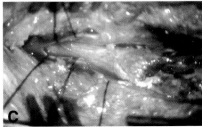

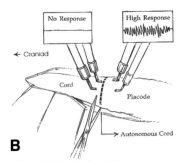

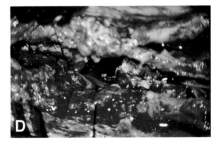

FIG. 6   Correction of late-onset spasticity following neonatal repair of myelomeningo-cele. (**A**) Drawing showing that the craniad electrode causes no response, indicating that those spinal roots do not subserve the lower extremities or anal sphincter. However, the more caudad electrode causes a high response in the lower extremities and anal sphincter, indicating the level of the autonomous cord (shown by black line perpendicular to the cord). (**B**) Drawing describes the level of the autonomous cord; the placode is then sectioned between these two points. (**C**) An intraoperative photograph before sectioning the placode. (**D**) An intraoperative photograph showing the sectioned placode, now retracted after the release of the tethering.

extremities and anal sphincter (Fig. 6A). Considering this to be the place where the "autonomous" placode begins, the authors then sectioned through the placode and, at this point, the ends retracted dramatically (Figs. 6C–E). The relief of spasticity is immediate.

DISCUSSION

This report describes the technique the authors have developed for IOM in tethered cord release procedures. The authors believe that this technique adds significantly to the safety and efficacy of the operation.

When used in most cases, the monitoring assumes a passive role. It is anticipatory: Something may happen to impair the neurophysiologic modality being monitored. If a change in the monitoring signals such an impairment, it is hoped that some change in the operation can be made to correct the injury.

The technique described here involves monitoring in a much more active fashion. The results of stimulation and recording are used to map innervation and guide the surgeon through the dissection of what is often substantially more complex anatomy than was anticipated. In a surprisingly high percentage of cases, the tissue involved in the tethering also contains active nerve. It has not been possible to distinguish nerve visually in many of these cases and, without the results of electrical stimulation for guidance, viable nerve would have been resected. The result would likely have been substantial denervation, particularly to the urethral and anal sphincters.

Although a number of IOM techniques have been described for this operation, only the report of Legatt *et al.* has been comparable to that of the authors (5). Legatt's group performed similar stimulation and recording on 25 patients undergoing cauda equina surgery, the majority of which were for tethered cord release. The group demonstrated nerve by stimulation that was not visually obvious in nine of the 25 cases (36%), including three in which nerve tissue was present in the filum terminale. The authors believe that our recording techniques, which differ from those of Legatt *et al.*, provide greater sensitivity. This was demonstrated by the higher percentage of cases in which active nerve was found in the filum or other tethering structures.

Our experience with this IOM technique has led us to modify the surgical approach to the problem on the tethered cord. The authors are most cautious in our dissections; however, the guidance of IOM allows for a more aggressive dissection in "safe" areas where electrical mapping demonstrates a lack of innervation. The authors recommend this technique to their colleagues for any procedure involving the cauda equina.

REFERENCES

1. Harner S, Daube JR, Ebersold MJ: Electrophysiologic monitoring of facial nerve during temporal bone surgery. **Laryngoscope** 96:65–69, 1986.
2. Harner S, Daube JR, Ebersold MJ, *et al.*: Improved preservation of facial nerve function with use of electrical monitoring during removal of acoustic neuromas. **Mayo Clin Proc** 62:92–102, 1987.
3. James HE, Mulcahy, JJ, Walsh JW, *et al.*: Use of anal sphincter electromyography during operations on the conus medullaris and sacral nerve roots. **Neurosurgery** 4:521–523, 1979.
4. Kothbauer K, Schmid UD, Seiler RW, *et al.*: Intraoperative motor and sensory monitoring of the cauda equina. **Neurosurgery** 34:702–707, 1994.
5. Legatt AD, Schroeder CE, Gill B, *et al.*: Electrical stimulation and multichannel EMG recording for identification of functional neural tissue during cauda equina surgery. **Child's Nerv Syst** 8:185–189, 1991.
6. Pang D, Casey K: Use of an anal sphincter pressure monitor during operations on the sacral spinal cord and nerve roots. **Neurosurgery** 13:562–568, 1983.

7. Phillips LH, Park TS: Electrophysiological studies of selective posterior rhizotomy patients, in Park TS, Phillips LH, Peacock WG (eds): *Management of Spasticity in Cerebral Palsy and Spinal Cord Injury.* Philadelphia, Hanley & Belfus, 1989, pp 486–496.

8. Phillips LH, Park TS: Electrophysiological monitoring during lipomyelomeningocele resection. **Muscle Nerve** 13:127–132, 1990.

9. Phillips LH, Park TS: Electrophysiological mapping of the segmental anatomy of the muscles of the lower extremity. **Muscle Nerve** 14:1213–1218, 1991.

10. Quencer RM, Montalvo BM, Naidich TP, *et al.*: Intraoperative sonography in spinal dysraphism and syringohydromyelia. **Am J Roentgenol** 148:1005–1003, 1987.

11. Ryken TC, Menezes AH: Intraoperative electrical and manometric monitoring in lumbosacral surgery, in Loftus CM, Traynelis VC (eds): *Intraoperative Monitoring Techniques in Neurosurgery.* New York, McGraw-Hill, 1994, pp 257–267.

12. Schneider SJ, Rosenthal AD, Greenberg BM, *et al.*: A preliminary report on the use of laser-Doppler flowmetry during tethered spinal cord release. **Neurosurgery** 32:214–218, 1993.

13. Shinomiya K, Fuchioka M, Matsuoka T, *et al.*: Intraoperative monitoring for tethered spinal cord syndrome. **Spine** 16:1290–1294, 1991.

11

Clinical Evaluation of Cutaneous Lesions of the Back: Spinal Signatures That Do Not Go Away

ROBIN P. HUMPHREYS, M.D., FRCSC, FACS

In what is becoming a classic editorial, Hendrick exhorted us not to "replace conversation with computer printouts" (3). This homily is vitally important when one assesses the various disorders of the child's spine. For if anything is certain, it is that the child will be singularly unyielding in terms of history and, during the physical assessment, will provide only a minimum of cooperation. All too frequently a child's visit to the consultant surgeon occurs after a very clear objective sign has made its presence known to the family. Yet, in many instances of spinal dysraphism, a cutaneous sign has been present from birth when it was dismissed as "just a cute little birthmark that will go away in a few years." If that little "birthmark" or "cutaneous signature" is located on the midline of the spinal axis, then neither the pediatrician nor neurosurgeon should trivialize its presence. These hallmarks—hemangioma, lipoma, dermal sinus, hairy patch, nevus, meningocele manqué or accessory appendage—are usually found in the lumbar segment of the spinal canal and lie directly on the midline (with the exceptions to be noted).

DEVELOPMENTAL BIOLOGY

The neuroectoderm is discernible at stage 7 of fetal development, when the columnar epithelium is taller than the surrounding cutaneous ectoderm (5). During the process of neurulation, there is apposition and fusion of first the cutaneous ectoderm and then later the neuroectoderm. The closure of the remaining neural tube continues through fetal stages 10 to 12.

Of this early intimacy between cell structures that are to form the cutaneous surface and others lying not so far beneath that will develop into the nervous system, it should not come as a surprise that anomalies of the former (ectoderm) act as a hallmark to a developmental disorder in the latter (neuroectoderm). In such a circumstance, the patient is described as having "spina bifida occulta," whose superficial features are far less flamboyant than those typical for the "open"

175

neural tube defect (*i.e.,* meningocele, myelomeningocele). The occult forms are more common than those which are "open," more frequent in girls, and show a greater variation in the associated symptoms and signs of neurologic upset. Fortunately, the occult developmental cord syndromes are not usually associated with hydrocephalus or the Chiari malformation. Thus, the spinal skin signatures represent dysplastic skin, spina bifida occulta, and intradural pathology.

CUTANEOUS SIGNATURES

Cutaneous Hemangioma

The cutaneous hemangioma or strawberry flare is of variable size and is almost always associated with something else. For example, it is frequently found at the dome of the skin raised over a subcutaneous lipoma. Alternatively, the hemangioma may form a small pink halo around a penetrating dermal sinus (Fig. 1). Sometimes, the hemangioma may be delayed in its appearance, coming on several months after the repair of an open neural tube defect. As that skin wound heals,

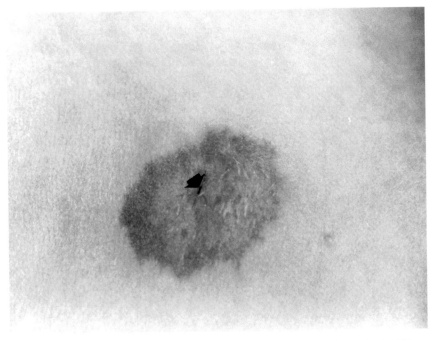

FIG. 1 A small pink hemangioma halo, lying directly on the lumbar spinal midline, encircles a dermal sinus opening (*arrow*).

the flush of the hemangioma begins to make its appearance, spreading centrifugally from the margins of the operative wound.

The midline spinal hemangioma is to be differentiated from those cutaneous hemangiomas that appear in the midline of the scalp. The latter, although located in the midline at the nasion or at the posterior hairline, are indeed very innocent and tend to show a distinct familial distribution.

Lipoma

A subcutaneous lipoma (Fig. 2) is usually but not always located in the midline of the lumbar or lumbosacral segments of the spinal axis.

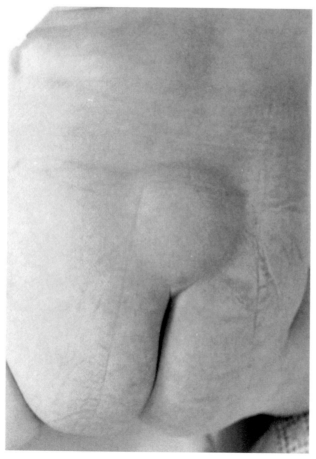

FIG. 2 Smooth otherwise unblemished skin is raised over the midline lumbosacral lipoma. The fat narrows as it passes deep through a fascial ring defect to enter the underlying dysraphic canal.

It ultimately represents spinal dysraphism as the fat penetrates and re-places components of the dural tube and also adheres to the spinal cord in a variety of fashions (1). The cord is thus effectively tethered for all time (4). While most lipomas are found in the midline, some can be lo-cated quite eccentrically, particularly in one or the other buttock (Fig. 3). The left buttock is more commonly involved than the right. In such a circumstance the entire mass of the subcutaneous lipoma may appear to reside well off the midline, but one must expect that eventually the fat will gain the midline structures to penetrate the dysraphic canal.

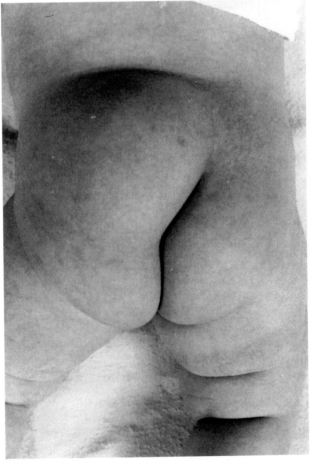

FIG. 3 The subcutaneous lipoma blends in with the left buttock. However, the fat does gain entry to the spinal canal in the midline.

Regardless of where the lipoma lies, the skin covering its dome may be completely unblemished, or it may show any combination of hemangioma discoloration, crinkling, or apparent penetration with a dermal sinus (which usually ends blindly in the morass of subcutaneous fat). On occasion, one may visualize a "caudal appendage" or a redundant skin tag that protrudes from the dome of the lipoma (Fig. 4). Rarely, one may be able to palpate small spicules of bone within the lipoma.

When the lipoma effectively anchors the spinal cord, neurologic disability is guaranteed if treatment is not undertaken. There is upward of a 50% risk of spontaneous deterioration by age 12 years (6).

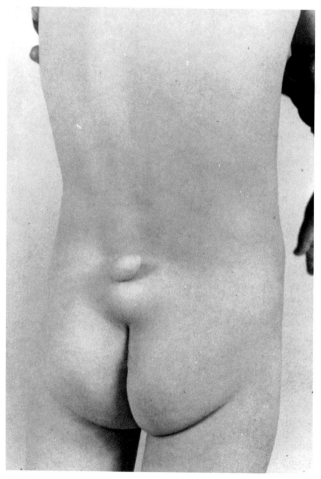

FIG. 4 An accessory skin tag is associated with a lipoma.

Dermal Sinus

It is a paradox that the significant dermal sinus that represents occult spinal dysraphism and the passage of a tract from the skin surface to the intradural space may be very difficult to spot in the midline spinal axis (Fig. 1). By contrast, the innocent "pilonidal sinus" found in the intergluteal cleft, can have a gaping opening and be very apparent (Fig. 5).

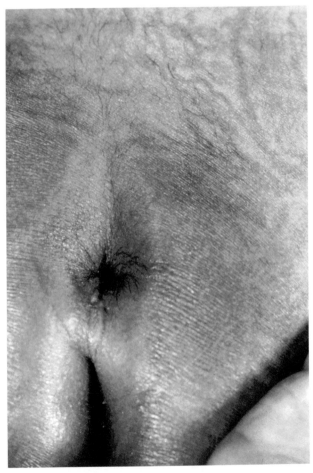

FIG. 5 This pilonidal or intergluteal sinus is buried in the interfluteal cleft and becomes apparent only after the buttocks have been eased apart. It runs progressively caudal and ends in deep fascia or on the surface of terminal coccygeal segments.

The true dermal sinus can be found anywhere in the spinal axis from the cervical hairline to the top of the intergluteal cleft. Most commonly, it is located over the lumbar segments of the spine and will show a very small ostium, surrounded by a pale pink hemangioma flare, and perhaps one or two fine blackened hairs. None of these are the features of the intergluteal pilonidal sinus, which is easily distinguished from the dermal sinus by the "traction test." The true dermal sinus runs in a rostral direction as it penetrates deeper tissues to gain the intradural space, so that it may end up two or three segment levels rostral to where it began on the skin surface. (On occasion, the reverse information may be given on a magnetic resonance imaging study for dermal sinuses located in the lumbosacral or sacral regions. In such circumstances the sinus appears to pass in a caudal direction before making a sharp rostral turn. This is a factor of crinkling of the patient's skin from lying on the imaging table). As a clinical test, the examiner's thumb is placed rostral to the dermal sinus opening, and as the skin is moved rostral, the course of the sinus tract is shortened, and there is the apparent feeling of "give" to the skin manipulation. The reverse is the case, should the sinus be taken in the caudal direction where there is no more "give," the skin appears under traction, and the opening of the sinus becomes creased. This simple maneuver can be carried out with the pilonidal sinus, where the findings are exactly the reverse, that is, the innocent intergluteal sinus that tends to end on deep fascia or the surface of the coccyx runs in a caudad direction, and so caudal traction will shorten its course and rostal traction will do the reverse.

The true dermal sinus must be sought in every instance of purulent meningitis that occurs in a child from a microorganism that is uncommon.

Hairy Patch

Unusual patterns of hair growth may be found along the midline spinal axis in association with the dysraphic condition. As indicated, a few fine blackened hairs may extend out from the opening of a tiny dermal sinus. However, a more luxurious tuft of hair may be found running horizontally across the midline of the spine at the thoracolumbar junction (Fig. 6). When the hair is shaved, the involved patch of skin is coarser than that which surrounds it. The hairy patch almost exclusively is associated with the diastematomyelia.

Nevus

The most infrequent cutaneous lesion is the pigmented nevus. This is not to be confused with the café-au-lait spot seen in patients with

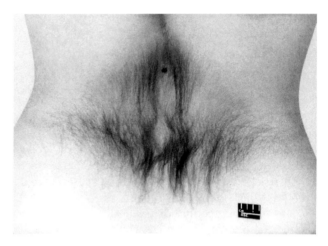

FIG. 6   This coarse hair growth is shaped in the form of an inverted triangle (apex up). Almost always, the hairy patch signifies a diastematomyelia.

neurofibromatosis. The cutaneous nevus is usually much larger, has a slightly darker brown color, and most commonly is found at the level of the thoracolumbar junction. Closer examination of the skin reveals the latter to have a somewhat rougher texture within the field of the nevus, and there may be coarse hair scattered across it. While such a nevus may be rarely associated with an intraspinal melanotic tumor, it is most usually associated in the dysraphic condition with diastematomyelia.

Meningocele Manque

This skin blemish is sometimes referred to as the "cigarette burn" as it resembles a small scarified loss of skin in the midline of the lumbar spine (Fig. 7). When obvious at birth, it is often feared that spinal fluid will leak through the thinned patch of skin. Seldom if ever does that happen. While its appearance otherwise seems to be quite innocent, and while attempts at its transillumination suggest that only the skin is involved, such is not the case. Characteristically this skin signature communicates to the intradural space by means either of an anomalous nerve root or a penetrating dermal sinus, both of which are capable of tethering the spinal cord.

Accessory Appendage

This rare cutaneous defect is sometimes known as the "caudal appendage" or the "accessory human tail" (Fig. 8). The anomaly is a finger-

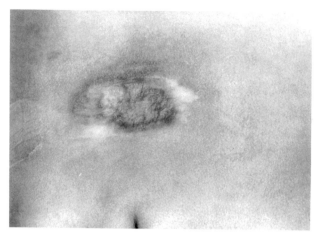

FIG. 7 The scarified "cigarette burn" is the appearance of the meningocele manqué. While it appears quite benign, there is a communication however small, from its deep surface to the intradural space.

like protrusion of skin usually at or caudal to the lumbosacral junction. It may rest anywhere over the dome of the skin raised by a subcutaneous lipoma. Whether or not the subcutaneous fat is so present, the appendage is associated in the intraspinal compartment with a penetrating lipoma that exerts its tethering effect on dura and cord structures. The suggestion that the appendage can easily be "nipped off" the skin ignores the fact that it is associated with underlying spinal dysraphism and cord tethering.

MANAGEMENT OF "SKIN SIGNATURES"

When asked for an opinion about these characteristic skin signatures, the neurosurgeon must first of all state that the problem is not the skin. The lesion is indicative of spina bifida occulta, and the attention must be on the spinal canal and its contents.

The clinical symptoms and signs associated with the occult dysraphic lesion may be present at birth. The obvious features are those of a unilateral small calf and foot, perhaps with a neurogenic posturing of the foot in the equinovarus position.

On other occasions, the symptoms and signs may appear much later. Regardless of when they do appear, the signs are slowly progressive. In rare instances acute deterioration may occur from the tethered cord in later years of life, after an otherwise innocent back injury, or in women during childbirth. Guthkelch has described the syndromes that characterize the examination of the patient with occult spinal dysraphism (2).

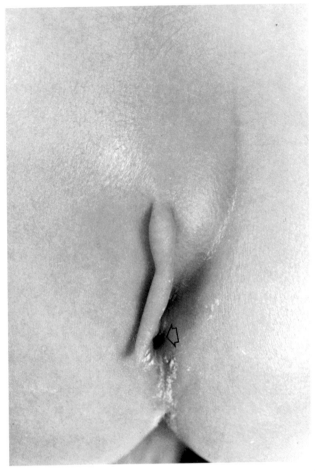

FIG. 8 This "caudal human tail" is an accessory skin tag sited just rostral to a sinus opening of the pilonidal type (*arrow*).

The *neurologic syndrome* features a wasted calf or foot, loss of ankle and/or foot power, an absent ankle reflex, sphincter incompetence, and diminished sensation to superficial stimulation in the L4-S2 dermatomes. The *orthopaedic syndrome* may feature any one or a combination of scoliosis, back stiffness, cavovarus feet, a cock-up toe, and failed skin nutrition. The diagnosis of a tethered spinal cord is thus made when these syndromic features are connected with the spinal skin signature.

The exact nature of the intradural pathology can now be well defined with various imaging studies. One must not be disappointed if the plain spine radiographs taken in the infant are deficient in the bony architectural details. The lack of maturity of the spinal skeleton at this early age, as well as the frequently accompanying overlying gas shadows, blur much of the bony detail for the surgeon.

Axial computerized tomographic imaging still plays an important role, particularly with the bone window images (Fig. 9). This is especially the case in the child with a diastematomyelia, in which the midline bony or cartilaginous septum separates two dural tubes. The attachment of the septum to the back of the vertebral body in front, its passage and direction between the tubes, and its union with more superficial overlying structures are all features that the surgeon should identify before contemplating a remedial operation.

The magnetic resonance images of the spinal cord will provide most of the detail required for the penetrating dermal sinus (Fig. 10), lipoma, thickened filum, as well as cord positioning and the level of the conus tip. Occasionally, the surgeon will be surprised to find that there are other add-ons that were not anticipated. These include hydromyelic

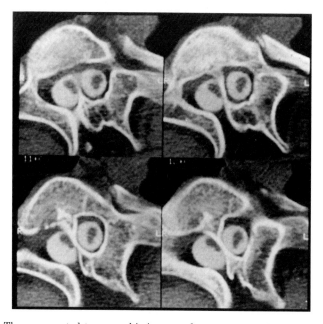

FIG. 9   These computed tomographic images of a contrast myelogram outline quite clearly the split spinal cords and enveloping dural sacs separated by the midline septum of bone. The latter arises from a slight flare on the dorsum of the vertebral body and then unites with the imperfect lamina on one side.

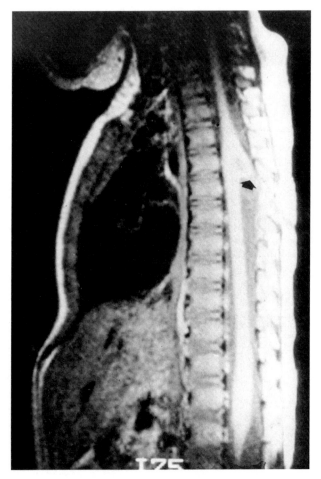

FIG. 10 This penetrating thoracic region dermal sinus (*arrow*) runs rostral as it reaches the dural sac.

cavitations, cord atrophy, ventral arachnoid cyst, and cord splitting within a single dural sac.

CONCLUSION

When the surgeon is asked for an opinion with regard to the spinal skin signature, the focus should be the intradural pathology and not the skin. Clearly, this "little birthmark" is neither "cute" nor will it "go away."

The focus is thus the intradural pathology and not the skin. The aim of the operative treatment is to prevent the inevitable neurologic deterioration. To be effective, the tethering effect must be operatively released and the anatomic tissue barriers reconstituted.

REFERENCES

1. Chapman PH: Congenital intraspinal lipomas: Anatomic considerations and surgical treatment. **Child's Brain** 9:37–47, 1982.
2. Guthkelch AN: Diastematomyelia with median septum. **Brain** 97:729–742, 1974.
3. Hendrick EB: Whatever mother says! (editorial) **Pediatr Neurosci** 12:193, 1986.
4. Humphreys RP: Review article: Current trends in spinal dysraphism. **Paraplegia** 29:79–83, 1991.
5. McLone DG, Dias MS: Normal and abnormal early development of the nervous system, in American Society of Pediatric Neurosurgeons, Section of Pediatric Neurosurgery of the AANS (eds): *Pediatric Neurosurgery: Surgery of the Developing Nervous System*. Philadelphia, W.B. Saunders, 1994, pp 3–30.
6. Pierre-Kahn A, Lacombe J, Pichon J, *et al.*: Intraspinal lipomas with spina bifida. *J Neurosurg* 65:756–761, 1986.

12

The Borderlands of the Primary Tethered Cord Syndrome

W. JERRY OAKES, M.D.

One of the most gratifying and important types of problems in medicine is the young patient who is found to have a lesion which, unattended, has a high likelihood of leading to a progressive neurologic deficit but can be maintained in a normal state by a single curative operation. The primary tethered cord syndrome (PTCS) with caudal fixation from a thickened filum terminale and/or dorsal fixation from aberrant nerve roots (meningocele manqué) (10) is such an entity. The primary problem with these conditions is not the technical aspects of disconnecting the band or bands fixating the spinal cord but in recognizing which patients are at risk of having these problems and what are the earliest possible symptoms and signs that would allow their discovery. The PTCS, if detected in early infancy and operated on, is likely to yield a neurologically intact child who will have the potential for a full and normal life.

WHAT COMPRISES THE PRIMARY TETHERED CORD SYNDROME?

Differentiating the extremes of normal from minimal pathologic states is one of the most difficult aspects of medicine (13). When the PTCS was first described clinically (8, 11, 23) clinically devastated patients with extreme caudal displacement of the conus medullaris into the sacrum from a thickened and unyielding filum terminale were easily differentiated from normal patients. Before the clinical observations, the normal anatomy and position of the distal spinal cord and filum terminale had been studied extensively (1, 15, 19, 23). The normal range in the termination of the spinal cord in these studies was seen to be from the midportion of the T12 vertebrae to the lower portion of L3. Of the 603 adult autopsies studied, only nine patients (1.5%) had the conus as low as over the body of the L3 vertebrae. This anatomic distribution has been confirmed more recently by magnetic resonance imaging (MRI) (30) with termination of the spinal cord over the body of L3 considered to be indeterminate with regard to pathologic significance. Barson (1) looked at the ascent of the spinal cord in relation to the spine in fetal development and early infancy. He found that the adult position of the conus above the body of L3 was achieved by 2 months of age, after term gestation. The position of the spinal cord in the last 15 weeks of normal *in utero* development showed progressive ascent from L4 to L2 (Fig. 1). Today, when premature delivery and survival are commonplace for neonates at 25 weeks' gestation, this more caudal position of the normal spinal cord must be kept in mind in routine clinical care. Figure 2 is the MRI of a neonate at 25 weeks of gestation rendered paraparetic from a lumbar puncture performed at L3–L4 with a resultant intramedullary hematoma.

It would be logical then to assume that tight fixation of the cord by the filum during *in utero* development would result in the most caudal position of the conus but that lesser degrees of tension would allow some cephalad migration. It might even be possible that mild tension on a relatively elastic cord could result in a relatively normal position of the conus, but with enough microtrauma over time that the patient might not become overtly symptomatic until adult life (20). The degree of caudal descent of the conus might be less impressive in this case and, yet, the patient could become symptomatic from intermittent traction and injury, especially spinal flexion, during normal daily activities (2,

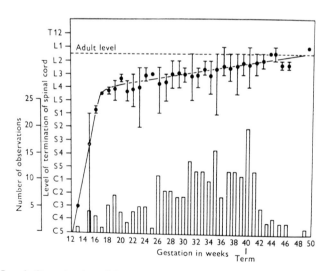

FIG. 1   Level of termination of the spinal cord plotted against gestational age. Ranges and mean values are indicated. The block graph represents the number of observations made in each gestational week. [Reproduced with permission from (1).]

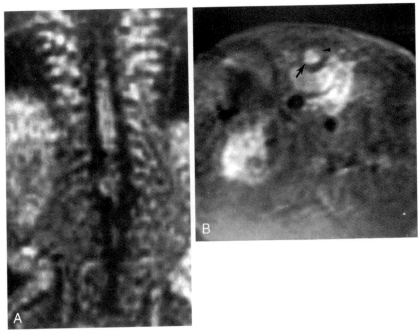

FIG. 2 **(A)** Coronal T1 MRI of the thoracic and lumbar spine, demonstrating a mass protruding from the lower spinal lumbar cord (*arrow*), representing a subacute intra-parenchymal hematoma. This neonate of 25 weeks' gestation received a lumbar puncture at L3–L4 for a "fever workup." The child was then found to be severely paraparetic several days later and was transferred for evaluation. At the time of operation, a hematoma within the substance of the spinal cord was appreciated, and the entry site through the dura was located directly over the hematoma. **(B)** Axial T1 MRI of the same patient. The large hematoma (*arrow*) and the displaced spinal cord (*arrowhead*) can be appreciated.

5). Could, then, a group of patients develop symptoms from caudal spinal cord tension and yet have the absolute position of the conus be in normal position (28, 29)? If that were the case, the clinician would have to look for additional factors other than simply conus position to assess the degree of traction intermittently applied to the distal spinal cord.

WHAT ARE LIKELY METHODS OF CLINICAL PRESENTATION TODAY?

The common methods of clinical presentation (Table 1) include the presence of a cutaneous signature (59%), neurogenic bladder with the development of primary or secondary incontinence or urinary tract infection (18%), leg or foot weakness (12%), leg or foot length discrepancy

TABLE 1
Primary Tethered Cord Syndrome: Patients Seen from 1992 to 1995

Patient	Age	Delay	Chief Complaint	Signs	SB	Skin	Associated Anomalies	F/U
BB	1 day	None	Cutaneous signature	WNL	+	Atretic meningocele	Meningocele manqué, AVM	6 mo
BH	1 day	None	Cutaneous signature	WNL	+	Meningocele	Meningocele manqué	2 mo
TM	3 wk	None	Cutaneous	None	+	Hirsutism	Meningocele manqué, dermal sinus, stem, no septum	3 mo
PW	5 mo	None	None Abdominal radiograph, done for other reason	WNL	+	Focal hirsutism, hemangioma	Meningocele manqué	18 mo
ZW	5 mo	None	WNL (elavuated for other anomalies)	WNL	+	WNL	Chromosomal anomaly 220	6 mo
EQ	9 mo	9 mo	Cutaneous mass (bone) + hemangioma	WNL GU-WNL	+	Mass + hemangioma	Meningocele manqué	2 mo
KS	1 yr	None	Cutaneous signature	WNL	+	"Dermal sinus" + focal hirsutism + hemangioma	Meningocele manqué, diastematomyelia, stem, no septum	2 mo
CB	1 yr	None	Weakness in left ankle	Weakness	+	WNL	Syrinx, meningocele manqué, diastematomyelia, no septum	3 mo

Table 1—*continued*

Primary Tethered Cord Syndrome: Patients Seen from 1992 to 1995

Patient	Age	Delay	Chief Complaint	Signs	SB	Skin	Associated Anomalies	F/U
CG	2 yr	2 yr	Cutaneous signature	WNL	+	Focal hirsutism	Meningocele manqué	5 mo
TL	3 yr	>2 yr	Cutaneous signature	Normal	+	Focal hirsutism	Diastematomyelia + bony septum and thick filum; all missed at initial surgery	15 mo
AR	7 yr	7 yr	Asymmetric leg weakness	Weakness	+	Hirsutism	Hemimyelia, previous myelomeningocele closure, syrinx, diastematomyelia, bony septum	2 yr
TP	9 yr	None	Subtle weakness Sibling with myelomeningocele	Mild leg weakness	+	WNL	Diastematomyelia with bony septum	16 mo
BC	10 yr	None	Foot length difference and weakness	WNL	+	WNL	Syrinx, meningocele manqué	16 mo
CP	11 yr	None	Pain	Paraplegia	+	WNL	Quadriparesis and spastic speech	2.5 yr
MH	17 yr	None	GU	GU only	+	WNL	None	8 mo
JV	18 yr	None	GU	GU only	+	WNL	Intramedullary lipoma L-2	
BT	18 yr	None	GU	GU only	+	WNL	Intramedullary dermoid resection × 3	2 mo

A Summary of the clinical and radiographic findings of all patients operated on within the last 3 years. *Delay* represents the time between the diagnosis of PTCS and referral; F/U, follow-up; WNL, within normal limits; AVM, arteriovenous malformation; GU, genitourinary.

(6%), foot deformity (Fig. 3) (pes cavus, claw toes), and nondermatomal back and leg pain (6%). Pain is by far the commonest chief complaint in adults with occult spinal dysraphism (OSD) but is much less frequent in childhood. When infants are symptomatic with pain, they may simply be more irritable then they would be normally. Differentiating this cause of irritability from more common causes can be quite difficult. Dorsal fixation of the cord by an aberrant nerve root may also be exquisitely sensitive, as demonstrated in Figure 4, (in which a 2-week-

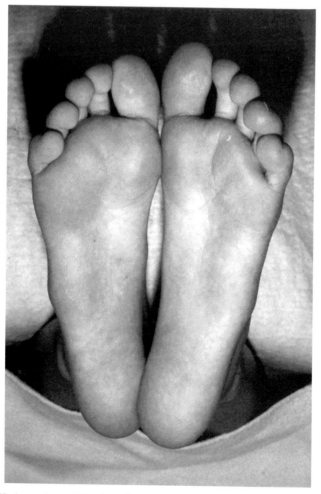

FIG. 3 Undersurface of the feet, demonstrating a foot length discrepancy and pes cavus.

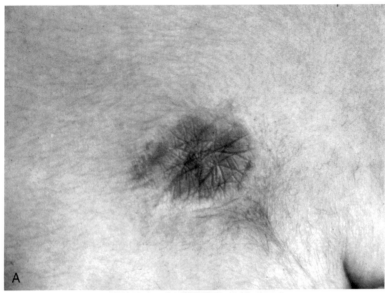

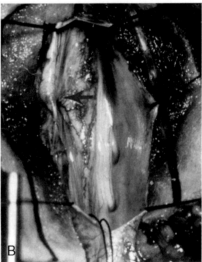

FIG. 4 (A)Photograph of the skin overlying the low back of a 2-week-old infant. There is evidence of a midline area of dermal hypoplasia that is exquisitely sensitive to pressure. Attached to the undersurface of this skin defect are aberrant roots (**B**) (*arrow*) that attach to the undersurface of this skin defect and through the dura, a connection to the dorsal aspect of the cord. They are responsible for this infant's pain syndrome. Section of these roots together with the thickened filum totally relieved this infant's pain.

old infant would not tolerate the prone position and even very light pressure within a 2-cm circumference around the lesion would awaken the baby from deep sleep. This was completely resolved with section of the dorsal bands and the filum terminale.

The weakness seen from primary distal spinal cord fixation usually has a combination of both upper and lower motor neuron signs. Typically, the patient might have decreased muscle bulk and increased or pathologic reflexes. The combination of both upper and lower motor neuron weakness in the legs should alert the examiner to the possibility of this clinical entity. Much later in the clinical course, rectal incontinence and the occurrence of insensitive foot ulceration may occur. Young children have difficulty describing dysesthesia, but with maturation this too may be described. Scoliosis in isolation is an unusual presentation for the PTCS.

With the increasing awareness of the association of the PTCS with other anomalies, a greater proportion of patients are studied and discovered at an earlier clinical stage. These recognized associations include anorectal atresia (10% incidence) (4) and the caudal regression syndrome (6, 27). With urodynamic testing, Kakizake et al. (12) studied 24 children with imperforate anus and found almost half to have detrusor-sphincter dyssynergia. In the subgroup with neurogenic bladder at least 67% had a neuroanatomic abnormality that explained the bladder dysfunction; most of these abnormalities were surgically correctable. With a more liberal definition of "abnormal," this proportion could be even higher and could be the cause of the high incidence of neurogenic bladder and probably be a contributing cause for perineal and rectal muscle weakness.

Also of importance is the common association of the PTCS with other forms of OSD. Lipomatous involvement of the distal cord runs the gamut from small accumulations of fat in an otherwise normal filum to extensive involvement of the distal spinal cord. Terminal syrinx, neurentic cyst, dermal sinus tract and intramedullary dermoid, and diastematomyelia with or without a median septum all may have an associated tight filum terminale, which must be sought at the time of surgical exploration. Dorsal tethering bands composed of aberrant nerve roots (meningocele manqué) (Fig. 5), usually coming from the medial aspect of an area of a split cord, can also fixate the cord and create an identical clinical picture of a tight filum terminale. Consideration should be given to surgical exploration of all patients with a split cord syndrome with or without a median septum in the search for these tethering bands.

Less clear but ultimately more interesting is the genetic predisposition for the occurrence of open neural tube defects (myelomeningocele,

FIG. 5 Intraoperative view of the dorsal surface of the spinal cord with the dura opened. At the *arrows* are multiple aberrant roots emanating from the medial surface of an area of disastematomyelia without a median septum. These roots then exit the dorsal dura and connect to the undersurface of the overlying laminae. They have no functional purpose and act simply to tether the spinal cord.

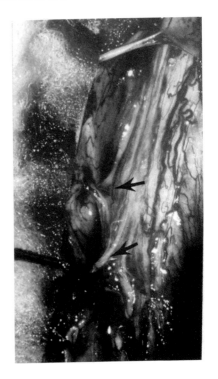

encephalocele, and anencephaly) with siblings who have one of the more occult forms of spinal dysraphism (3). It has also been reported that multiple siblings with PTCS (14) have been discovered together with parents who both were shown to have bony spina bifida occulta (SBO) in the lumbosacral area. The expression of this genetic predisposition is intriguing and is currently under investigation. Of interest is the answer to this question: Is the bony SBO, seen in approximately 4% of the population, a recessive expression of the predisposition to form these spinal cord malformations?

HOW DOES ONE OBTAIN CONFIRMATION OF THE CLINICAL SUSPICION OF PTCS?

Ideally, spinal cord tension and elasticity could be measured and assessed in an objective manner. Currently that is not technically possible in a noninvasive clinical manner (24, 25). Therefore, we must rely on more indirect measures. Dynamic visualization of the spinal cord can be accomplished by real-time ultrasound in young infants (22) and by cine MRI (16) in patients without an acoustical window in the dorsal spine. These methods allow us to watch the motion of the cord, but only a qualitative assessment can be made. More indirect than dynamic studies is an assessment of the cord position with MRI (18, 21). If the position of the conus is indeterminate (L3) or even above the L2–L3 disc space, one can still look for other associated findings to help explain clinical symptoms. Small accumulations of fat within the filum (Fig. 6 **A** and **B**) may be seen in 6% of the normal population but in > 90% of patients symptomatic from the PTCS (17). This finding alone should alert the clinician. Almost all patients with PTCS will have bony SBO in the low lumbar and/or sacrum. This finding, too, is seen in a small percent of the normal population but when present in a symptomatic patient, PTCS must again be entertained. Cutaneous signatures of OSD (midline capillary hemangioma, subcutaneous lipoma, dermal sinus tract, epithelial appendage, focal hirsutism, and dermal hypoplasia with an atretic meningocele) (Fig. 7 **A–C**) are strong evidence of an underlying problem. Unfortunately, these are present in only about half of isolated PTCS patients from a tight filum terminale. Of particular interest are the capillary hemangioma and epithelial appendage, which are more likely to have a PTCS from a tight filum ter-

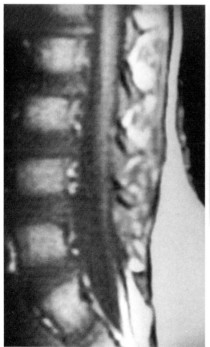
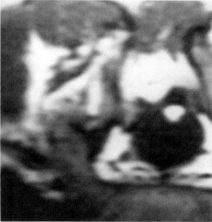

FIG. 6 **(A)** MRI taken sagittally with evidence of fat infiltrating the filum. The conus is displaced into the lumbar spine. **(B)** Axial T1 MRI of the same patient, demonstrating an enlarged fatty infiltrated filum.

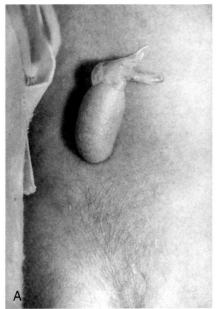
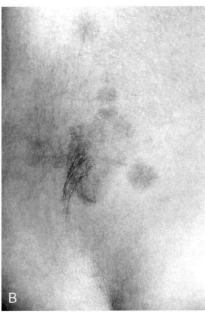
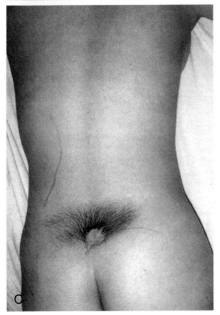

FIG. 7 (**A**) Photograph of the skin overlying the lumbar and sacral spine of an infant, demonstrating an epithelial tag. The patient had a fatty infiltrated, low-lying filum. The filum was sectioned prophylactically, and the patient has remained normal. Tags like this should not be removed without also investigating the intradural anatomy. (**B**) Photograph of the low back of an infant with a small area of hirsutism on a bed of capillary hemangioma. Infant had both caudal and dorsal spinal cord fixation. (**C**) Back of an adolescent girl with nondermatomal pain and normal neurologic function. At exploration, dorsal tethering bands coming from the median aspect of an area of diastematomyelia without a median septum were cut, and the pain was resolved.

minale seen in isolation. Dorsal bands or meningocele manqué (10) have more of a predilection to be seen with focal hirsutism in association with the split cord syndrome or with an atretic meningocele without the split cord.

WHEN SHOULD OPERATION BE OFFERED OR "CAN'T WE JUST WATCH AND SEE WHAT HAPPENS?"

The natural history of a low lying conus from a fatty infiltrated and thickened filum terminale is now accepted to be progressive loss of neurologic function usually over years. This knowledge, together with the low risk of surgical intervention and high likelihood of cure with a single procedure, justify an operation. When framed in this context, no other conclusion seems reasonable.

When the patient presents with progressive symptoms possibly attributable to spinal cord traction but the conus is indeterminate or normal in position, the clinician must look for associated findings (other congenital malformations, fat in the filum, bony SBO, other expressions of OSD, or a cutaneous signature). If many of these are present, then the rationale to proceed with the very low risk procedure of section of the filum should be considered. The timing of that operative intervention would make little sense in being delayed months to years for fear of incurring additional sacral nerve injury, making damage irreversible (urogenic bladder); consideration should be given to proceeding electively directly after diagnosis.

By far the most difficult patients are infants or young children without symptoms who had their MRI performed because of an overtly affected sibling, a cutaneous signature, or an associated clinical condition (anorectal atresia or caudal regression syndrome) and in whom the conus is above the L2–L3 disc space, but there is fat in the filum and a bony SBO is present. The families of these patients want to know the natural history of their child's condition and to be reassured as to the infant's long-term normal functioning. Unfortunately, the first symptom likely to occur is the irreversible development of a neurogenic bladder. Even with normal urodynamic testing done in infancy, deterioration remains a concern (7). Without available data the clinician is left to discuss the options with the family and outline further conservative follow-up, as contrasted with operative intervention. The obvious negative aspect of simple observation is the development of a fixed deficit that could have been avoided, although suggesting even a relatively safe operation without clear evidence is also unappealing. Hopefully, long-term observation of the natural history of these patients at risk will allow a more rational approach in the future.

WHAT EXACTLY IS DONE IN THE OPERATION?

The purpose of operation is to release the neural tissue from all points of fixation without damaging any functional neural tissue.

Section of the filum terminale can most safely be done through a sacral laminectomy over the cul-de-sac of the subarachnoid space. With the subarachnoid space usually ending in the area of S2 or lower, this is the area to be exposed. A limited two-level laminectomy is performed and the dura opened in the midline. The filum is identified immediately before it exits the dura dorsally. All roots are separated from the filum just prior to it exiting the dura. Nodes of Ranvier are visible under high magnification as parallel bands occurring along nerve roots approximately every millimeter. The filum lacks these bands, exits the midline dorsally, and has a slightly bluish hue. Fat is also commonly seen within the filum of this patient population at this level, as previously noted. Removal of a section of filum for histologic examination is commonly performed. One should recognize that there are normally scattered nerve elements within the filum in interpreting the pathologic report (9, 26). Care should be taken to section the filum as low as possible. The S5 nerve roots in infants are quite small, and their section results in a significant fixed deficit of the perineum.

In exploring for dorsal tethering bands, remember that these are composed of neural tissue with visible nodes of Ranvier. They exit dorsally and terminate in the dura or undersurface of the laminae. Care should be taken in removing the laminae in an area of a split cord malformation just for that reason. Realizing that traction and movement on the aberrant root applies direct traction on the spinal cord will help make the laminectomy safer. The fixating aberrant roots are cut intradurally adjacent to the spinal cord and removed along with their point of exit from the dura. The pia mater of the dorsal cord is manipulated as little as possible to minimize refixation of the cord by scar. Dorsal root ganglions elements are frequently distributed near the dorsal dural exit site. It is important to open the dura over the entire length of the split cord malformation to visualize all of the fixating bands.

WHAT'S THE OUTLOOK?

Children with normal function who are at significant risk of neurologic deterioration should be maintained without a deficit. The likelihood of serious neurologic injury from the sectioning of a tough filum terminale or dorsal tethering bands is very small (<1%). Unfortunately, not all patients present neurologically intact. Those with moderate scoliosis not associated with segmental bony anomalies are likely to stabilize or improve. Foot and leg length discrepancy and other bony deformities of the foot from long-standing neural injury will not improve and may even worsen despite full relief of intradural tension. Leg weakness that is not profound is likely to improve as is any sensory disturbance. Lost muscle mass implies a more severe neurologic impairment and will not improve.

Of primary interest in childhood is the ability of a neurogenic bladder to normalize. Patient and family expectation in this regard almost always runs high, but the surgeon's ability to restore the complex integration of detrusor and sphincter motor function is quite limited, making operation primarily a prophylactic procedure.

A bright spot in the prognostic horizon is the almost universal elimination of pain in childhood and in the normally motivated adult.

SUMMARY

The PTCS is easily dealt with surgically with little risk of additional injury. The likelihood of some improvement in neurologic function and the elimination of pain is high, with the exception of the neurogenic bladder. In the patient with the position of the conus over the L3 vertebral body of below, the rationale of therapeutic or prophylactic surgery is clear. As for the patient with progressive symptoms attributable to the PTCS, and in the young asymptomatic child or infant if the conus is above the L2–L3 disc space, the patient should be assessed in the context of the other associated anomalies present.

REFERENCES

1. Barson AJ: The vertebral level of termination of the spinal cord during normal and abnormal development. **J Anat** 106:489–497, 1970.
2. Breig A: Overstretching of and circumscribed pathological tension in the spinal cord—A basic cause of symptoms in cord disorders. **J Biomech.** 3:7–9, 1970.
3. Carter CO, Evans KA, Till K: Spinal dysraphism: Genetic relation to neural tube malformations. **J Med Genet** 13:343–350, 1976.
4. Davidoff AM, Thompson CV, Grimm JK, *et al.:* Occult spinal dysraphism in patients with anal agenesis. **J Pediatr Surg** 26:1001–1005, 1991.
5. Editorial: Tethered spinal cord. *The Lancet:*549–550, 1986.
6. Estin D, Cohen AR: Caudal agenesis and associated caudal spinal cord malformations. **Neurosurg Clin North Am** 6:377–391, 1995.
7. Fukui J, Kakizaki T: Urodynamic evaluation of tethered cord syndrome including tight filum terminale: Prolonged follow-up observation after intraspinal operation. **Urology** 16:539–552, 1980.
8. Garceau GJ: The filum terminale syndrome. **J Bone Joint Surg Am** 35:711–716, 1953.
9. Harmeier JW: The normal histology of the intradural filum terminale. **Arch Neurol Psych** 29:308–316, 1933.
10. James CCM, Lassman LP: *Spina Bifida Occulta,* Butterworth London, 1982, ed 2.
11. Jones PH, Love JG: Tight filum terminale. **Arch Surg** 73:556–566, 1956.

12. Kakizaki H, Nonomura K, Asano Y, *et al.:* Preexisting neurogenic voiding dysfunction in children with imperforate anus: Problems in management. **J Urol** 151:1041–1044, 1994.
13. Köhler A, Zimmer EA: *Borderlands of the Normal and Early Pathologic in Skeletal Roentgenology,* Transl. by SP Wilk, New York, Grune & Stratton, 1968.
14. Love JG, Daly DD, Harris LE: Tight filum terminale: Report of condition in three siblings. **JAMA** 176:31–33, 1961.
15. McCotter RE: Regarding the length and extent of the human medulla spinalis. **Anat Rec** 10:559–564, 1916.
16. McCullough DC, Levy LM, DiChiro G, *et al.:* Toward the prediction of neurological injury from tethered spinal cord: Investigation of cord motion with magnetic resonance. **Pediatr Neurosurg** 16:3–7, 1990–91.
17. McLendon RE, Oakes WJ, Heinz ER, *et al.:* Adipose tissue in the filum terminale: A computed tomographic finding that may indicate tethering of the spinal cord. **Neurosurgery** 22(5):873–876, 1988.
18. Moufarrij NA, Palmer JM, Hahn JF, *et al.:* Correction between magnetic resonance imaging and surgical findings in the tethered spinal cord. **Neurosurgery** 25(3): 341–346, 1989.
19. Needles JH: The caudal level of termination of the spinal cord in American whites and American negroes. **Anat Rec** 63:417–424, 1935.
20. Pang D, Wilberger JE Jr: Tethered cord syndrome in adults. **J Neurosurg** 57:32–47, 1982.
21. Raghavan N, Barkovich AJ, Edwards M, *et al.:* MR imaging in the tethered spinal cord syndrome. **Am J Roentgenol** 152:843–852, 1989.
22. Raghavendra BN, Epstein FJ, Pinto RS, *et al.:* The tethered spinal cord: Diagnosis by high-resolution real-time ultrasound. **Radiology** 149:123–128, 1983.
23. Reimann AF, Anson BJ: Vertebral level of termination of the spinal cord with report of a case of sacral cord. **Anat Rec** 88:127–138, 1944.
24. Sarwar M, Crelin ES, Kier EL, *et al.:* Experimental cord strechability and the tethered cord syndrome. **Am J Neuroradial** 4:641–643, 1983.
25. Tani S, Yamada S, Knighton RS: Extensibility of the lumbar and sacral cord: Pathophysiology of the tethered spinal cord in cats. **J Neurosurg** 66:116–123, 1987.
26. Tarlov IM: Structure of the filum terminale. **Arch Neurol Psych** 40:1–17, 1938.
27. Towfighi J, Housman C: Spinal cord abnormalities in caudal regression syndrome. **Acta Neuropathol** 81:458–466, 1991.
28. Warder DE, Oakes WJ: Tethered cord syndrome and the conus in a normal position. **Neurosurgery** 33(3):374–377, 1993.
29. Warder DE, Oakes WJ: Tethered cord syndrome: The low-lying and normally positioned conus. **Neurosurgery** 34(4):597–600, 1994.
30. Wilson DA, Prince JR: MR imaging determination of the location of the normal conus medullaris throughout childhood. **Am J Roentgenol** 152:1029–1032, 1989.

CHAPTER

13

The Adult with a Tethered Cord

DAVID G. McLONE, M.D., PH.D.

Adults with tethered spinal cords are arguably the most neglected individuals in the population with neurosurgical disease. Over the past several decades major pediatric neurosurgical clinics have developed programs to manage tethered cords in children (2–4, 6, 7). Because this entity has developed primarily as a pediatric problem, most of the expertise resides within the pediatric neurosurgical community. Unfortunately, large numbers of adults have deteriorated over the years from tethered cords and have not been recognized as patients who could be helped by a neurosurgical procedure.

In this paper, I am going to argue that only through awareness of the problem of tethered cord will it be recognized, and when recognized, it should be treated aggressively. I feel quite strongly that individuals who have the cutaneous manifestations of a tethered cord should be studied and operated on as soon as is reasonable. This situation, in my opinion, is urgent but not emergent. I would argue strongly that even individuals who are neurologically intact and have escaped deterioration during childhood are at significant risk and should be operated on and the spinal cord released prophylactically (1).

Obviously, if you are going to offer prophylactic surgery to prevent the onset of a neurologic deficit, you must offer a procedure that has an extremely low morbidity and essentially, a zero mortality. However, it must be kept in mind that every neurosurgical procedure carries some risk.

The number of tethered cords in the general population could be as high as 300,000 of our fellow Americans. These statistics are arrived at based on the birthrate and the incidence of neural tube defects such as myelomeningoceles and lipomyelomeningoceles and a variety of other abnormalities of the caudal spinal cord that can lead to tethered cord.

At the present time, at Children's Memorial Hospital in Chicago, a large multidisciplinary clinic, is following 1400 individuals with known neural tube defects who remain at risk for tethered cord. Half of these individuals are adolescents and young adults. Only about 50 are individuals who are more than 30 years of age.

It is important to remember that this wave of young children is moving toward adulthood and will graduate from these multidisciplinary pediatric neurosurgery clinics across the United States. Their care will then shift to those neurosurgeons who care primarily for adults. If they are not conversant with the problems and nuances of tethered cord, this population will deteriorate over time and will go from being independent to being individuals with significant handicaps and dependence.

It is interesting that we have for years believed that if an individual has a congenital abnormality of the spinal cord and we can prevent deterioration before puberty, that patient would then enjoy a stable life from that point onward. It is now quite clear that individuals who have congenital abnormalities of their spinal cord are at risk for subtle deterioration at essentially every decade of adult life (1, 5). We have now operated on individuals in every decade up to and including the seventh.

CHARACTERISTICS OF ADULTS WITH TETHERED CORD

One unfortunate characteristic of the adult with a tethered cord is that he or she often comes late for care. It is quite obvious that if the child complains of pain or limps, the mother will have the child seen by a pediatrician or some specialist within 24 hours. An adult with pain or a minor neurologic deficit, such as some slight numbness or weakness, will take analgesics and avoid seeking care, often for months. He or she will deny problems with urinary retention for long periods of time. Unfortunately, delay in making the diagnosis of tethered cord makes the possibility of retrieval of lost function unlikely. This is especially true of bladder and bowel function. In our series, once bladder and bowel function has been lost for a few months, the chances of returning that function to normal is 15% or less.

Pain is a particularly difficult problem in the adult. In childhood, when the child complains of pain you can almost guarantee the parents that, after untethering of the cord, the pain will be relieved. This is not true of adults. Pain has usually been present for a long time, which makes the problem of relief of any of the complications of tethered cord less likely. It is important to inform the adult patient who arrives with pain as his or her major complaint of tethered cord, that is possible that the pain will not be altered by untethering of the cord. It is probable that it will; however, the pain may be the same, it may be less, or there may be a new pain present after untethering of the spinal cord. I have only seen this occur in adults and have not seen it in children. Therefore, informed consent about this possibility is extremely important for the neurosurgeon and the neurosurgeon's relationship with his patient during the postoperative period.

Adults with a tethered cord can be divided into three groups. One group is the so-called "occult" group, with known cutaneous markers but, who have been neglected. These individuals have lipomas located at the lumbosacral junction, hairy patches, or other markers located over the lower part of their spine. They have been seen by physicians and told that these markers were simply birthmarks and that they really indicated no underlying problem. Or, worse yet, these markers are recognized as being related to an underlying abnormality of the nervous system, but patients are told by an uninformed physician or surgeon that surgery is likely to make them worse (8, 9).

Another large group is comprised of patients with the truly occult spinal dysraphism. These individuals have no cutaneous manifestations, appear to be intact over a number of years and then, as adolescents or young adults, begin to develop progressive foot deformities or problems with urinary tract infections, ultimately leading to a neurogenic bladder, scoliosis, or another deficit. Only when these things are recognized as possibly having a neurogenic origin is the diagnosis of a truly occult lesion made. With the use of the MR these underlying, low-lying tethered cords with intramedullar lipomas are discovered and can be dealt with.

The third and largest group is the postrepair stable population at risk for deterioration secondary to a retethered cord. This large group of adolescents and young adults that is graduating from pediatric neurosurgical centers into adult care is going to require lifelong monitoring by multidisciplinary groups, including neurosurgeons, orthopaedic surgeons, and urological surgeons.

It is important to remember that the spinal cord untethered at the time of the primary repair remains at risk for deterioration throughout the life of the individual. Therefore, lifelong follow-up by an informed group of multidisciplinary medical care individuals is critical to maintaining the quality of these individuals' lives.

Lesions that tether the adult cord include the following. (a) Myelomeningocele represents probably the single largest group. These individuals are obviously diagnosed at birth. The majority of them have hydrocephalus and require lifelong monitoring of their shunts, but they remain at risk for deterioration from a retethered cord. The survival rate now is nearly 90%. Eighty percent of these individuals will have intelligence within the normal range and are likely to be independent. Only through neglecting them as adults will the majority of these individuals deteriorate into a condition of dependency. (b) The second largest group represents those individuals who have lipomas, either of the cord itself or of the filum terminale. These individuals, once untethered, have a low incidence of retethering, but it exists and,

therefore, as in the population with the myelomeningocele, lifelong follow-up is critical to preserving their function. (c) Dermal sinus tracts,
diastematomyelia, and myelocystoceles are some of the other lesions
that are rare but, again, they leave these individuals at risk for insidious deterioration as adults.

CASE HISTORIES

To better illustrate the problems of the adult with a tethered cord, a
few case histories are included. In the 50 individuals that we are following who are 30 years of age or older, these stories are typical.

Case 1

A 38-year-old businessman has a dimple located over the lumbosacral area of his spine. In high school he played athletics but always
was noted to have smaller calves than any of the other individuals on
the team. In his mid-20s, he had a series of urinary tract infections. Ultimately, by the end of his 20s he became incontinent. He was told by
a neurologist that the neurogenic bladder was the result of his recurrent urinary tract infections; that was completely the opposite of what
was the case. He now presents with numbness in his lower extremities
and progressive distal weakness. He is incontinent and on intermittent
catheterization at this time. An MR scan done at the time shows a
lipoma that is attached to the distal end of the spinal cord, tethering
into the sacrum (Fig. 1). A good example of preventable disease.

Case 2

A 35-year-old engineer working, ironically, on the development of
the MRI scanner for General Electric. He was apparently normal until his mid-teens, at which time he began to develop progressive distal
weakness. He has a fatty mass located over his lumbosacral spine. He
saw a series of neurosurgeons who told him that operating on this mass
on his back would likely make him worse, not better. He, therefore, was
left untreated and gradually deteriorated to the point of paraplegia
and bladder incontinence. He now has only flicker quadriceps function.
He continues to work out of a wheelchair as an engineer, and he is an
outstanding marathon wheelchair racer. Again, this is a young man
with profound deficits that were preventable.

Case 3

A physician, internist, in his mid-30s, has three children and has had
a known mass located over the lumbosacral spine. He had bilateral

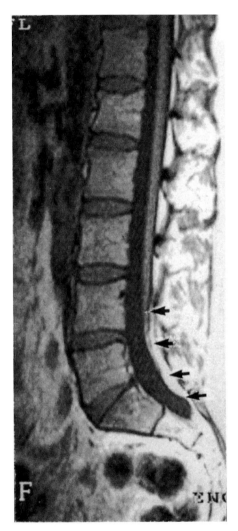

FIG.1 The spinal cord extends down to the level of L4-L5 interspace and is attached to a lipoma (*arrows*) that extends to the end of the thecal sac.

triple arthrodesis done as a teenager. He was sent to us by a urologist because of complaints of intermittent incontinence and numbness on one side of his penis. His main concern was the loss of sexual function. An MR was done that again showed a lipoma inserting into the caudal end of the spinal cord, which was tethered at the lower lumbosacral region. After untethering of his spinal cord, his sexual function returned to normal, and his incontinence improved.

Case 4

A 40-year-old accountant who played racquetball and jogged had always been known to have small, asymmetric calves. He had been followed for a number of years by urologists because of intermittent urinary retention. Finally, the diagnosis of a neurogenic bladder led to the performing of an MRI, which showed a low-lying cord with a thickened fatty filum. He has remained stable since the untethering of his cord.

Case 5

The next patient is in his early 30s. He was apparently an outstanding college athlete. He had a series of urinary tract infections and then developed urinary retention. It is interesting that he was operated on as an infant for a congenital anomaly of urinary bladder. It is important to recognize the association of urogenital or rectal anomalies with developmental abnormalities of the caudal end of the spinal cord. Any child with an abnormality of the genitalia or of the anorectal area deserves to be studied for the possibility of an underlying lesion of their spinal cord. With untethering of his spinal cord, the patient has remained stable.

These are a few stories from the adult population that reflect the problems in the medical community in dealing with individuals with tethered cord. Only through an awareness of the problem and an understanding of its manifestations can the early diagnosis be made. The insidious deterioration that occurs with tethered cord can be prevented.

In conclusion, tethered cord is a major problem. It is an opportunity for the neurosurgeon to offer stability to our fellow citizens with these congenital abnormalities. There also needs to be some educational process to inform orthopaedic and urologic surgeons, as well as the physicians who are most likely to interact initially with people who have a tethered cord.

REFERENCES

1. Bassett RC: The neurologic deficit associated with lipomas of the cauda equina. **Ann Surg** 131:109–116, 1950.
2. Bruce DA, Schut L: Spinal lipomas in infancy and childhood. **Childs Brain** 5:192–203, 1979.
3. Hendrick EB, Hoffman HJ, Humphreys RP: The tethered spinal cord. **Clin Neurosurg** 30:457–463, 1983.
4. Hoffman HJ, Taecholarn C, Hendrick EB, *et al.*: Management of lipomyelomeningoceles. **J Neurosurg** 62:1–8, 1985.
5. Love JG, Daly DD, Harris LE: Tight filum terminale: Report of condition in three siblings. **JAMA** 176:31, 1961.
6. McLone DG, Mutluer S, Naidich TP: Lipomeningoceles of the conus medullaris, in *Concepts in Pediatric Neurosurgery*. Basel, S. Karger, 1982, vol 3, pp 171–177.

7. McLone DG, Naidich TP: Laser resection of fifty spinal lipomas. **Neurosurgery** 18:611–615, 1986.

8. Naidich TP, McLone DG, Harwood-Nash DC: Spinal dysraphism, in Newton TH, Potts DG (eds): *Modern Neuroradiology: Computed Tomography of the Spine and Spinal Cord*. San Anselmo, CA, Clavadel Press, 1983, vol 1, pp 299–254.

9. Naidich TP, McLone DG, Mutleur S: A new understanding of dorsal dysraphism with lipoma (lipomyeloschisis): Radiological evaluation and surgical correction. **AJNR Am J Neuroradial** 4:103, 1983.

10. Yamada S, Zinke DE, Sanders D: Pathophysiology of "tethered cord syndrome." **J Neurosurg** 54:494–503, 1981.

14

Decade of the Brain Lecture:
Congress of Neurological Surgeons*

ZACHARY W. HALL, PH.D.

I am deeply honored to receive the Decade of the Brain Award from the Congress of Neurological Surgeons. Those of us who are concerned with the brain are privileged to live in an unprecedented time of exploration and discovery in brain research. I feel more privileged than most, having worked for over two decades as a basic researcher in neuroscience, and now having the pleasure and responsibility of directing the National Institute of Neurological Disorders and Stroke, the preeminent institution in conducting and sponsoring research on the brain and its disorders. It is a particular pleasure for me to receive this award from the Congress of Neurological Surgeons, a group that represents the present and future leaders of neurosurgery. As we stand midway within the Decade of the Brain, we can look back to see what we have achieved. However, most importantly, especially with an audience that represents the future of neurological surgery, we can look forward to the future of neurological research and to neurosurgery's role.

What have we already accomplished in brain research? Over the last 30 years, astonishing progress has been made in fundamental neuroscience, progress which has come about through the availability of remarkable tools. Of these, perhaps the most important is molecular biology. Our ability to manipulate molecules and cells through recombinant DNA technology has allowed us to identify an increasing number of the molecules that do the business of the nervous system. This technology has particularly benefited brain research, because so many of our most important molecules—receptors, growth factors, ion channels—occur in minute quantities. Using the techniques of molecular biology, we can now often bypass the painstaking biochemical work required of previous generations and go directly to the gene. Once we have found the gene, it

---

*Delivered on October 17, 1995, at the 43rd Meeting of the Congress of Neurological Surgeons, San Francisco, California.

can be expressed in cells that can produce large amounts of protein for research and for therapy.

Molecular biology has been particularly important within the context of human genetics. The study of genetic diseases has been literally revolutionized with a large payoff for understanding disorders of the brain. Because the brain expresses more genes than any other organ of our bodies, 25–30% of all genetic diseases are estimated to be brain diseases. The genes responsible for over 40 disorders of the brain have now been identified, with many more to come within the next decade. These include many of our most significant diseases, such as Alzheimer's disease, Huntington's disease, and amyotrophic lateral sclerosis (ALS). Just within the last year, for example, NINDS-sponsored researchers have identified two genes for early onset Alzheimer's disease, one on chromosome 14 and one on chromosome 1; the gene responsible for Batten's disease, which is the primary neurodegenerative disease of childhood; and the gene for ataxia-telangiectasia, an autosomal recessive disease that is not only of interest as a brain disease but also because carriers of the altered gene, estimated at 1% of the population, may be at an increased risk for cancer. Identification of the gene responsible for a disease leads to new ideas, new tools and, eventually, to new therapies. Perhaps the most important immediate result of a new gene discovery is the possibility of producing transgenic animal models of the disease, which can be used for investigating mechanisms of pathogenesis and testing new therapies.

Other important techniques have contributed knowledge at a different level. New biophysical techniques that allow electrical recording from cells in slices from the brain and the imaging of single cells to allow the spatial localization of biologically important molecules have brought new precision to our understanding of intracellular and intercellular signaling in the nervous system. New computational techniques, coupled in some cases with cellular imaging, now allow us to follow the behavior of large populations of neurons, whose circuitry must be understood if we are to delve into the complex functions of the brain. Our increasing sophistication about higher functions of the nervous system—learning, memory, cognition, language—are inextricably linked to these new techniques.

Finally, new techniques of imaging the intact, functioning brain have literally given us a new anatomy of the nervous system. Computer-assisted tomography (CT), magnetic resonance imaging (MRI), positron emission tomography (PET), and now, functional MRI and magnetoencephalography (MEEG) allows us to detect lesions in the disease brain and to follow function in both normal and diseased brains. These have proved to be powerful tools for research and medicine. We can now examine the precise localization of regions of the brain that become activated during movements, during sensory stimulation, or, most remarkably, even during thought processes.

Against this background of progress, what do we see for the future? Basic research will continue to progress, as there is much yet that we need to know. One of the most important basic areas for future research, in my view, is to delineate the interrelated, intracellular pathways in neurons that control growth and cell death. These pathways are important both for understanding and devising therapies for disorders that are as apparently unrelated as brain tumors and neurodegenerative diseases. There is a growing conviction and increasing body of evidence that neurons have one or more intrinsic cell death pathways that can be activated by ischemic or traumatic injury, by neurodegenerative disease, or by environmental or infectious agents. We must understand more about these pathways so that we can intervene appropriately to help neurons fight injury and avoid death. A complex set of pathways also controls cell division, a pathway that goes awry during cancer. Interestingly and mysteriously, the two sets of pathways, controlling cell death and cell division, may be linked, as illustrated by the disease of ataxia-telangiectasia, a single gene defect that causes both Purkinje cell degeneration and increased susceptibility to cancer.

Although basic research will continue to thrive, I believe that the most exciting area of progress in the next 15 to 20 years will be in areas related to clinical research. Application of the new tools and insights provided by basic research to human disease have the power to transform the clinical treatment of brain disorders. Much of that work is already underway. The aggressive and acute treatment of stroke with the thrombolytic agents made available by recombinant DNA technology, for example, promises to revolutionize the treatment of that disease. New growth factors are available and are being tested in the clinic. The use of myotrophin as a treatment for ALS and the testing in animals of implanted cells that have been engineered to produce dopamine as a possible treatment for Parkinson's disease are current examples of new therapies that could not have been imagined 15 years ago. As we look further ahead, we can see the possibility of gene therapy, in which DNA is introduced into specific brain regions, either to correct defects or to cause the expression of proteins that will help neurons recover from trauma or from degenerative processes. Alternatively, new cells, derived from stem cells, or engineered to produce specific substances, may be introduced to replace injured cells or to provide a continuing source of missing proteins. In addition to the introduction of new genes or new cells, we also hope to develop small molecules as agents that can intervene in the intracellular pathways that control growth and injury. Finally, not all of our solutions will be high-tech. As we learn more about how the nervous system develops or responds to injury, we find that substances as simple as aspirin or magnesium or folic acid are able to serve as powerful preventive agents to prevent brain disorders.

What will be the role of neurosurgery in this new era? Neurosurgeons will clearly contribute to the mainstream of fundamental and clinical research related to neurological disease, particularly with respect to brain tumors, stroke, and traumatic brain injury. In addition, I see two special roles that neurosurgeons will fill; perhaps you see others as well. First, in a phrase borrowed from your current President, Dr. Ralph Dacey: "Neurosurgeons in a new era of brain treatment will be the ones who deliver the goods." Many of the agents that one wishes to deliver to the brain, whether genes, gene products, peptides, or genetically engineered cells, will have to be given locally to affect specific populations of neurons. In many cases, local delivery will be desirable both for reasons of efficiency and because particular treatments may be dangerous when generally applied to cells of the nervous system. Proteins (such as bcl-2) that block cell death, for example, might be useful in injured regions of the nervous system but can cause lymphomas when overexpressed in lymphocytes. The increasing need for precise delivery of therapeutic agents to specific populations of neurons or particular regions of the brain will put a premium on the development of techniques for guiding delivery and for assessing the exact position of the instruments of delivery. In addition to delivering substances and cells, neurosurgical procedures will be key in bringing tumor cells and pathologic material out of the brain and into the laboratory.

A second important area concerns clinical trials. Clinical research for neurosurgeons is not new, but the design and implementation of the appropriate clinical trials in relation to delivery of newer therapeutics will tax your ingenuity in the future. Neurosurgery already has an impressive record of accomplishment in this area. Neurosurgeons were in the forefront of the controlled perspective randomized clinical trials carried out for many years in the treatment of malignant glioma. Neurosurgeons, along with their radiotherapy colleagues, first put to test the value of radiation therapy for the treatment of malignant glioma and clearly demonstrated its efficacy. Neurosurgeons played a pivotal role in two of the largest clinical trials ever run by the National Institute of Neurological Disorders and Stroke: the North American Symptomatic

Carotid Endarterectomy Trial (NASCET), which examined the value of carotid endarterectomy in symptomatic patients, and the Asymptomatic Carotid Atherosclerosis Study (ACAS), which evaluated the value of endarterectomy in asymptomatic patients. These trials have clearly demonstrated the utility of careful and appropriate surgical intervention in preventing stroke. Neurosurgeons and the basic investigators who work with them were responsible for demonstrating the first drug treatment that ameliorates the serious consequences of spinal cord injury. Although these studies were difficult, those which you will need to design for the future will be an order of magnitude more complex. Your second major challenge, then, will be to develop, in laboratories and clinics, germane research hypotheses and potential therapeutic maneuvers, as well as to conduct the necessary clinical trials to establish their effacy.

Given the exciting future that we see for both basic and clinical research, what are the prospects for funding? Here, the picture becomes paradoxically somber. Large changes are sweeping across the landscape of biomedical research funding that will fundamentally affect how we do our business. The most important of these is that Government support for biomedical research is likely to remain flat or to actually decrease over the remaining years of this century and perhaps into the beginning years of the next. Both the Administration and the Congress have read the last election as a strong desire on the part of the American people to have less Government and to spend less for it. Although the budget for FY 1996 is not yet decided, the most optimistic projection is that the National Institutes of Health (NIH), which apparently will fare better than most Government agencies, will have a budget that will keep us even with inflation; more pessimistic projections see us as losing money. It is important to emphasize that this is not an idiosyncratic year, after which business as usual will continue. Rather, there will continue to be strong pressure to decrease Government spending. In addition to reduced Government support, changes in the economics of health care will have enormous effects on research in academic institutions. It is estimated that approximately $1 billion per year now generated by clinical income that now flows into medical research, either directly or indirectly, will be lost as economic competition for the health care dollar increases. Finally, public institutions that sponsor biomedical research are coming under increasing pressure as states reduce their financial commitments, a process that is likely to increase as expensive federal programs are turned back to the states. Two possible sources are often mentioned as filling the void: private foundations and pharmaceutical companies. Neither will provide the substantial help required to make up the deficit in support of biomedical research. Although support from private foundations is increasing, the funds are modest when viewed in terms of the total biomedical research budget. The Howard Hughes Medical Institute, for example, which is perhaps the largest private supporter of biomedical research, spends about $250 million per year, less than 3% of the total NIH budget. As for pharmaceutical companies, they are facing pressure to downsize just like the rest of us. While some companies may be growing, the larger ones are cutting research budgets and scientific personnel. We must look then, to a prolonged period of reduced funding for biomedical research.

The decreased funding available for biomedical research means that we will have to rethink many of the ways in which we do business. More and more, the phrase "science in the steady state" is being heard in Washington. This refers to a growing perception that the long expansionary phase of biomedical research that began after World War II is now coming to a close and that the size of the total enterprise of biomedical research is likely to remain approximately constant for a period of time. This phrase implies that the number of scientists entering the field can only equal those who are leaving and that the funding for any new projects will only come at the expense of those already funded.

What are we to do with this dichotomy—with the stark contrast between our perception that neuroscience is more exciting and more promising than it has ever been and, therefore, more deserving of new funds and new investigators, and with the austere realities of an enterprise that is apparently frozen in size? I have no answers, but to tell you that it will be a challenge for us to maintain our sense of excitement and dedication, even as we think of how we can do more with less. Despite the difficulties, I remain convinced that we are privileged to be part of the amazing narrative of biological and medical progress that is taking place before our very eyes. The Decade of the Brain is just the beginning.

III

General Scientific Session III—Lumbar Disc Disease: Current Trends in Management

15

Neurotrophin Infusion Improves Cognitive Deficits and Decreases Cholinergic Neuronal Cell Loss After Experimental Brain Injury

GRANT SINSON, M.D., MADHU VODDI, B.A.,
EUGENE S. FLAMM, M.D., AND TRACY K. McINTOSH, PH.D.

An estimated 420,750 people per year are discharged alive from hospitals in the United States after sustaining a head injury (13). Approximately 20% of these people have residual neurologic disabilities after their injury (13). Even subtle alterations in cognitive function can affect those who have otherwise made good recoveries (3, 15, 20). The lateral fluid-percussion (FP) model of brain injury has been extensively studied because of the pathologic and behavioral similarities it shares with clinical head injury (6, 19). Cognitive deficits persist for months after this model of brain injury (24, 30).

Administration of various growth (neurotrophic) factors have been shown to support neuronal cells in a variety of models of CNS injury (12, 16). Nerve growth factor (NGF) remains the most extensively studied neurotrophic factor, and treatment with NGF has been shown to attenuate cell death after ischemic, excitotoxic, or hypoglycemic injury and after axonal transection (2, 4, 5, 8, 26, 28). Patterson *et al.* have demonstrated the presence of NGF in the cerebrospinal fluid of brain injured human patients (23). Previously, we have shown that NGF infusion can significantly improve the cognitive deficits normally associated with FP brain trauma (29). However, the cognitive benefits identified in that study were measured during continuous infusions of NGF, and no histopathologic differences were noted to correlate with these improvements. This study was performed to evaluate the presence of lasting cognitive improvements induced by NGF infusion after FP brain injury in rats and to identify the histologic correlates of these behavioral changes.

MATERIALS AND METHODS

Surgical Procedures

The lateral (parasagittal) FP model of brain injury utilized has been described previously (19). The injury was delivered after attaching a male Sprague-Dawley rat to the FP device, which rapidly injects a bolus of saline into the epidural space. All animals received brain injury of moderate severity (2.1 to 2.3 atm). Twenty-four hours after brain injury, animals underwent placement of an osmotic minipump connected to an indwelling brain cannula, which delivered 0.5 ul/hr infusate for 14 days directly into the region of maximal cortical injury (29). Animals in group 1 ($n = 12$) received infusions containing NGF (artificial cerebrospinal fluid, 0.1 mg/ml rat serum albumin, 25 µg/ml 7S NGF, and 0.05 mg/ml gentamycin); group 2 animals received infusion of the same solution without NGF. Two weeks after injury, the brain cannula and pump were removed. Procedures in all groups were performed under sterile conditions, and normothermia was maintained with warming pads. Brain temperature was not directly monitored, because it has previously been shown that use of warming pads maintains normal brain temperature in this model of brain injury (21).

Evaluation of Motor and Cognitive Function

The evaluation of memory and motor function in rats undergoing a FP brain injury has been previously described in detail (19, 29, 31, 32). All animals received training in the Morris Water Maze (MWM) 4 weeks after injury. Uninjured, sham animals ($n = 12$) were also trained using the same paradigm. Each animal learned to locate a submerged platform using external visual cues. Latency to find the platform was recorded for each of 20 trials. At 48 hours after training, animals in all groups were assessed for their ability to remember the learned task of locating the platform in the MWM. For this evaluation the platform was removed from the maze, and the animals' swimming pattern was recorded with a computerized video system that generates a numerical memory score (10, 21, 31, 32). Animals also underwent evaluation of neurologic motor function by a blinded investigator at 1, 2, and 4 weeks after injury using previously described paradigms (19, 32). A composite motor score (0 to 36) was generated by combining the scores for each of nine tests.

Histologic Evaluation

Animals were sacrificed, perfused with 4% paraformaldehyde, and brains were sectioned (50 µm) on a vibratome. The regions of cortical injury and hippocampal CA3 cell loss were assessed with Nissl stain (toludine blue). Acetylcholinesterase staining was performed on sections through the hippocampus (9). Choline acetyltransferase immunohistochemistry was used to count cholinergic cells in the medial septal nucleus (8). Measurements of the area of the septal nuclei were performed using image analysis.

RESULTS

The learning latencies, memory scores, motor scores, and septal nucleus cell counts are illustrated in Figures 1 to 3 and Table 1. Two animals from each group were euthanized before completion of the study because of a failure to thrive. NGF-treated animals learned significantly more quickly than the vehicle controls (P < .05). A significant difference was also noted with respect to memory scores (P < .05). There was no significant motor differences between the injured groups. A significant loss of septal nuclei volume and cholinergic cells was identified in all injured animals (P < .05). The NGF-treated animals had less cholinergic cell loss than vehicle-treated animals. The difference was statistically significant only when comparing cell loss on the side contralateral to the injury (P < .05). Histologic evaluation of the cortical injury cavity (Fig. 4) did not demonstrate differences between the

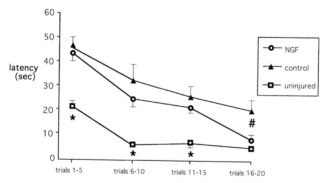

FIG. 1 Comparison of latencies to find the water maze platform during learning trials. Average latencies for each set of five trials are shown. During the first three sets (trials 1 to 15), all injured animals had latencies that were significantly longer than uninjured animals (*=P < .05). Though the latencies of animals that had received NGF were better than injured controls during these sets, the difference was not significant. The last set of trials shows that the latencies for NGF-treated animals improved and are not significantly different from those of uninjured, sham animals. The latencies of the NGF-treated animals are significantly better than the control, injured animals during this last set of trials (# = P <.05).

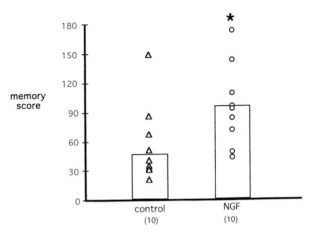

FIG. 2 Comparison of memory scores (48 hours after completing the MWM training) of vehicle-treated, NGF-treated, and uninjured animals. The NGF-treated animals had significantly higher memory scores, compared with those of vehicle-treated control animals (* = $P < .05$). Number of animals tested is in parentheses.

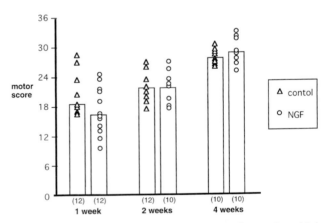

FIG. 3 Neurologic motor scoring in injured, vehicle-treated controls and injured, NGF-treated animals at 1, 2, and 4 weeks after injury. There is a gradual improvement in motor scores over time in both groups and no significant differences between these groups. Number of animals tested is in parentheses.

TABLE 1

Measured Septal Nucleus Area and ChAT-positive cells in NGF-treated (Injured), Control (Injured), and Sham (Uninjured) Rats

Animal	Septal Area (mm²)	Mean Area (mm²)	ChAT + Cells (Ipsilateral)	Mean Cells (Ipsilateral)	ChAT + Cells (Contralateral)	Mean Cells (Contralateral)	ChAT + Cells (Total)	Mean Cells (Total)
NGF 1	7.73	6.8	56	57.6	55	64.8†	111	122.3
NGF 2	6.51		53		69		122	
NGF 3	7.96		47		58		105	
NGF 4	7.78		42		61		103	
NGF 5	6.39		56		68		124	
NGF 6	6.20		72		65		137	
NGF 7	6.77		69		63		132	
NGF 8	5.81		38		68		106	
NGF 9	5.86		85		76		161	
Control 1	7.35	7.2	54	51.2	60	50.3	114	101.5
Control 2	7.77		49		44		93	
Control 3	6.69		58		59		117	
Control 4	7.57		57		40		97	
Control 5	7.38		40		50		90	
Control 6	6.21		49		49		98	
Sham 1	8.12	8.4*	111	109.0*	106	118.3*	217	227.3*
Sham 2	8.51		97		111		208	
Sham 3	8.20		119		138		257	
Sham 4	8.00							
Sham 5	9.21							

*P < .05 compared to both groups of injured animals; †P < .05 compared to control (injured) animals.[a]

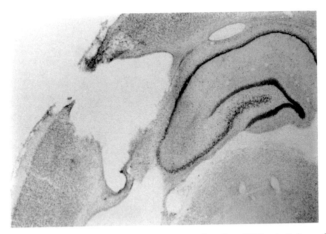

FIG. 4 Coronal 50-μm Nissl-stained section 4 weeks after FP brain injury. Cavitation of the parietal injury region is evident, and necrotic tissue has been cleared. The breach in the superficial portion of the cavity represents the site of entrance for the infusion cannula. Cellular loss in the CA3 pyramidal layer in the hippocampus is also apparent.

vehicle-treated or NGF-treated animals (data not shown). Qualitative assessment of acetylcholinesterase staining of the hippocampus suggested an attenuation of the loss of staining in animals treated with NGF (Fig. 5).

DISCUSSION

Previous studies have characterized the cognitive deficits that result after FP brain injury in the rodent (10, 30, 31). Leonard et al. have proposed that these deficits may be, in part, the result of damage to the septal-hippocampal pathway (14). To our knowledge the current study is the first to correlate neuronal loss in the septal nucleus with impaired cognitive function after FP brain injury. We have also demonstrated the ability of NGF to decrease this neuronal loss and, in doing so, result in improved cognitive outcomes.

An increased understanding of the biomechanics of human head injury has provided valuable information about the relationship between diffuse axonal injury (DAI) and poor cognitive outcomes (1, 7, 33). However, the cumbersome nature of assessing cognitive changes in animal models of head injury and the paucity of histopathologic specimens from human patients who have a well-defined cognitive deficit after a head injury have made further correlation of neuronal damage and specific types of cognitive dysfunction difficult. For instance, in a series of classic monographs on the pathology of human head injury, Strich

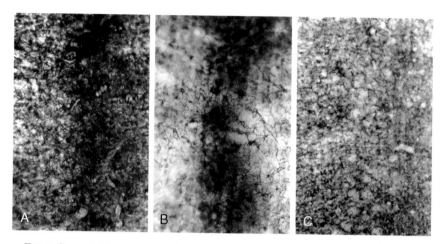

FIG. 5 Coronal 50-μm sections through the caudal hippocampus ipsilateral to the side of injury stained for acetylcholinesterase-containing fibers (black). Photomicrographs represent the CA3 region of the hippocampus with the pyramidal cell layer forming a vertical line in the center of the field and the stratum oriens to the right of this layer (original magnification = 400×). (**A**) Uninjured animal with diffuse, robust acetylcholinesterase staining of cholinergic afferents to the hippocampus. (**B**) Injured, NGF-treated animal also has a significant amount of acetylcholinesterase staining. (**C**) Injured, vehicle-treated animal demonstrates much fewer acetylcholinesterase-containing processes.

notes only that the presence of axonal degeneration in the fornices is a common occurrence (33–35). Also, in a review of a series of head injury patients who developed a post-traumatic dementia, Hillbom and Jarho summarize that lesions causing memory disturbances ". . . are always bilateral and damage the limbic system and their connections with the frontal lobes" (11). More recently, known links between Alzheimer's disease and head trauma have been identified and defined on a molecular scale (17, 18, 25). The loss of cholinergic neurons in Alzheimer's disease has long been known and has even resulted in a clinical trial of NGF administration to treat Alzheimer's disease (22, 27).

These data demonstrate that damage to the septal-hippocampal pathway results in cognitive deficits in the clinically relevant model of FP brain injury in the rat. Infusion of NGF starting 24 hours after injury results in improvements in post-traumatic learning deficits that persist after halting of the NGF treatment. This model of NGF infusion into traumatic brain-injured animals suggests that neurotrophin therapy may be a useful option for the prevention of post-traumatic cognitive deficits, and further evaluation of this hypothesis is warranted.

ACKNOWLEDGEMENTS

This work was supported, in part, by Grants NS26818 and NS08803 from the National Institutes of Health.

REFERENCES

1. Adams J, Graham D, Murray L, *et al.*: Diffuse axonal injury due to nonmissile head injury in humans: An analysis of 45 cases. **Ann Neurol** 12:557–563, 1982.
2. Cheng B, Mattson MP: NGF and bFGF protect rat hippocampal and human cortical neurons against hypoglycemic damage by stabilizing calcium homeostasis. **Neuron** 7:1031–1041, 1991.
3. Dacey RG, Vollmer D, Dikmen SS: Mild head injury, in Cooper PR (ed): *Head Injury.* Baltimore, Williams and Wilkins, 1993, pp 159–182.
4. Dekker AJ, Fagan AM, Gage FH, *et al.*: Effects of brain-derived neurotrophic factor and nerve growth factor on remaining neurons in the lesioned nucleus basalis magnocellularis. **Brain Res** 639:149–155, 1994.
5. Frim DM, Short MP, Rosenberg WS, *et al.*: Local protective effects of nerve growth factor-secreting fibroblasts against excitotoxic lesions in the rat striatum. **J Neurosurg** 78:267–273, 1993.
6. Gennarelli TA: Animate models of human head injury. **J Neurotrauma** 11:357–368, 1994.
7. Gennarelli TA, Thibault LE, Adams JH, *et al.*: Diffuse axonal injury and traumatic coma in the primate. **Ann Neurol** 12:564–574, 1982.
8. Hagg T, Manthorpe M, Vahlsing HL, *et al.*: Delayed treatment with nerve growth factor reverses the apparent loss of cholinergic neurons after acute brain damage. **Exp Neurol** 101:303–312, 1988.
9. Hedreen JC, Bacon SJ, Price DL: A modified histochemical technique to visualize acetylcholinesterase-containing axons. **J Histochem Cytochem** 33:134–140, 1985.
10. Hicks RR, Smith DH, Lowenstein DA, *et al.*: Mild experimental brain injury in the rat induces cognitive deficits associated with regional neuronal loss in the hippocampus. **J Neurotrauma** 10:405–414, 1993.
11. Hillbom E, Jarho L: Posttraumatic Korsakoff syndrome, in Walker AE, Caveness WF, Critchley M (eds): *The Late Effects of Head Injury.* Springfield, IL, Charles C Thomas, 1969, pp 98–109.
12. Korsching S: The neurotrophic factor concept: A reexamination. **J Neurosci** 13: 2739–2748, 1993.
13. Kraus JF: Epidemiology of head injury, in Cooper PR (ed): *Head Injury.* Baltimore, Williams & Wilkins, 1993, pp 1–25.
14. Leonard JR, Maris DO, Grady MS: Fluid percussion injury causes loss of forebrain choline acetyltransferase and nerve growth factor receptor immunoreactive cells in the rat. **J Neurotrauma** 11:379–392, 1994.
15. Levin HS, Benton AL, Grossman RG: *Neurobehavioral Consequences of Closed Head Injury.* New York, Oxford University Press, 1982, pp 63–72.
16. Maness LM, Kastin AJ, Weber JT, *et al.*: The neurotrophins and their receptor: Structure, function, and neuropathology. **Neurosci Biobehav Rev** 18:143–159, 1994.
17. Mayeux R, Ottman R, Maestre G, *et al.*: Synergistic effects of traumatic head injury and apolipoprotein-e4 in patients with Alzheimer's disease. **Neurology** 45:555–557, 1995.

18. Mayeux R, Ottman R, Tang MX, *et al.*: Genetic susceptibility and head injury as risk factors for Alzheimer's disease among community-dwelling elderly persons and their first-degree relatives. **Ann Neurol** 33:494–501, 1993.
19. McIntosh TK, Vink R, Noble L, *et al.*: Traumatic brain injury in the rat: Characterization of a lateral fluid percussion model. **Neuroscience** 28:233–244, 1989.
20. Oddy M, Humphrey M: Social recovery during the year following severe head injury. **J Neurol Neurosurg Psychiatry** 43:798–802, 1980.
21. Okiyama K, Smith DS, Thomas MJ, *et al.*: Evaluation of the novel calcium channel blocker (S)-emopamil on neurochemical, cognitive, and behavioral function after experimental brain injury. **J Neurosurg** 77:605–615, 1992.
22. Olson L: NGF and the treatment of Alzheimer's disease. **Exp Neurol** 124:5–15, 1993.
23. Patterson SL, Grady MS, Bothwell M: Nerve growth factor and a fibroblast growth factor-like neurotrophic activity in cerebrospinal fluid of brain injured human patients. **Brain Res** 605:43–49, 1993.
24. Pierce JES, Smith DS, Eison MS, *et al.*: The nootropic compound BMY 21502 improves spatial learning ability in brain injured rats. **Brain Res** 624:199–208, 1993.
25. Roberts GW, Gentleman SM, Lynch A, *et al.*: B-Amyloid protein deposition in the brain after severe head injury. **J Neurol Neurosurg Psychiatry** 57:419–425, 1994.
26. Schumacher JM, Short MP, Hyman BT, *et al.*: Intracerebral implantation of nerve growth factor-producing fibroblasts protects striatum against neurotoxic levels of excitatory amino acids. **Neuroscience** 45:561–570, 1991.
27. Seiger A, Nordberg A, vonHolst H, *et al.*: Intracranial infusion of purified nerve growth factor to an Alzheimer patient: The first attempt of a possible future treatment strategy. **Behav Brain Res** 57:255–261, 1993.
28. Shigeno T, Mima T, Takakura K, *et al.*: Amelioration of delayed neuronal death in the hippocampus by nerve growth factor. **J Neurosci** 11:2914–2919, 1991.
29. Sinson G, Voddi M, McIntosh TK: Nerve growth factor administration attenuates cognitive but not neurobehavioral motor dysfunction or hippocampal cell loss following fluid-percussion brain injury in rats. **J Neurochem,** in press, 1995.
30. Smith DH, Lowenstein DL, Gennarelli TA, *et al.*: Persistent memory dysfunction is associated with bilateral hippocampal damage following experimental brain injury. **Neurosci Lett** 168:151–154, 1994.
31. Smith DH, Okiyama K, Thomas M, *et al.*: Evaluation of memory dysfunction following experimental brain injury using the Morris Water Maze. **J Neurotrauma** 8:259–269, 1991.
32. Smith DH, Okiyama K, Thomas MJ, *et al.*: Effects of the excitatory amino acid receptor antagonists kynurenate and indole-2-carboxylic acid on behavioral and neurochemical outcome following experimental brain injury. **J Neurosci** 13: 5383–5392, 1993.
33. Strich S: Diffuse degeneration of the cerebral white matter in devere dementia following head injury. **J Neurol Neurosurg Psychiatry** 19:163–185, 1956.
34. Strich S: Shearing of nerve fibers as a course of brain damage due to head injury. **Lancet** 2:443–448, 1961.
35. Strich SJ: Cerebral trauma, in Blackwood W, Corsellis JAN (eds): *Greenfield's Neuropathology.* Chicago, Year Book Medical Publishers, 1976, pp 327–360.

16

Lumbar Discectomy Microdiscectomy: "The Gold Standard"

PAUL J. APOSTOLIDES, M.D., RONALD JACOBOWITZ, PH.D., AND VOLKER K. H. SONNTAG, M.D.

The "gold-standard" of surgical management for appropriately selected patients with symptomatic lumbar disc herniation who have failed an adequate trial of conservative therapy is open discectomy with the aid of either loupes and a headlamp (*i.e.* conventional lumbar discectomy) or the operating microscope (lumbar microdiscectomy). Treatment alternatives include microlumbar discectomy as described by Williams (37–39), chemonucleolysis with chymopapain, percutaneous lumbar discectomy, and open discectomy with fusion.

Unfortunately, the lack of large prospective, randomized, well-controlled studies comparing these various treatment alternatives makes meaningful comparison of reported surgical results difficult. In fact, there are no prospective, randomized studies comparing traditional open discectomy techniques (conventional lumbar discectomy and lumbar microdiscectomy) with the minimalistic microlumbar discectomy technique. Four studies compare open discectomy and chemonucleolysis, two studies compare open discectomy and percutaneous lumbar discectomy, and one study compares open discectomy via laminectomy with and without instrumentation and fusion. This chapter reviews the pooled results from these comparison studies to evaluate which surgical procedure is most effective in treating appropriately selected patients with symptomatic lumbar disc herniation who have failed conservative therapy. The χ^2 test for homogeneity and the odds ratio were calculated for each group using a 2×2 table.

SURGICAL INDICATIONS AND PATIENT SELECTION

The most common cause of failure after lumbar disc surgery remains poor patient selection (4, 12). Only 5 to 10% of patients with sciatica will eventually require an operation (15). In these patients, the clinical diagnosis of lumbar disc herniation must be confirmed by careful correlation of the patient's signs and symptoms with specific pathology documented on appropriate imaging studies. The indications for lumbar disc excision include cauda equina syndrome, significant motor weakness, and intractable recurrence of radicular pain. However, the success of the operation will depend on a variety of definitive and well-documented factors.

In 1991, Abramovitz and Neff (2) reported the results of the Prospective Lumbar Discectomy Study sponsored by the Joint Section on Disorders of the Spine and Peripheral Nerve of the American Association of Neurological Surgeons and the Congress of Neurological Surgeons to evaluate the indications and efficacy of lumber discectomy. This study showed that the absence of back pain, absence of work-related injury or insurance claim, absence of back pain on the straight leg-raise examination, and presence of reflex asymmetry were factors independently predictive of successful outcome after lumbar disc surgery. Not surprisingly, the success rate was directly correlated with the number of factors present.

CONVENTIONAL DISCECTOMY/MICRODISCECTOMY VERSUS MICROLUMBAR DISCECTOMY

The introduction of the operating microscope for lumbar disc surgery by Caspar (5) and Yasargil (41) has allowed for a natural refinement of open discectomy. Despite the plethora of articles comparing the differences between conventional discectomy and lumbar microdiscectomy, assimilation of these two techniques has been slowly occurring over the past 18 years. At present, both procedures require a small skin incision, limited soft-tissue dissection, adequate removal of bone, excision of the ruptured fragment, and generous evacuation of the disc space material. In addition, both procedures often must be customized for each patient to obtain a safe and satisfactory decompression of the neural elements. The primary difference between these two techniques is whether the surgeon uses loupes and a headlamp (*i.e.,* conventional lumbar discectomy) or the operating microscope (*i.e.,* lumbar microdiscectomy). We believe that the advantages of the operating microscope (*i.e.,* improved vision and lighting, variable magnification, and allowing the co-surgeon to observe and assist during the procedure) are extremely beneficial during open discectomy, particularly in the setting of a teaching institution. Despite this personal preference, it is our contention that conventional lumbar discectomy and lumbar microdiscectomy represent simple variations of open discectomy. However, these techniques are not the same as microlumbar discectomy.

Microlumbar discectomy represents an extremely conservative microsurgical procedure for the treatment of lumbar disc herniation, which was first reported in 1978 by Williams (37). This minimalistic technique consists of no bone removal, no electrocautery use in the spinal canal, preservation of all extradural fat, blunt perforation of the annulus fibrosus, and preservation of nonherniated disc material (37–39). In 1993, Williams (39) surveyed his experience with microlumbar discectomy in 1051 patients over a 20-year period and reported a surgical "cure" rate of 84% after initial operation and a 7.0% rate of recurrent disc herniation with 5.5% occurring at the site of the initial surgery, 1.2% occurring at the same level but opposite side and 0.3% representing missed discs.

No prospective, randomized studies compare traditional open discectomy (conventional lumbar discectomy and lumbar microdiscectomy) with microlumbar discectomy. The reported success and complication rates in prospective series of open discectomy (1, 2, 21, 34, 35) appear similar to the reported success and complication rates in retrospective series of microlumbar discectomy (16, 39). However, the rate of recurrent disc herniation when using minimal (*i.e.,* Williams technique) versus generous disc excision remains controversial. On one hand, Rogers (28) reviewed 68 patients who underwent microsurgical discectomy with either minimal ($n = 33$) or generous ($n = 35$) disc excision and follow-up varying from 11 to 30 months. He reported a 21% rate of recurrent disc herniation in patients undergoing only fragment removal as compared with a 0% rate in patients undergoing generous disc removal. On the other hand, Balderston *et al.* (3) reviewed 83 patients who underwent conventional discectomy with either minimal ($n = 43$) or generous ($n = 40$) disc excision and a follow-up of at least 2 years. They reported a 5% rate of recurrent disc herniation in patients undergoing only fragment removal as compared to a 4.7% rate in patients undergoing generous disc removal.

Table 1 lists a number of articles that have reported the specific type of disc excision (generous or minimal) and the rate of recurrent disc herniation. The pooled results of these studies reveal a 3.7% rate of recurrent disc herniation after generous disc excision as compared with 7% after minimal disc excision ($P < 0.001$). The odds of recurrent disc herniation were 1.9 times as great after minimal disc excision than after generous disc excision. Based on these studies, generous disc excision is significantly more effective in preventing recurrent disc herniation than minimal disc excision.

Chemonucleolysis Versus Placebo

Chemonucleolysis with chymopapain has been surrounded by controversy regarding its therapeutic efficacy since its clinical introduction by Smith in 1964 (31). There are currently four published prospective, randomized clinical trials of chemonucleolysis with chymopapain versus a placebo for the treatment of lumbar disc herniation (Table 2)

(8, 13, 18, 29). The pooled results of these studies reveal a 69% success rate for chymopapain compared to 46% for the placebo ($P < 0.0001$). The odds of successful outcome were 2.6 times as great after chymopapain than after the placebo. Thus, chemonucleolysis with chymopapain appears to be significantly more effective than the placebo in treating lumbar disc herniation. These findings confirm those previously reported by Haines (17) in his critical review of the first three published clinical trials comparing chemonucleolysis with chymopapain and placebo (13, 18, 29) in 1985.

Chemonucleolysis Versus Open Discectomy

There are four published prospective, randomized clinical trials comparing chemonucleolysis with chymopapain and open discectomy for the treatment of lumbar disc herniation (Table 3) (7, 11, 26, 33). The pooled results of these studies reveal an 87% success rate for open discectomy compared to 62% for chymopapain ($P < 0.0001$) and a 2.5% reoperation rate for open discectomy compared with 29% for chymopapain ($P < 0.0001$). The odds of a successful outcome were 4.0 times as

TABLE 1
Generous Versus Minimal Disc Excision
(Reported Rate of Recurrent Disc Herniation)

Study	Generous Disc Excision		Minimal Disc Excision	
Williams (37)	—		74/1051	(7%)
Balderston *et al.* (3)	2/43	(4.7%)	2/40	(5%)
Caspar *et al.* (6)	10/299	(3.3%)	—	
Rogers (28)	0/35	(0.0%)	7/33	(21%)
Silvers (30)	9/270	(3.3%)	—	
Ebeling *et al.* (10)	22/485	(4.5%)	—	
Maroon and Alba (23)	5/120	(4.0%)	—	
Wilson and Harbaugh (40)	2/100	(2.0%)	—	
Goald (16)	—		28/477	(6%)
Total	50/1352	(3.7%)	111/1601	(7%)

TABLE 2
Chemonucleolysis Versus Placebo
(Reported Success Rates in Prospective Comparison Series)

Study	Chymopapain		Placebo	
Dabezies *et al.* (8)	37/54	(69%)	32/70	(46%)
Javid *et al.* (18)	40/55	(73%)	22/53	(42%)
Fraser (13)	23/30	(77%)	16/30	(53%)
Schwetschenau (29)	18/31	(58%)	17/35	(49%)
Total	118/170	(69%)	87/188	(46%)

TABLE 3
Chemonucleolysis Versus Discectomy/Microdiscectomy
(Reported Success Rate and Reoperative Rates in Prospective Comparison Series)

Study	Chymopapain		Discectomy/Microdiscectomy	
	Success Rate	Reoperation Rate	Success Rate	Reoperation Rate
Muralikuttan et al. (26)	35/44 (80%)	9/44 (20.5%)	66/78 (85%)	1/42 (2.4%)
van Alphen et al. (33)	46/73 (63%)	18/73 (25.0%)	41/42 (98%)	2/78 (3.0%)
Crawshaw et al. (7)	11/24 (46%)	11/24 (46%)	23/26 (88%)	1/26 (4.0%)
Ejeskär et al. (11)	5/15 (33%)	8/15 (53.0%)	9/14 (64%)	0/14 (0.0%)
Total	97/156 (62%)	46/156 (29.5%)	139/160 (87%)	4/160 (2.5%)

great after open discectomy than after chymopapain injection. The odds of reoperation were 16.3 times as great after chymopapain injection than after open discectomy. In addition, open discectomy was found to be more cost-effective than chemonucleolysis because of its significantly lower rate of reoperation (26). Thus, the open discectomy was significantly more effective than chemonucleolysis for the treatment of lumbar disc herniation. However, these differences were no longer significant 1 year after the final treatment (11, 26, 33).

Percutaneous Discectomy (Prospective Series)

There are currently six published prospective series that evaluate the potential therapeutic efficacy of percutaneous lumbar microdiscectomy for the treatment of lumbar disc herniation in the English literature (Table 4) (9, 19, 20, 22, 25, 27). The pooled results from these studies reveal a success rate of 79% and a reoperation rate of 12% when treating patients with "contained" or small subligamentous lumbar disc herniations. However, the results of these studies cannot be generalized beyond those patients with small focal disc bulges or protrusions because of the extremely stringent radiographic inclusion criteria required for percutaneous discectomy. Unfortunately, there are no prospective, randomized studies that compare the results of percutaneous discectomy and prolonged conservative therapy in this carefully selected group of patients. Perhaps patients with similar radiographic findings represented the majority of the 60% of patients who were cured with conservative management in Weber's classic study (34), meaning that they may not have required any surgical intervention.

Percutaneous Discectomy Versus Open Discectomy

There are only two published prospective, randomized clinical trials that compare percutaneous discectomy and open discectomy for the treatment of lumbar disc herniation (Table 5) (24, 32). The pooled results

TABLE 4
Percutaneous Discectomy
(Reported Success and Reported Rates in Prospective Series)

Study	Success Rate (%)		Reoperation Rate (%)	
Mochida and Arima (25)	54/85	(64%)	22/85	(26.0%)
Luft *et al.* (22)	53/68	(78%)	4/68	(6.0%)
Davis *et al.* (9)	439/518	(85%)	38/518	(7.0%)
Onik *et al.* (27)	246/327	(75%)	41/327	(13.0%)
Kahanovitz *et al.* (19)	21/38	(55%)	13/38	(34.0%)
Kambin and Schaffer (20)	81/93	(87%)	12/93	(13.0%)
Total	894/1129	(79%)	130/1129	(12.0%)

TABLE 5
Percutaneous Discectomy Versus Discectomy/Microdiscectomy
(Reported Success and Reoperation Rates in Prospective Comparison Series)

Study	Percutaneous Discectomy				Discectomy/Microdiscectomy			
	Success Rate		Reoperation Rate		Success Rate		Reoperation Rate	
Stevenson et al. (32)	11/31	(35%)	20/31	(65%)	39/40	(98%)	1/40	(3.0%)
Mayer and Brock (24)	14/20	(70%)	3/20	(15%)	13/20	(65%)	0/20	(0.0%)
Total	25/51	(49%)	23/51	(45%)	52/60	(87%)	1/60	(1.7%)

of these studies reveal an 87% success rate for open discectomy compared with 49% for percutaneous discectomy ($P < 0.0001$), and a 1.7% reoperation rate for open discectomy compared to 45% for percutaneous discectomy ($P < 0.0001$). The odds for successful outcome were 6.8 times as great after open discectomy than after percutaneous discectomy. The odds of reoperation were 48.5 times as great after percutaneous discectomy than after open discectomy. In addition, open discectomy was found to be more cost-effective than percutaneous discectomy because of its significantly lower rate of reoperation (32). Thus, open discectomy appears to be significantly more effective than percutaneous discectomy for the treatment of lumbar disc herniation.

Fusion Versus No Fusion

No prospective, randomized studies compare lumbar discectomy/microdiscectomy with and without fusion, and only one such study compares open discectomy *via* laminectomy with and without instrumentation and fusion (36). In this study, the success rates for patients with and without fusion were 53 and 71%, respectively; and only 11% of fused patients had "excellent" results compared with 29% of nonfused patients. There were no specific data regarding rates of reoperation for these two groups.

Table 6 includes data from the above prospective study as well as from one large retrospective review that compared open discectomy *via* laminectomy with and without fusion (14). The pooled results of these studies reveal a success rate of 67% with fusion compared with 65% without fusion ($P = 0.79$) and a reoperation rate of 14% with fusion and 18% without fusion ($P = 0.41$). In addition, patients receiving fusion took significantly longer to return to work than those not receiving fusion (14, 36). Thus, fusion appears to provide no significant benefit over nonfusion in the treatment of lumbar disc herniation.

TABLE 6
Fusion Versus No Fusion
(Reported Success and Reoperation Rates)

Study	Fusion		No Fusion	
	Success Rate	Reoperation Rate	Success Rate	Reoperation Rate
White *et al.* (36) (prospective)	20/38 (53%)	—	22/31 (71%)	—
Frymoyer *et al.* (14) (retrospective)	116/166 (70%)	23/166 (14%)	49/78 (63%)	14/78 (18%)
Total	136/204 (67%)	23/166 (14%)	71/109 (65%)	14/78 (18%)

CONCLUSION

The lack of large prospective, randomized, well-controlled studies that compare various surgical alternatives for the treatment of lumbar disc herniation make meaningful comparison of reported surgical results difficult. However, the available data indicate that open discectomy (conventional lumbar discectomy and lumber microdiscectomy) has a significantly lower rate of recurrent disc herniation than microlumbar discectomy and is significantly more effective than chemonucleolysis and percutaneous discectomy. In addition, the significantly higher rates of reoperation with chemonucleolysis and percutaneous discectomy make them less cost-effective than open discectomy. Finally, fusion provides no significant additional benefit than open discectomy alone and therefore is not justified on a routine basis. Based on this analysis, the "gold-standard" of surgical management for appropriately selected patients with symptomatic lumbar disc herniation who have failed an adequate trail of conservative therapy remains open discectomy.

REFERENCES

1. Alaranta H, Hurme M, Einola S, Falck B, Kallio V, Knuts L-R, Lahtela K, Törmä T: A prospective study of patients with sciatica. A comparison between conservatively treated patients and patients who have undergone operation, Part II: Results after one year follow-up. **Spine** 15:1345–1349, 1990.
2. Abramovitz JN, Neff SR: Lumbar disc surgery: Results of the Prospective Lumbar Discectomy Study of the Joint Section on Disorders of the Spine and Peripheral Nerves of the American Association of Neurological Surgeons and the Congress of Neurological Surgeons. **Neurosurgery** 29:301–308, 1991.
3. Balderston RA, Gilyard GG, Jones AAM, Wiesel SW, Spengler DM, Bigos SJ, Rothman RH: The treatment of lumbar disc herniation: Simple fragment excision versus disc space curettage. **J Spinal Disord** 4:22–25, 1991.
4. Burton CV, Kirkaldy-Willis WH, Yong-Hing K, Heithoff KB: Causes of failure of surgery on the lumbar spine. **Clin Orthop** 157:191–199, 1981.
5. Caspar W: A new surgical procedure for lumbar disc herniation causing less tissue damage through a microsurgical approach. **Adv Neurosurg** 4:74–77, 1977.
6. Caspar W, Campbell B, Barbier DD, Kretschmmer R, Gotfried Y: The Caspar microsurgical discectomy and comparison with a conventional standard lumbar disc procedure. **Neurosurgery** 28:78–87, 1991.
7. Crawshaw C, Frazer AM, Merriam WF, Mulholland RC, Webb JK: A comparison of surgery and chemonucleolysis in the treatment of sciatica. A prospective randomized trial. **Spine** 9:195–198, 1984.
8. Dabezies EJ, Langford K, Morris J, Shields CB, Wilkinson HA: Safety and efficacy of chymopapain (discase) in the treatment of sciatica due to a herniated nucleus pulposus. Results of a randomized, double-blind study. **Spine** 13:561–565, 1988.
9. Davis GW, Onik G, Helms C: Automated percutaneous discectomy. **Spine** 16:359–363, 1991.
10. Ebeling U, Reichenberg W, Reulen H-J: Results of microsurgical lumbar discectomy. Review on 485 patients. **Acta Neurochir** 81:45–52, 1986.

11. Ejeskär A, Nachemson A, Herberts P, Lysell E, Andersson G, Irstam L, Peterson L-E: Surgery *versus* chemonucleolysis for herniated lumbar discs. A prospective study with random assignment. **Clin Orthop** 174:236–242, 1983.
12. Fager CA, Freidberg SR: Analysis of failures and poor results of lumbar spine surgery. **Spine** 5:87–94, 1980.
13. Fraser RD: Chymopapain for the treatment of intervertebral disc herniation. A primary report of a double-blind study. **Spine** 7:608–612, 1982.
14. Frymoyer JW, Hanley E, Howe J, Kuhlmann D, Matteri R: Disc excision and spine fusion in the management of lumbar disc disease. A minimum ten-year followup. **Spine** 3:1–6, 1978.
15. Frymoyer JW: Back pain and sciatica. **N Engl J Med** 318:291–300, 1988.
16. Goald HJ: Microlumbar discectomy: Follow-up of 477 patients. **J Microsurg** 2:95–100, 1980.
17. Haines SJ: The chymopapain clinical trails. **Neurosurgery** 17:107–110, 1985.
18. Javid MJ, Nordby EJ, Fort LT, Hejna WJ, Whisler WW, Burton C, Millett DK, Wiltse LL, Widell EH, Jr., Boyd RJ, Newton SE, Thisted R: Safety and efficacy of chymopapain (chymodiactin) in herniated nucleus pulposus with sciatica: Results of a randomized double-blind study. **JAMA** 249:2489–2494, 1983.
19. Kahanovitz N, Viola K, Goldstein T, Dawson E: A multicenter analysis of percutaneous discectomy. **Spine** 15:713–715, 1990.
20. Kambin P, Schaffer JL: Percutaneous lumbar discectomy. Review of 100 patients and current practice. **Clin Orthop** 238:24–34, 1989.
21. Lewis PJ, Weir BKA, Broad RW, Grace MG: Long-term prospective study of lumbosacral discectomy. **J Neurosurg** 67:49–53, 1987.
22. Luft C, Weber J, Horvath W, Pürgyi P: Interventional radiology. Automated percutaneous lumbar discectomy (APLD)—Method and 1-year follow-up. **Eur Radiol** 2:292–298, 1992.
23. Maroon JC, Abla AA: Microlumbar discectomy. **Clin Neurosurg** 33:407–417, 1986.
24. Mayer HM, Brock M: Percutaneous endoscopic discectomy: Surgical technique and preliminary results compared to microsurgical discectomy. **J Neurosurg** 78:216–225, 1993.
25. Mochida J, Arima T: Percutaneous nucleotomy in lumbar disc herniation. A prospective study. **Spine** 18:2063–2068, 1993.
26. Muralikuttan KP, Hamilton A, Kernohan WG, Mollan RAB, Adair IV: A prospective randomized trail of chemonucleolysis and conventional disc surgery in single level lumbar disc herniation. **Spine** 17:381–387, 1992.
27. Onik G, Mooney V, Maroon JC, Wiltse L, Helms C, Schweigel J, Watkins R, Kahanovitz N, Day A, Morris J, McCullough JA, Reicher M, Croissant P, Dunsker S, Davis GW, Brown C, Hochschuler S, Saul T, Ray C: Automated percutaneous discectomy: A prospective multi-institutional study. **Neurosurgery** 26:228–233, 1990.
28. Rogers LA: Experience with limited versus extensive disc removal in patients undergoing microsurgical operations for ruptured lumbar discs. **Neurosurgery** 22:82–85, 1988.
29. Schwetschenau PR, Ramirez A, Johnston J, Wiggs C, Martins AN: Double-blind evaluation of intradiscal chymopapain for herniated lumbar discs. Early results. **J Neurosurg** 45:622–627, 1976.
30. Silvers HR: Microsurgical versus standard lumbar discectomy. **Neurosurgery** 22:837–841, 1988.
31. Smith L: Enzyme dissolution of the nucleus pulposus in humans. **JAMA** 187:137–140, 1964.

32. Stevenson RC, McCabe CJ, Findlay AM: An economic evaluation of a clinical trial to compare automated percutaneous lumbar discectomy with microdiscectomy in the treatment of contained lumbar disc herniation. **Spine** 20:739–742, 1995.

33. van Alphen HAM, Braakman R, Bezemer PD, Broere G, Berfelo MW: Chemonucleolysis versus discectomy: A randomized multicenter trial. **J Neurosurg** 70: 869–875, 1989.

34. Weber H: Lumbar disc herniation. A controlled, prospective study with ten years of observation. **Spine** 8:131–140, 1983.

35. Weir BKA, Jacobs GA: Reoperation rate following lumbar discectomy. An analysis of 662 lumbar discectomies. **Spine** 5:366–370, 1980.

36. White AH, Von Rogov P, Zucherman J, Heiden D: Lumbar laminectomy for herniated disc: A prospective controlled comparison with internal fixation fusion. **Spine** 12:305–307, 1987.

37. Williams RW: Microlumbar discectomy. A conservative surgical approach to the virgin herniated lumbar disc. **Spine** 3:175–182, 1978.

38. Williams RW: Microlumbar discectomy. A 12-year statistical review. **Spine** 11:851–852, 1986.

39. Williams RW: Lumbar disc disease. Microdiscectomy. **Neurosurg Clin North Am** 4:101–108, 1993.

40. Wilson DH, Harbaugh R: Microsurgical and standard removal of the protruded lumbar disc: A comparative study. **Neurosurgery** 8:422–427, 1981.

41. Yasargil MG: Microsurgical operation of herniated lumbar disc. **Adv Neurosurg** 4:81, 1977.

CHAPTER

17

Is There a Future for
Percutaneous Intradiscal Therapy?

JOSEPH C. MAROON, M.D., MATTHEW R. QUIGLEY, M.D.,
P. LANGHAM GLEASON, M.D.

Minimally invasive techniques have become the standard treatment for many common disorders. Laparoscopic abdominal procedures, transluminal angioplasty, endovascular occlusion of aneurysms, and stereotactic endoscopic brain surgery are but a few examples. In 1963, Lyman Smith introduced percutaneous intradiscal therapy with chymopapain (CHY) for the treatment of herniatic lumbar disks. Over the ensuing 30 years, other forms of intradiscal therapy (IDT) have evolved. These have included percutaneous manual discectomy (PMD), automated percutaneous discectomy (APD), percutaneous laser discectomy (PLD), and more recently microendoscopic spinal endoscopy (MSE). Despite hundreds of papers dealing with both basic and clinical aspects of these procedures, there still is no unanimity as to the efficacy and in some cases the safety of intradiscal therapy.

These techniques, however, enjoy many theoretical advantages compared with conventional open surgery: (a) avoidance of general anesthesia; (b) brief hospital stay; (c) lack of postoperative epidural scar formation; (d) preservation of spinal stability; and (e) unencumbered ability to subsequently perform conventional open disc surgery.

Although they are less morbid, intradiscal methods are less successful than open techniques. Furthermore, only a small percentage of disc patients are eligible for these noninvasive methods. Review of the radiographs from patients with herniated discs within our own practice indicated only 20% would be considered for an IDT procedure based on radiographic CT or MRI criteria alone. However, during the same time, only 4% of these patients underwent a percutaneous operation. The discrepancy between these statistics can be ascribed to patient exclusion by further diagnostic studies and surgeon preference.

Finally, intradiscal methods remain controversial. Critics assert that intradiscal techniques cannot be used to treat an extruded disc fragment (11). In addition, clinical response does not appear to be related to the mass of disc material removed (28), nor do postoperative scans generally show a reduction in disc material or herniation (2). Proponents argue that the clinical response after intradiscal therapy is related to improved disc compliance under load (5, 24), as well as the phenomenon of "sucking" the herniation back into the disc space (17), although there is little evidence to support these claims.

Although many clinicians remain skeptical about the value of IDT therapies and unsure as to their indications, it is difficult to deny the wealth of clinical studies attesting to their efficacy. Scrutiny of this literature would indicate there probably exists a small population of carefully selected individuals in whom IDT therapies are efficacious.

In this report, we will review the history and development of these various procedures, the general indications for intradiscal therapy, the published results, and introduce new neuroimaging techniques that may have a profound affect on the future development of intradiscal therapy.

CHEMONUCLEOLYSIS

In 1941, Jansen isolated chymopapain from crude papain. Thomas, in 1956, first injected it intravenously and showed a reversible softening of the ear and tracheal cartilage of rabbits. Subsequently, Lyman Smith, after extensive animal experiments, first performed chemonucleolysis in a human lumbar disc in 1963 using fluoroscopic guidance, thus setting the stage for all future intradiscal therapy (45).

In 1994, Javid and Nordby provided an up-to-date review on the current status of chymopapain for herniated lumbar discs (22). Despite initial enthusiasm (21, 32), the introduction of chymopapain to the orthopedic and neurosurgical community was an invitation to subsequent problems. In 1981, a seven-center study of 108 patients demonstrated satisfactory results (12). In 82% of patients receiving chymopapain and in 41% of those receiving a placebo, no complications were observed. Following the approval of chymopapain for clinical use in 1982, 6,214 orthopedic and neurologic surgeons participated in 1-day training sessions in Chicago and Los Angeles. Although emphasized as a "practical course," these sessions consisted of lectures, slide presentations, and only the minimum use of mannequins at times without x-ray control to learn proper needle placement. Subsequently, thousands of patients were injected with chymopapain at times with disastrous results frequently due to poor surgical technique and indications (15, 49).

Anaphylactic reactions were the first to be observed (16). Between 1983 and 1987, these ranged from 0.4% for Caucasians to 1.7% in black females (21). Recent blood tests (RAST and chymofast) may reduce this problem by excluding sensitive patients, but they do not have the sensitivity or specificity to eliminate it. In addition to anaphylaxis, major neurological complications have been reported in 0.05% (1 in 2,000) of cases with chemoneurolysis. Furthermore, disastrous results may occur due to intrathecal injection because of its direct proteolytic effect on nervous structures. Unexplained transverse myelitis, although rare, may occur in a delayed fashion and be irreversible. Finally, severe postoperative back spasm in 20–30% of patients may increase the morbidity of the procedure.

Despite these problems, investigators in Europe, Canada, and Australia continue to use chymopapain in a selective fashion and maintain that it is a safe, effective and practical alternative to laminectomy at approximately half the cost.

PERCUTANEOUS MANUAL DISCETOMY

Following chemoneucleolysis, the next innovative procedure for intradiscal therapy was devised by Hijikata, an orthopedic surgeon in Japan. He first used instrumentation for the percutaneous manual removal of lumbar discs in 1975. He initially reported a 70% success rate. He used a 5-ml diameter cannula through which disc material was removed by the use of specially designed cutting and grasping instruments. In 1989, he reported his 14-year experience with a 72% success rate (17). There was one major vascular injury and one case of discitis. The procedure was limited by the size of the instruments and also the limited ability to perform the procedure at L5 S1.

Subsequently, Schreiber et al. used an 8-mm cannula and different instrumentation coupled with an endoscope placed from the opposite side of the disc to actually visualize the percutaneous removal of disc material using bilateral portals (41, 42). He reported a success rate of 85% but had seven cases of discitis as well as a major vascular injury. Schreiber's modifications to Hijikata's technique increased the complication rate without expanding the scope of the patient population.

In 1973, Schaffer and Kambin further modified Hijikata's technique, used a 7-mm cannula and developed their own unique set of instrumentation. In 1991, they analyzed 100 patients and found an 88% success rate and had no permanent major complications with the exception of one case of discitis. As with previous investigators, Kambin acknowledged that free and extruded disc fragments were still beyond the capability of existing intradiscal techniques (24, 25).

In 1993, Mayer and Brock compared percutaneous endoscopic discectomy with microsurgical discectomy and concluded that this technique offered an alternative to microdiscectomy for patients with "contained" and small subligamentous herniations (31). Two years after percutaneous endoscopic discectomy, sciatica had disappeared in 80% (16 of 20 patients). Two years after microdiscectomy, only 65% (13 of 20 patients) had an absence of sciatica.

AUTOMATED PERCUTANEOUS DISCECTOMY

In 1985, Onik, in collaboration with engineers, designed an automated percutaneous discectomy system that used a reciprocating suction-cutter for removing disc material (35). The instrument consisted of a 2-ml blunt-tipped device with a single side port and a guillotine-like knife that morselized disc material as it was aspirated through the side port and amputated at approximately 180 times per minute by the cutter. This smaller-sized instrumentation that was automated eliminated the major drawbacks of other percutaneous techniques. Maroon and Onik published their initial series in 1987 and reported a 79% success rate.

Following their initial series, over 100,000 patients have had APLD as primary treatment for herniated lumbar discs. Over 3,000 surgeons have participated worldwide in instructional courses. In more than 20 studies from different institutions in the United States and Europe, the success rate remains between 60–80% (3, 4, 18, 23, 28, 29, 35).

In a retrospective review of our own series, we assessed the results in 86 patients with a followup ranging from 2.3 years to 9.4 years and the average being 6.3 years. The excellent and good results were 59% and there were no significant complications. APLD appears then to be the safest procedure for the intradiscal removal of selected lumbar discs, although two cases of cauda equina injury have been reported secondary to improperly placed instrumentation (10, 36).

PERCUTANEOUS LASER DISCECTOMY

In 1991, Choy, et al. introduced the Nd: YAG laser to vaporize the nucleus pulposus for percutaneous laser discectomy (6). They performed the procedure on 377 patients with a good-to-fair response in 78.4% and a poor response in 21%. Although other investigators have continued to use different forms of laser energy for internal disc decompression (7, 43), the spread of heat beyond the confines of the laser tip and the relatively small amount of disc vaporized has limited use of this procedure. Recently, two channel endoscopes of 2-mm diameter are being evaluated to further define the potential use of lasers for intradiscal therapy.

MICROENDOSCOPIC ENDOSCOPY

All of the above procedures have relied on internal decompressions of the disc for their efficacy. Free or extruded fragments of disc in the epidural space are considered beyond the confines of all of these procedures. In 1993, Mathews, an orthopedic surgeon in Virginia, introduced spinal endoscopy with a flexible catheter system to obtain real time visualization of the epidural space. Technologically this represented a marked improvement over the system first introduced by Poole 50 years ago. Special instrumentation was also designed to probe, deflect, and extract disc material from the neural foramen and epidural space. Experience thus far is too limited to comment on its long-term applicability. Its efficacy, however, in a small number of highly selected cases appears to be satisfactory.

RATIONALE FOR INTRADISCAL THERAPY

The pathophysiology of low back and radicular pain from herniated lumbar discs is variably described to biochemical and/or mechanical factors. Investigators have demonstrated nociceptive substances released from the disc space that have a direct inflammatory reaction on nerve roots. It is further well recognized that mechanical compression by protruding or herniated disc fragments causes radicular symptoms. The efficacy of percutaneous intradiscal procedures is attributed to reducing the intradiscal pressure in discs that are still contained by the posterior longitudinal ligament and thus mechanically decompressing the nerve root (5, 21, 27, 47). Kambin et al. showed a marked decrease in the mean level of intradiscal pressure after percutaneous discectomy under loading conditions (5). Other studies have shown a significant decrease in pressure under static as well as loading conditions after automated percutaneous discectomy.

A less emphasized mechanism but one suggested by the efficacy of chymopapain is that biochemical substrates that result in inflammatory responses of the nerve(s) are reduced or eliminated by various dissolving, aspirating, grasping, sucking or laser techniques. Remarkably, virtually all of the intradiscal forms of therapy have similar results in the 60–80% range.

PATIENT SELECTION

Patient selection is the key to success with all forms of intradiscal therapy. Clinically, the most important symptoms are radicular leg pain greater than back pain in patients who have failed all conservative therapy and remain significantly disabled by pain. A history of paresthesias of specific dermatome is significant. Physical findings should include a positive straight leg raising sign, slight weakness of the extensor halluces longus or planter flexures of the foot, mild to moderate sensory disturbances, and reflect alterations. Posterior leg pain that does not radiate below the knee is viewed with suspicion particularly if not associated with other physical findings. Marked weakness of any muscle group, bowel or bladder disturbances, or profound sensory loss are contraindications to the procedure. Also a cross-positive straight leg raising sign usually indicated a sequestered fragment that would not be relieved by percutaneous techniques.

Radiographically, a herniation at the level of the disc space should be visualized on CT, MR, or intrathecally enhanced CT and myelography and correlate with the patient's physical findings. The ideal candidate is one who has a small-to-moderate focal herniation at the disc level consistent with the patient's symptomatology. Patients with marked degenerative disc disease, diffuse annular bulging, lateral recessed stenosis, calcified disc herniations, or focal or diffuse spinal stenosis are contraindicated for most intradiscal therapies. Patients with evidence of instability such as spondylolisthesis are also not candidates for the procedure.

The most difficult decision is determining whether or not there is a sequestered disc fragment. It has been shown that herniations that compromise by 50% or more the thecal sac have a 90% correlation with sequestration (13). The angle of the herniation also has some relevance in that is should not be obtuse (20). Acute angulations suggest extrusions and contraindicate most intradiscal forms of therapy.

Although controversial, CT discography adds useful information to the planning of intradiscal therapy (9). We employ the following morphologic description: (a) normal—dye contrast confined entirely within the nucleus, (b) contained herniation—contrast tracking through an annular tear and collecting within the herniation and posterior longitudinal ligament, (c) free herniation—contrast extending into the epidural space above and below the posterior longitudinal ligament.

RESULTS

The reported outcome following all types of intradiscal treatment is in general quite good and remarkably consistent among the different therapies. Documented success rates of APD vary from 55–85% with higher failure rates among patients not fitting the classic "radicular" clinical patterns or those harboring radiographic evidence of disc fragmentation. Most literature concerning PMD reports success within the 70–80% range, although a recent report from Mayer and Brock documents the most optimistic experience yet whereby 80% had total symptom relief and 95% returned back to work following their bilateral approach with "discoscopy." The large experience following CHY injection discloses a positive outcome from 67.6–86.5% with a reported 86.5% success rate at 4 years and 77% success rate at 10 years following a double-blind trial.

Results following percutaneous laser discectomy (PLD) are dependent on the laser employed. Choy et al. analyzed 333 patients treated with both the 1.06 μm and 1.32 μm Nd: YAG lasers (1.32 μm Nd: YAG not PDA approved) and reported 78.4% good or fair response (6). Davis, employing 532 nm KTP® laser says 85% of patients had "minimal residual discomfort and return to gainful employment" (7). Using a self-reported pain scale as an outcome measure, Sherk could not detect a treatment effect versus control group in 47 patients subjected to 2.1 μm Ho: YAG laser discectomy, although patient selection into treatment or control groups was not randomized (43).

A review of the comparative trials pitting one form of IDT versus another or IDT versus traditional microdiscectomy clearly fails to establish any consensus on these issues and in some series, appears more to reflect the inclinations of the investigators as opposed to the superiority of one method over another.

COMPLICATIONS

The difficulties encountered with IDT methods may be classified as those specific to each method and those secondary to the extradural posterior-lateral approach employed. Complications following CHY are now well known and have probably contributed to its virtual abandonment in this country. Enzyme anaphylaxis may occur in 0.2–0.67% of patients and appears heightened among women and when general anesthesia is employed. Preoperative testing for chymopapain specific IgE immunoglobulin is useful in screening those who are positive, but many false negatives do occur. Delayed neurologic complications, such as transverse myelitis are even rarer still (2/29, 075) and are believed to be secondary to the technical lapse of subarachnoid enzyme injection.

The complications of PMD have been tabulated by Mayer and Brock and they report a 0.3% incidence of abdominal vascular injury and a 0.6% rate of root injury, the majority of these complications occurring at L5-S1. There was a 1.5% discitis rate. As indicated earlier, entry into L5-S1 was the most cumbersome level with some one-third of such cases technically impossible to perform.

Discitis has also complicated a single case of PLD among 333 patients studied by Choy. He also relates anecdotal evidence of two bowel perforations during PLD (Choy DSF, personal communication, 1993).

APD may have the best safety record of all. Major complications include only a 0.2% risk of discitis and there have been two reports of severe cauda equina injury in one heavily sedated and in another anesthetized patient.

MR AND CT INNOVATIONS FOR INTRADISCAL THERAPY

Presently, all forms of intradiscal therapy rely on conventional fluoroscopic images for correct localization and instrument placement. Fluoroscopy does not provide images of soft tissue structures, such as the actual herniation, the nerve roots, the dura or intradural contents. Furthermore, the required radiation results in small, but concerning, risk to the patient and occasionally the surgeon, especially with prolonged imaging.

Recently, engineers from the General Electric Corporation and physicians from the Brigham and Women's Hospital of Boston have collaborated in the development of a new intraoperative MR imaging guidance system. A unit was constructed that provides direct access to patients and permits interactive MR guided interventional procedures (Fig. 1) (40). This use of an open configuration, with near real time imaging and interactive image control for the first time allows immediate visualization of the effects of intradiscal therapy (Fig. 2).

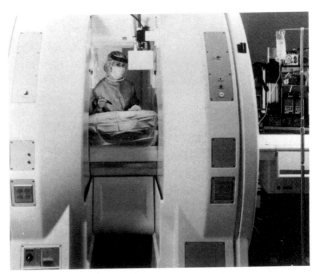

FIG. 1 View of surgeon standing within open configuration magnet MRT system. Note the probe in the surgeon's right hand. This probe uses a light emitting diode-charge coupled device camera (LED-CCD) tracking system to prescribe the scan plane, thereby showing the operator the trajectory of any instrument attached to the probe.

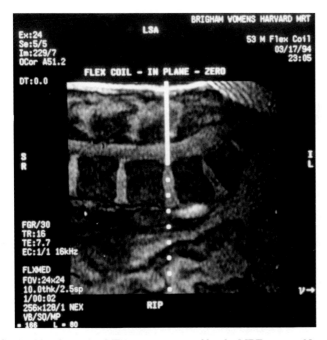

FIG. 2 Sagittal lumbar spine MR image generated by the MRT system. Note the white line on the image indicating the position of a needle attached to the scan-controlling probe. The dotted white line indicates the trajectory of the needle should it be inserted further.

With this system, the potential for complications should be virtually eliminated in terms of injury to nerve root and/or the cauda equina. The actual visualization of the herniation and the subsequent reduction size may be seen in real time during intradiscal therapy. The absence of radiation makes the procedure safe from both a patient and a physician viewpoint.

Finally, since it is possible to place the position in an actual sitting position, axial loading with three dimensional visualization is possible and may contribute significantly to removing discs that are symptomatic only during axial loading (Fig. 3).

The primary impediment to use of such instrumentation is the necessity to avoid the use of any ferro magnetic materials because such objects are strongly attracted by the magnetic field. Instead, non-ferro magnetic materials, such as aluminum, titanium, and ceramic must be used.

In addition to tremendous advances in MR technology, the Toshiba Company recently reported new CT applications that may revolutionize

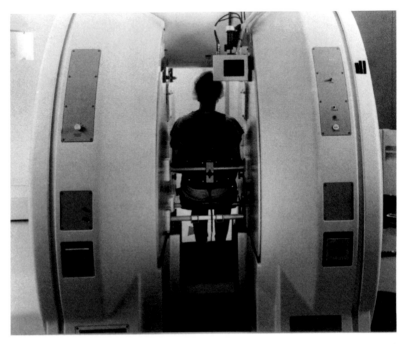

FIG. 3 Patient seated in the MRT system for imaging of the loaded lumbar spine. Note the wire leading from the backrest, which contains the built-in surface radiofrequency coils used for imaging.

intradiscal therapy, as well as other forms of interventional treatments. In 1993, engineers from the Systems Design Group of Toshiba began developing CT fluoroscopy and real time helical scan CT with the combination of a newly developed array processor and a new reconstruction algorithm (26). These features resulted in the development of a system that permitted instantaneous reconstruction of CT images at a speed of six images per second with a delay time of approximately 0.6 seconds. Using this system, essentially real time viewing of CT images has become possible. Although it does not have the resolution of MR, this system certainly visualizes the disc herniation and intraspinal contents in such a way that percutaneous puncture and manipulation could be effected in a much more efficient manner than with fluoroscopy alone.

The challenges facing CT fluoroscopy include: radiation exposure, metallic artifact, artifact resulting from reconstruction, the delay time, and restricted puncture directions. With time, however, it is anticipated that these challenges will be overcome.

CONCLUSION

Over the last 30 years, surgeons have been persistent in seeking more minimally invasive techniques for relieving the incapacitating pain associated with herniated lumbar discs. Various types of enzyme dissolution, grasping, sucking, and aspirating devices, and more recently the application of laser energy have all been used with relative success. The "relative success" seems to be largely dependent on patient selection and the degree of disc herniation and its configuration.

With the recent introduction of near real time MR and CT fluoroscopic imaging, we may now be on the threshold of major advancements in the application of intradiscal forms of therapy. By combining the various intradiscal and imaging modalities, absolutely precise needle placement with the marked reduction in the possibility of complications and the actual real time visualization of what is happening with the disc herniation is possible.

We believe we are on the threshold of using intradiscal therapies in a most precise, accurate and meaningful manner relative to application, as well patient selection.

REFERENCES

1. Agre K, Wilson RR, Brim M, *et al.*: Chymodiactin post marketing surveillance. **Spine** 9:479, 1984.
2. Bernhardt M, Gurganious L, Bloom DL, *et al.*: MRI analysis of percutaneous discectomy. **Spine** 18:211, 1993.
3. Bocchi L, Ferrata P, Passarello F, *et al.*: La nucleoaspirazione secondo Onik nel trattamento del'ernia discale lumbare analisi multicentrica dei risultati su oltre 650 trattamenti. **Riv Neuroradiol** 2 (Suppl 1):119, 1989.
4. Castro WHM, Jerosch J, Hepp R, *et al.*: Restrictions of indication for automated percutaneous lumbar discectomy based on CT discography. **Spine** 17:1239, 1992.
5. Castro WHM, Jerosch J, Rohdhuis J, *et al.*: Biomechanical changes of the lumbar intervertebral disc after automated and non automated percutaneous discectomy: An *in vitro* investigation. **Eur Spine J** 1:96, 1992.
6. Choy DSJ, Ascher PW, Saddekni S, *et al.*: Percutaneous laser disc decompression. **Spine** 17:949, 1992.
7. Davis JK: Early experience with laser disc decompression. **J Florida M A** 79:37, 1992.
8. Day PL: Lateral approach for lumbar discogram and chemonucleolysis. **Clin Orthop** 67:90, 1969.
9. Edwards WC, Orme TJ, Orr-Edwards G: CT discography: Prognostic value in the selection of patients for chemonucleolysis. **Spine** 12:792, 1987.
10. Epstein NE: Surgically confirmed cauda equina and nerve root injury following percutaneous discectomy at an outside institution: A case report. **J Spinal Dis** 3:380, 1990.
11. Fager CA: Percutaneous discectomy. **J Neurosurg** 67:150, 1987 (letter).

12. Fraser RD: Chymopapain for the treatment of intervertebral disc herniation. A preliminary report of a double-blind study. **Spine** 7:608, 1982.
13. Freis J, Abodely D, Vijungo J, et al.: CT of herniated and extruded nucleus pulposus. **J Comput Assist Tomogr** 6:874, 1982.
14. Garvin PJ, Jennings RB, Smith L, et al.: Chymopapain: A pharmacologic and toxicologic evaluation in experimental animals. **Clin Orthop** 42:204, 1965.
15. Grogan WJ, Fraser RD: Chymopapain. A ten-year double-blind study. **Spine** 17:388, 1992.
16. Hal BB, McCulloch JA: Anaphylactic reactions following the intradiscal injection of chymopapain under local anesthesia. **J Bone Joint Surg** 65A:1215, 1983.
17. Hijikata S: Percutaneous nucleotomy. A new concept technique and 12 years' experience. **Clin Orthop** 238:9, 1989.
18. Hoppenfeld S: Percutaneous removal of herniated lumbar discs. 50 cases with ten-year follow-up periods. **Clin Orthop** 238:92, 1989.
19. Hopper K, Sherman J, Kuethke J, et al.: The retrorenal colon in the supine and prone patient. **Radiology** 162:443, 1987.
20. Jackson RP, Cain JE, Jacobs RR: Neuroradiographic diagnosis of lumbar herniated nucleus pulposus. **Spine** 14:1362, 1989.
21. Javid MJ, Norby EJ, Ford LT, et al.: Safety and efficacy of chymopapain (Chymodiactin) in herniated nucleus pulposus with sciatica. **JAMA** 249:2489, 1983.
22. Javid, M: A 1- to 4-year follow-up review of treatment of sciatica using chemonucleolysis or laminectomy. **J Neurosurg** 76:184, 1992.
23. Kahanovitz N, Viola K, Goldstein T, et al.: A multi-center analysis of percutaneous discectomy. **Spine** 15:713, 1990.
24. Kambin P, Sampson S: Posterolateral percutaneous suction-excision of herniated lumbar intervertebral discs. **Clin Orthop** 107:37, 1986.
25. Kambin P, Schaffer JL: Percutaneous lumbar discectomy. Review of 100 patients and current practice. **Clin Orthop** 238:24, 1989.
26. Katada K: Further innovations in CT technology—CT fluoroscopy and real-time helical scan CT. **Toshiba Med Rev** 53:1, 1995.
27. MacNab I, McCulloch HA, Weiner DS, et al.: Chemonucleolysis. **Can J Surg** 14:280, 1971.
28. Maroon JC, Allen RC: A retrospective study of 1,054 APLD cases: A twenty-month clinical follow-up at 35 US centers. **J Neurol Orthop Med Surg** 10:335, 1989.
29. Maroon JC, Onik G, Quigley MR, et al.: Automated percutaneous lumbar discectomy. Indications, techniques and results, in Hardy RW (ed): *Lumbar Disc Disease*. New York, Raven Press, 1993, pp 147–153.
30. Mayer HM, Brock M: Complications of percutaneous discectomy, in Tarlov EC (ed): *Complications of Spinal Surgery Neurosurgical Topics*. Park Ridge, American Association of Neurological Surgeons, 1991, pp 115–127.
31. Mayer MM, Brock M: Percutaneous endoscopic discectomy: Surgical technique and preliminary results compared to microsurgical discectomy. **J Neurosurg** 78:216, 1993.
32. McCulloch JA: Chemonucleolysis: Experience with 2,000 cases. **Clin Orthop** 146:128, 1980.
33. Morris J, Onik GM: Percutaneous nucleotomy, in White A, Rothman RH, Ray CD (eds): *Lumbar Spine Surgery*. St. Louis, CV Mosby, 1987, pp 141–147.
34. Onik G, Helms CA, Ginsberg L, et al.: Percutaneous lumbar discectomy using a new aspiration probe. **AJNR** 6:290, 1985; **AJR** 144: 1137, 1985.

35. Onik G, Mooney V, Maroon JC, *et al.*: APD: A prospective multi-institutional study. **Neurosurgery** 26:228, 1990.

36. Onik G, Maroon JC, Jackson R: Cauda equina injury from percutaneous discectomy. **Neurosurgery** 20:412, 1992.

37. Pappas CTE, Harrington T, Sonntag VKH: Outcome analysis in 654 surgically treated lumbar disc herniations. **Neurosurgery** 30:862, 1992.

38. Ramirez LR, Thisted R: Complications and demographic characteristics of patients undergoing lumbar discectomy in community hospitals. **Neurosurgery** 25:226, 1989.

39. Sachs BL, Vanharanta H, Spivey MA, *et al.*: Dallas discogram description. A new classification of CT/discography in low-back disorders. **Spine** 12:287, 1987.

40. Schenck JF, Jolesz FA, Roemer PB, *et al.*: Superconducting open-configuration MR imaging system for image-guided therapy. **Radiology** 195:805, 1995.

41. Schreiber A, Suezawa Y: Transdiscopic percutaneous nucleotomy in disc herniation. **Orthop Rev** 15:75, 1986.

42. Schreiber A, Suezawa Y, Leu H: Does percutaneous nucleotomy with discoscopy replace conventional discectomy? **Clin Orthop** 128:35, 1989.

43. Sherk HH, Rhodes A, Black J, *et al.*: Results of percutaneous lumbar discectomy with lasers, in Sherk HH (ed): *Spine: State of the Art Reviews Laser Discectomy.* Philadelphia, Henley & Belfus, 1993, vol 7; pp 141–150.

44. Silvers HR: Microsurgical versus standard lumbar discectomy. **Neurosurgery** 22:837, 1988.

45. Smith L: Enzyme dissolution of the nucleus pulposus in humans. **JAMA** 187:137, 1964.

46. Stolke D, Sollmann WP, Seifert V: Intra- and postoperative complications in lumbar disc surgery. **Spine** 14:56, 1989.

47. Suezawa Y, Jacob HAC: Percutaneous nucleotomy. An alternative to spinal surgery. **Arch Orthop Trauma Surg** 105:287, 1986.

48. Vanharanta H, Sachs BL, Spivey MA, *et al.*: Relation of pain provocation to lumbar disc deterioration as seen by CT/discography. **Spine** 12:295, 1987.

49. Watts C: Complications of Chemonucleolysis for lumbar disc disease. **Neurosurgery** 1:2, 1977.

18

The Case for Posterior Lumbar Interbody Fusion

CHARLES L. BRANCH, JR., M.D.

The role of lumbar fusion in the treatment of degenerative lumbar disc disease remains somewhat controversial, even in the face of an apparent increase in its popularity over the last decade. Improvements in diagnostic imaging, the development of new spinal instrumentation systems, and possibly changing perceptions with regard to lumbar disc disease have all contributed to a more widespread belief that, in selected patients, fusion may be superior to nonsurgical therapy or discectomy alone. Posterior lumbar interbody fusion has emerged as a technique that combines discectomy and neural decompression, using the traditional posterior approach with an interbody fusion that may be biomechanically superior to a fusion of the laminae or transverse processes.

HISTORY AND DEVELOPMENT

The concept of lumbar interbody fusion probably should be attributed to Mercer (42), who mentioned it in 1936 but suggested that the surgical difficulties would make it technically impossible. By 1943, the technical difficulties proved not to be insurmountable, and Cloward developed the technique of posterior lumbar interbody fusion (PLIF) using iliac crest grafts after discectomy. He presented his early results at various meetings between 1945 and 1951 and first published his technique and results in 1953 (12). For a series of 321 cases, he reported limited complications and satisfactory results in "over 85 per cent." Concurrent with Cloward's early operation (using iliac crest bone,) Ovens and Williams (45) in 1945 and Jaslow (29) in 1946 reported using bone from the spinous process or the posterior element as the preferred graft material for PLIF after diskectomy. Variations of both techniques evolved over the next 40 years.

Pedicle screw plate fixation as an adjunct to the PLIF was reported by Steffee and Sitkowski (54) in 1988 and was the first major alteration of the earlier PLIF techniques. Immediate internal fixation was hailed by some as an advantage over PLIF alone, and experience using different fixation techniques has since been reported (58). Routine use of segmental internal fixation appears to be of value for some indications, as it may enhance fusion potential.

More recent advances include the development of metallic and carbon fiber implants for use as interbody grafts or struts in addition to, or in lieu of, a cancellous bone graft (7,55). The proposed value of this adjunct is a standardized interbody support material that will eliminate or diminish graft settling or retropulsion. Electromagnetic field stimulation appears to be a fusion enhancement technique. A randomized double-blind study of the use of a brace with an electromagnetic field stimulator in interbody fusion patients has shown a significant increase in fusion rate over that in a placebo group (43).

NATURAL HISTORY OF DEGENERATIVE LUMBAR DISC DISEASE

The case for PLIF begins with the natural degenerative process of the lumbar disc and intervertebral motion segment. The process of disc degeneration is complex and affects not only the disc itself but also the surrounding vertebrae, facets, and supporting ligaments. Chronic or repeated elevation of intradiscal pressure results in narrowing of the disc space with a decrease in intradiscal water concentration and an increase in the concentration of collagen (1, 21, 33).

As illustrated here the disc becomes dessicated, with fissures in the cartilaginous plates and annulus. There is mucoid degeneration; an accumulation of gas in the disc, an ingrowth of fibrocartilage; and ultimate obliteration of the nucleus pulposus. From this condition arises annular tension and bulging with reactive bone formation (osteophytes) and ultimate disc space collapse and arthrodesis.

It appears, then, that the natural history or process of spinal degeneration involves a period of dysfunction that progresses to instability, then, ultimately, to stabilization, the concept of which is illustrated in the chart from Kirkaldy-Willis (31). If one ascribes to this concept, which appears to be valid, then there is a point in time at which, for the treatment of symptomatic degenerative disease, a stabilizing fusion becomes advantageous. When and where along this continuum, and for what particular pathologic entities, is still subject to much debate.

The first argument in the case for PLIF is summarized by the concept that the natural progression of disc degeneration is toward collapse and arthrodesis, with the interval between early mildly symptomatic dysfunction and ultimate arthrodesis punctuated by symptomatic dysfunction and/or instability. Surgically accelerated arthrodesis may complete the natural progression and provide symptomatic relief.

BIOMECHANICS

Biomechanically, one may determine or postulate the vector forces acting upon the lumbar spine. Kummer suggests that there are two major vector forces, the muscle force and gravity. The resultant force acting upon the lumbar spine passes through the disc (34). Schlegel and Pon, in their analysis of this concept in spondylolisthesis, suggest that additional translational forces create an environment in which the interbody graft that places the anterior and posterior ligaments in tension and occupies a significant surface area of the end plate is the optimal fusion construct (49).

INDICATIONS

The reported indications for PLIF include those for both surgical and nonsurgical treatment of degenerative lumbar spine disease. Cloward's global indication was "the treatment of low back pain with or without sciatica due to lumbar disc disease" (12). This attitude was in all likelihood responsible for much of the controversy that initially surrounded this technique; yet Cloward's reported results are enviable. Efforts by others to refine the indications have created lengthy lists of more "specific" conditions but have not significantly narrowed the scope of Cloward's indications. Keim (30) included in his list an unstable joint complex associated with a long history of low back pain, facet resection from previous surgery, heavy labor or sports activity associated with simple disc herniation, bilateral or massive midline disc herniation, previous disc surgery, failed back surgery syndrome, obesity with a lateral disc herniation, and focal spinal stenosis, spondylolisthesis, or other symptomatic congenital anomaly. Lin and Gill (22), Farfan and Kirkaldy-Willis (19), and others (17, 51) have proposed similar indications, most of which were based on the ill-defined term "segmental instability." Frymoyer (20), in his review, gave this definition: "Segmental instability is an abnormal response to applied loads, characterized by motion in motion segments beyond normal constraints." However, with the exception of an obvious instability seen radiographically, it is often difficult to determine the specific origin of symptoms in a spine with degenerative changes at a single level or at multiple levels. Likewise, with the exception of the multiple recurrent disc herniations at the same level, it is difficult to determine, in the majority of patients with a simple disc herniation or spinal stenosis, who will and who will not enjoy protracted relief of symptoms after a simple discectomy or decompression.

The value of discography of a diagnostic tool has long been debated (44). Although recent evidence indicates that it may be a reliable means of assessing pain originating from the intervertebral disc (60), whether it also is reliably predictive of a good outcome with fusion has been difficult to determine (23).

The theoretical advantages of PLIF have been discussed by Cautilli (9), who listed them as: (a) a wide area of bone surface; (b) adequate blood supply through the cancellous portion of the vertebral body, once the cortical plate has been perforated or removed; (c) a fusion proximate to the centers of motion and of compression forces; (d) complete visualization of the area of nerve root compression and complete access for removal of areas of compression both centrally and laterally; and (e) preservation or restoration of the interbody distance so that there will be no further disc-space collapse or possible lateral stenosis as a sequela of the disc excision.

The intervertebral surface area that must be occupied by graft to prevent failure under a 600-N load in a thoracic spine model has been studied and appears to be 30%, according to Closkey and colleagues (11). This minimum or critical area appears to increase with increased load or decreased trabecular bone density in the adjacent vertebral bodies. Evans reinforces the concept of the biomechanical superiority of the interbody fusion with a comparison to a tripod or flagpole with supporting wires or cables. The axial force along the pole is supported by the interbody graft with the annulus, facet, and posterior spinous ligaments acting as tension bands or guide wires (18). In contrast, Stambough (52) contends that PLIF is biomechanically unsound, because it disrupts the posterior and middle columns and a portion of the anterior column in an attempt to achieve long-term stability by means of interbody fusion. In the absence of these posterior supporting elements, a segmental internal fixation device, such as the pedicle screw and VSP device of Steffee, restores this posterior tension band and enhances the likelihood of successful fusion (53).

A second argument derives from the evidence that the interbody graft is a biomechanically superior construct when the posterior supporting structures remain competent or are substituted with a segmental internal fixation device. The disc space height and foraminal area are restored. The graft is in compression between vascular vertebral bodies, and the annular and posterior ligamentous tissues are placed in tension-resisting rocking or translational motion.

Magnetic resonance imaging (MRI), with and without enhancement with gadolinium, has improved the capacity to visualize the degenerated disc and the reactive changes in the adjacent vertebral bodies. It also reliably differentiates postoperative epidural fibrosis from recurrent disc herniation with neural compression. These findings, coupled with an appropriate clinical presentation, often provide the most valuable information with which to make a decision regarding a PLIF.

It is very difficult to develop a scientifically derived set of indications for PLIF. Inability to determine or to image symptomatic segmental instability, clouded by psychosocioeconomic factors in both patients and physicians, contributes to this difficulty.

The available literature, personal experience, and advice from colleagues with extensive experience combine to suggest that the set of indications for PLIF ranges from strong to mild. "Strong" indications are present in the patient who is unlikely to obtain even temporary symptomatic relief with return to normal activity unless a PLIF or comparable stabilizing fusion is performed. These are also the patients in whom internal fixation will enhance fusion potential. "Mild to moderate" indications are found in patients who may obtain symptomatic relief with nonsurgical or decompressive surgical therapy alone, but in whom this relief may be incomplete or short-lived, once the patient returns to reasonably normal activity.

The indications for which I now routinely consider PLIF without internal fixation include: recurrent lumbar disc herniation and nonoperated or virgin broad-based or centrally herniated discs with significant loss of disc space height. Internal fixation is generally used with PLIF in patients with pseudoarthrosis, postlaminectomy spondylolisthesis, and degenerative or lytic spondylolisthesis and for patients with stenosis adjacent to a previous fusion.

A significant deficiency in the reported experience with PLIF is the lack of uniform analysis of the outcome on the basis of specific indications. Although several large series have been reported with analyses of outcome for specific indications (15, 27, 38), differences in technique, differences in outcome, and a relative vagueness in the description of the indication for PLIF, as opposed to a decompressive procedure or an alternative fusion technique, make it somewhat difficult to apply this information to the development of a list of special indications in which PLIF will be the superior procedure.

Recurrent Herniated Lumbar Disc Disease

The incidence of symptomatic recurrent lumbar disc herniation is still somewhat difficult to ascertain. Reported incidence requiring reoperation ranges from 1.3 to 21%. Criteria for reoperation vary but reherniations occur, and are generally associated with a less favorable outcome with each recurrence. Tria et al. (57) and Vaughan et al. (58) have reported substantially decreased reoperation rates if fusion is used in conjunction with discectomy.

While the strength of the indication is mild to moderately strong, conceptually it makes sense that if the PLIF can be done quickly and safely, with satisfactory fusion rates, it will eliminate the potential for reoperation at that level and effectively decompress neural elements. The strength of the indication increases if there have been multiple same-side, same-level disc herniations.

Lin *et al.* (38) reported the results with PLIF for 143 patients who had recurrent disc herniation with at least 1-year of follow-up. A satisfactory outcome was reported in 74% of all patients (106 of 143) and in 80% when the compensation group was omitted. Satisfactory fusion was reported at 149 levels (92%). Branch and Branch (6) reviewed 46 cases, 50% of which were compensation cases, with a mean follow-up interval of 12 months and an average of 1.4 prior operations. A satisfactory outcome was documented in 35 patients (76%), which compared favorably with the outcome in similar patients treated by the senior author with laminectomy alone (40% satisfactory outcome) or with laminectomy and lateral fusion (66% satisfactory outcome). Our experience over the last 5 years with 125 patients indicates that a satisfactory outcome can be achieved in 75%.

Central or Midline Lumbar Disc Herniations

A more troublesome situation is encountered with the broad-based midline protrusion or frank midline herniation in the patient who has not been previously operated on. Walker *et al.* reported a substantially worse outcome in these patients, as compared to those who had more lateral disc herniations, and suggested that a more generous decompression was warranted (59). The author personally agrees with part of this concept and will attempt to illustrate the rationale behind that agreement.

Most likely, the midline disc herniations are associated with greater annular disruption with destabilization of the disc. Therefore, a simple laminectomy and discectomy or percutaneous discectomy may decompress the neural elements but does not repair and, in fact, may worsen this substantial disruption of the posterior annulus and longitudinal ligaments. This situation, in the author's opinion, is ideally treated with a PLIF that restores disc space height, supports axial load, and resists torsional or shear stress and, in addition, prevents a recurrence at that level.

Degenerative Spondylolisthesis

Although still somewhat controversial, evidence is mounting to indicate that decompression and fusion are superior to decompression alone in the treatment of symptomatic degenerative spondylolisthesis.

Mardjetko *et al.*, in their meta-analysis of the literature for degenerative spondylolisthesis from 1970 to 1993 found the composite of satisfactory outcome to be 69% without fusion and 90% with fusion with or without internal fixation (41). Herkowitz and Kurz, in their randomized study, demonstrated similar outcomes (25).

As the PLIF appears to be equivalent or superior to lateral fusion techniques, there is a case for the use of PLIF in the treatment of degenerative spondylolisthesis. The canal is decompressed, and the pathologic disc space is restored to its premorbid height and alignment. The bone graft is placed in compression, enhancing fusion potential, and may be successful with or without internal fixation, depending on the integrity of the residual posterior supporting structures.

This case in a 54-year-old woman with neurogenic claudication illustrates this concept. MRI shows the degenerative slip with resultant canal and lateral recess stenosis. The outcome at 1 year with PLIF and segmental internal fixation was excellent.

Postlaminectomy Spondylolisthesis

It appears that there may be an increasing incidence of postlaminectomy spondylolisthesis or symptomatic instability without radiographic slip. The presence of an aging population with several decades of nonfused decompressive laminectomy patients makes this a potentially sizeable group in the future.

In the radiographically obvious slip group, the indication for fusion and even internal fixation is almost noncontroversial. Hutter's experience (27) with PLIF in 124 patients with spinal stenosis who had been previously operated on reveals a satisfactory clinical outcome in 78%, with a fusion rate of 91%.

Posterior lumbar interbody fusion and segmental internal fixation with pedicle screw-plate devices appears to be ideal, as the foraminal and central canal area is restored, and the missing posterior tension band is recreated with the fixation device. In selected cases, the PLIF alone or in conjunction with lateral transverse process and facet fusion may provide satisfactory treatment as has been reported by Hutter, Lin and others (6, 15, 38). An illustrative case is of a 50-year-old woman who had undergone a laminectomy for the removal of a cauda equina ependymoma and experienced a significant slip that occurs with chronic erosive changes of the vertebrae. Standing or even sitting in an upright position had become exquisitely painful in both the back and legs. Decompression of the reparative pannus, incompetent facets, and scar with PLIF and pedicle screw-plate fixation resulted in both dramatic and rapid relief of her symptoms.

Adjacent Segment Degeneration

Another group in which PLIF may play an increasing role is in the operative treatment of the degenerated segment adjacent to a lumbar fusion. Whitecloud et al. in their small series found that in the five patients with adjacent segment stenosis subsequently treated with an uninstrumented lateral fusion to include that level, only the patient who also had an interbody fusion went on to solid arthrodesis, whereas 10 of 12 patients with instrumented lateral fusions fused (61). Biomechanically, PLIF is a superior fusion construct and may prevent the need for internal fixation if preservation of adequate posterior elements is possible.

This is illustrated in the case of a 52-year-old meat cutter who returned to work after his first PLIF for recurrent lumbar disc herniations. He once again developed disabling pain and his CT postmyelogram and conventional myelogram study revealed a stenosis at L3–L4, the segment adjacent to the previous PLIF. The posterior elements were sufficient to allow for a PLIF at the symptomatic level without internal fixation.

In most cases, though, the existence of adjacent internal fixation probably increases the potential for pseudoarthrosis with PLIF alone, and the author routinely revises the internal fixation to include the adjacent segment in addition to PLIF. A 70-year-old patient with a long segment fusion and internal fixation developed adjacent degeneration and instability over 2 years. Decompression and revision of internal fixation to cross the thoracolumbar junction provided significant symptomatic relief.

TECHNIQUES

Cloward's technique requires an interlaminar exposure of the affected disc space with removal of the disc and cortical endplate using a variety of curettes and osteotomes. An interlaminar spreader is used to facilitate exposure and to provide distraction for graft insertion. Once the space has been prepared to a depth of 3 cm, the cortical endplate is perforated or removed to create bleeding surfaces. Three or four bicortical or tricortical iliac crest grafts are inserted into the space and manipulated medially using Puka chisels until all grafts are seated in the space. A complete illustration and description of the technique by Cloward is reproduced in the Codman technical manual (14).

Lin (37) modified this technique with the "unigraft" concept of filling the disc space with cancellous bone in addition to the cortical grafts. Lin's goal was to have the cancellous bone appear radiographically as dense as the cortical bone and thereby to facilitate more rapid fusion. Cloward (35) was somewhat critical of this modification, claiming that it did not improve upon his already satisfactory success rate.

Variations in the shape or size of the iliac crest graft material have been developed by others. Hutter (26, 28) used a reverse wedge graft to diminish the potential for graft extrusion. Wiltberger (62) and

Blume (2, 3) described dowel graft techniques. Modifications of the instrumentation to facilitate safer, more rapid, and more standardized preparation of the disc space or graft placement also have been proposed. Ma (39, 40) described a mortise chisel device for both disc and endplate removal and for graft placement. The Total Disc Replacement system of Collis (15, 16) uses progressively larger disc space shapers for the rapid removal of the disc and cortical endplates. In all of these techniques, both autogenous and banked bone grafts have been used with similar success rates.

The major variation from the Cloward technique and its modifications is the use of posterior bony elements as the interbody graft material. As previously noted, Owens and Williams (45) first placed the spinous process in the disc space as a graft material. Briggs and Milligan (8) described the use of posterior elements cut into corticocancellous chips and impacted into the interspace. This technique was modified by Simmons (50, 51) using the Ma instrumentation for vigorous impaction of the bone chips. A larger piece of the lamina and facet complex was used as the graft by Christoferson (10).

Branch (4, 5) developed the keystone wedge technique, in which smaller chips or matchstick fragments are impacted anteriorly in the disc space, and the larger corticocancellous midline laminar arch is impacted posteriorly as a keystone-shaped wedge.

The addition of an internal fixation device to the PLIF has been hailed by some as an advantage over the previously described techniques, especially when there is removal or disruption of the posterior bony elements (18, 53, 56). A variety of fixation devices is available, and all provide rigid internal segmental fixation (32). However, the indications for this additional internal fixation remain controversial, but the addition of internal fixation appears to consistently increase the fusion rate. Satisfactory results with the PLIF technique without internal fixation, even when the posterior element is removed, have been reported in large series.

COMPLICATIONS

The potential for significant complications with PLIF should be considered and may be cited as a reason to consider an alternative, potentially less effective technique. Surgeons experienced with the PLIF technique generally acknowledge that it is technically demanding and that it requires a thorough knowledge of the regional anatomy and careful attention to detail (14, 37, 51)

In Lin's review (37) of PLIF complications and their avoidance in five collected series involving over 2,000 patients, the symptomatic graft retropulsion rate ranged from 0.3 to 2.4%. Lin also noted that that rate was 1.6% in other series with 60 to 700 patients, whereas it was 9% in series with only 3 to 60 patients, thus showing a correlation between the complication rate and the experience of the surgeon. Lin also listed the technical details that must be adhered to in order to prevent graft retropulsion.

The incidence of clinically significant pseudoarthrosis is very difficult to determine. Flexion-extension films, tomography, MRI, technetium bone scanning, and computed tomography (CT) all may reflect stability of the graft, but they do not determine the fusion or graft incorporation endpoint or detect a subtle lack of integrity of the fusion (36). The author is currently investigating the value of SPECT (single photon emitted computed tomography) in the diagnosis of pseudoarthrosis. Prolo (46) reviewed an extensive experience with the physiology of bone fusion, placing particular emphasis on posterior interbody fusion. However, his clinical paradigm for the evaluation of the success of interbody fusion was not physiological, but rather the anteroposterior and lateral radiographic appearance of the fusion (47). Mooney (43), after describing an elegant method for the quantitative analysis of new bone formation in the laboratory, still relied on the radiographic appearance of the fusion to analyze the rate of fusion augmented by pulsed electromagnetic stimulation.

RESULTS

The reported rate of successful fusions ranges from 50 to 94% (13, 15, 16, 26, 37, 43, 48), with most authors reporting an 85 to 90% successful fusion rate. However, any scientific assessment of the outcome or results of a technique based upon retrospective reviews would be unsound. In fact, it may be that even with a prospective randomized study it will be extremely difficult to make a scientifically valid broad or general assessment of outcome due to the many indications, technical variations, and patient variables involved. A global review of results gleaned from the PLIF literature is found in Simmons' recent review (51), which reported satisfactory clinical outcomes ranging from 54 to 94%.

Cloward's (13) series of 100 patients with lytic spondylolisthesis had documented "long-term" follow-up (exact interval not noted) in 97 patients. At the time of follow-up or death, 95 patients had an excellent or good outcome, and 94 had a radiographically apparent fusion. Three patients had a pseudoarthrosis but had not undergone reoperation. Hutter (27) reviewed 142 patients with spinal stenosis, 124 (87%) of whom had had one or more prior operations. The follow-up interval was at least 3 years, and the fusion rate was 91%. Clinical outcome was excellent or good in 78% of the entire group, and in 98% of patients who had not undergone a prior operation. Hutter compared this technique with conventional decompressive therapy, using reports indicating a 15 to 20% short-term failure and a 50% long-term failure as the standards against which PLIF for this indication was compared. These above reports, like many in the literature, document the experience with PLIF and report good clinical outcomes with this technique, but contain significant deficiencies that hinder the application of this experience to certain questions or to specific clinical statistics.

In patients with spondylolisthesis and stenosis, it is difficult to document an obvious superiority of the PLIF technique over other fusion techniques. However, when PLIF is performed by a careful, experienced surgeon, it does not appear to carry undue hazard, and a satisfactory outcome can be anticipated in the majority of cases. With recurrent disc disease, the reported satisfactory outcome at the second operation is 40 to 50% with laminectomy and discectomy alone, this incidence dropping by 50% with each similar subsequent operation (24). In view of these findings, PLIF may have a significant advantage for this indication.

An analysis of PLIF failures by Wetzel and LaRocca indicates that clinical outcome may not correlate with fusion in the presence of a chronic radiculopathy. The author has found this to be especially true in the recurrent disc herniation group. Another observation from this report confirms the role of adjacent segment degeneration in recurrent or persistent symptoms after a successful fusion at one level. The report by Verlooy may be a good example of the importance of preservation of the posterior tension band, of placing the graft in compression, and maximizing the graft vertebral interface, as their failure to do this in this group of spondylolisthesis patients resulted in what appears to be a 50% fusion rate.

The author's experience over the past 5 years with this groups of patients has been increasingly favorable. In all, 355 patients have been treated with PLIF with or without internal fixation. Those with traumatic or neoplastic lesions are not included. Patients in each diagnostic category had satisfactory outcomes ranging from 66 to 88%.

By and large these are challenging patients who have been previously operated upon. Operative time is not exorbitant and has steadily decreased, helping to control both cost and complication rates. Mean operative time in the 40 patients treated most expeditiously was 4 hours in 1992 to 1993 and 3 hours, 10 minutes in 1994 to 1995. Both the outcomes and the ability to perform this technique expeditiously certainly add to the arguments for PLIF.

SUMMARY

The accumulated experience with PLIF over more than four decades seems to validate this technique and the described variations as reasonably safe and efficacious. It is difficult to determine the indications for which PLIF is a superior procedure, although there is evidence that for recurrent lumbar disc herniation it may be superior to discectomy or decompression alone. The indications for which supplementing the PLIF or any fusion technique with internal fixation is superior have yet to be determined. In the presence of gross instability, the addition of internal fixation for more rapid resolution of symptoms and to enhance fusion rate appears to be reasonable, but routine or indiscriminant augmentation of lumbar fusion with instrumentation is not supported by the literature. Theoretically, PLIF is advantageous in the absence of, or with disruption of, the posterior elements, but experience indicates that this is not always true. In the patient with intractable, posturally related back pain and degenerative disc disease or segmental instability in whom a fusion appears to be indicated, PLIF theoretically appears to be superior to lateral fusion. The difficulties in reliably identifying symptomatic segmental instability force this indication into the arena of judgment on the part of the surgeon experienced with this technique and knowledgeable about the natural history and outcomes of alternative surgical procedures for lumbar spinal disorders. Yet, it also potentiates the misapplication or misuse of PLIF when a nonsurgical or less morbid technique might have resulted in an equivalent, or even superior, outcome.

There are in fact some significant arguments in the case against PLIF or any fusion as Deyo et al. propose. With an extensive review of literature reporting lumbar spine fusion, they could not determine a general consensus on indications for fusion. In a population of Medicare patients, they could not find a significant advantage over nonfusion. Their conclusion is that variations in methodology for the determination of indications and subsequent outcome assessment in addition to the fusion techniques have made it difficult to retrospectively show a benefit with fusion in this large, tremendously varied population.

For global indications for PLIF, a recent review by Rish (48) of his own experience with 455 patients is of interest. These patients showed no significant difference in clinical outcome between patients treated with PLIF and patients treated with laminectomy and discectomy alone. Yet the technique appeared to reduce the number of recurrent problems requiring repeat surgery. This should serve as a reminder that PLIF may be superior only if used for specific indications.

The inadequacy of historical or retrospective reviews to identify uniformly applicable results with specific indications contributes to the persistent controversy surrounding this technique. Rapid developments in and indiscriminate use of internal fixation to augment, or to use in lieu of, PLIF may, in fact, delay or prevent the resolution of certain basic questions, i.e., which PLIF techniques are equivalent therapy and for which indications is PLIF a consistently superior alternative therapy. The results of prospective uniform analysis to resolve these basic questions are desirable. These are but a few of the arguments that have been raised against not only the PLIF, but against fusions in general, and even against spine surgery in general! The close of the decade of the brain may in fact herald the dawn of the decade of the outcome study when some of these questions about indications may be answered.

A major difficulty in standardization of technique remains the quality of the bone graft itself. The thought of promoting another implant seems unwise in the light of the current implant atmosphere. Yet, the carbon fiber or titanium interbody grafts or spacers appear to have biomechanically uniform and testable qualities that are superior to bone graft (7). They have performed well in clinical trials. But will elimination of the bone graft-quality variable in favor of an interbody implant truly eliminate a variable or introduce more?

Without a doubt, PLIF and fusion in general have their unanswered questions, just like every other intellectually and technically demanding area of our specialty. As with skull base, cerebrovascular, and other highly specialized procedures, a satisfactory outcome with this technique is very surgeon- or operator-dependent. If as neurosurgeons we abandon and criticize theoretically sound, but technically demanding, techniques after a few less than satisfactory attempts, will we continue to elevate the standard of care beyond its current level? Our heritage is doing what most others can't or won't do, and doing it well through persistence and a desire to be the best.

Is there a case for the PLIF? I believe there is for the reasons that I have presented, and there may be others that I've overlooked or omitted. As indications and techniques are refined, I believe that the concept of interbody fusion has stood and will continue to stand the test of time as the superior spinal arthrodesis.

REFERENCES

1. Benzel EC: *Biomechanics of Spine Stabilization, Principles and Clinical Practice.* New York, McGraw-Hill, 1995.
2. Blume HG: Unilateral posterior lumbar interbody fusion: Simplified dowel technique. **Clin Orthop** 193:75–84, 1985.

3. Blume HG. Unilateral lumbar interbody fusion (posterior approach) utilizing dowel grafts, in Lin PM, Gill K (eds): *Lumbar interbody fusion.* Rockville, MD, Aspen, 1989, pp 201–209.

4. Branch CL, Branch CL Jr: Posterior lumbar interbody fusion with the keystone graft: Technique and results. **Surg Neurol** 27:449–454, 1987.

5. Branch CL, Branch CL Jr: Posterior lumbar interbody fusion: The keystone technique, in Lin PM, Gill K (eds): *Lumbar Interbody Fusion.* Rockville, MD, Aspen, 1989, pp 211–219.

6. Branch CL, Branch CL Jr: Operative management of the failed back syndrome, in Youmans JL (ed): *Neurological Surgery,* 3rd ed. Philadelphia, WB Saunders, 1990, pp 2731–2748.

7. Brantigan JW, Steffee AD, Geiger JM: A carbon fiber implant to aid interbody lumbar fusion. Mechanical testing. **Spine** 16(S):S277–S282, 1991.

8. Briggs H, Milligan PR: Chip fusion of the low back following exploration of the spinal canal. **J Bone Joint Surg Am** 26:125–130, 1944.

9. Cautilli RA: Theoretical superiority of posterior lumbar interbody fusion, in Lin PM (ed): *Posterior Lumbar Interbody Fusion.* Springfield, IL, Charles C. Thomas, 1982, pp 82–93.

10. Christoferson LA, Selland B: Intervertebral bone implants following excision of protruded lumbar discs. **J Neurosurg** 42:401–405, 1975.

11. Closkey RF, Parsons JR, Lee CK, *et al:* Mechanics of interbody spinal fusion, analysis of critical bone graft area. **Spine** 18(8):1011–1015, 1993.

12. Cloward RB: The treatment of ruptured lumbar intervertebral discs by vertebral body fusion. I. Indications, operative technique, after care. **J Neurosurg** 10:154–168, 1953.

13. Cloward RB: Spondylolisthesis: Treatment by branch-laminectomy and posterior interbody fusion. Review of 100 cases. **Clin Orthop** 154:74–82, 1981.

14. Cloward RM: Posterior lumbar interbody fusion (P.L.I.F.), in *Surgical Techniques.* Randolph, MA, Codman, 1990.

15. Collis JS: Total disc replacement: A modified posterior lumbar interbody fusion. Report of 750 cases. **Clin Orthop** 193:64–67, 1985.

16. Collis JS: The technique of total disc replacement: A modified posterior lumbar interbody fusion, in Lin PM, Gill K (eds): *Lumbar Interbody Fusion.* Rockville, MD, Aspen, 1989, pp 221–226.

17. Crock HV: *The Practice of Spinal Surgery.* New York, Springer-Verlag, 1983.

18. Evans JH. Biomechanics of lumbar fusion. **Clin Orthop** 193:38–46, 1985.

19. Farfan HF, Kirkaldy-Willis WH: The present status of spinal fusion in the treatment of lumbar intervertebral joint disorders. **Clin Orthop** 158:198–214, 1981.

20. Frymoyer JW: Segmental instability: overview and classification, in, Frymoyer JW *et al.* (eds): The adult spine. Principles and practices. New York, Raven Press, 1991, pp 1873–1891.

21. Frymoyer JW, Moskowitz RW: Spinal degeneration: Pathogenesis and medical management, in Frymoyer JW (ed): *The Adult Spine.* New York, Raven Press, 1991, pp 611–634.

22. Gill K: Clinical indications for lumbar interbody fusion, in Lin P, Gill K (eds): *Lumbar Interbody Fusion.* Rockville, MD, Aspen, 1989, pp 35–53.

23. Hanley EN Jr, Phillips ED, Kostuik JP: Who should be fused? in Frymoyer JW *et al.* (eds): *The Adult Spine. Principles and Practices.* New York, Raven Press, 1991, pp 1893–1917.

24. Hardy RW: Repeat operation for lumbar disc, in Hardy RW (ed): *Lumbar Disc Disease.* New York, Raven Press, 1982, pp 193–202.

25. Herkowitz HN, Kurz LT: Degenerative lumbar spondylolisthesis with spinal stenosis. **J Bone Joint Surg** 73A:802–808, 1991.
26. Hutter CG: Posterior intervertebral body fusion. A 25 year study. **Clin Orthop** 179:86–96, 1983.
27. Hutter CG: Spinal stenosis and posterior lumbar interbody fusion. **Clin Orthop** 193:103–114, 1985.
28. Hutter CG: A technique for posterior lumbar interbody fusion, in Lin PM, Gill K (eds): *Lumbar Interbody Fusion.* Rockville, MD, Aspen, 1989, pp 227–232.
29. Jaslow IA: Intercorporal bone graft in spinal fusion after disc removal. **Surg Gynecol Obstet** 82:215–218, 1946.
30. Keim HA: Indications for spine fusions and techniques. **Clin Neurosurg** 25: 266–275, 1978.
31. Kirkaldy-Willis WH: *Managing Low Back Pain.* New York, Churchill Livingstone, 1983.
32. Krag MH: Spinal fusion. Overview of options and posterior internal fixation devices, in Frymoyer JW *et al.* (eds): *The Adult Spine. Principles and Practices* New York, Raven Press, 1991, pp 1919–1945.
33. Kramer J: *Intervertebral Disc Disease: Causes, Diagnosis, Treatment and Prophylaxis,* 2nd ed. Stuttgart, George Thieme Verlag, 1990, pp 14–47.
34. Kummer B: Funktionelle und pathologische Anatomie der Lendenwirbelsaeule. **Orthop Praxis** 2:84, 1982.
35. Lin PM: A technical modification of Cloward's posterior lumbar interbody fusion. **Neurosurgery** 1:118–124, 1977.
36. Lin PM: Radiographic evidence of posterior lumbar interbody fusion with an emphasis on computed tomographic scanning. **Clin Orthop** 242:158–163, 1989.
37. Lin PM: Technique and complications of posterior lumbar interbody fusion, in Lin PM, Gill K (eds): *Lumbar Interbody Fusion.* Rockville, MD, Aspen, 1989, pp 171–199.
38. Lin PM, Cautilli RA, Joyce MF: Posterior lumbar interbody fusion. **Clin Orthop** 180:154–168, 1983.
39. Ma GWC: Posterior lumbar interbody fusion with specialized instruments. **Clin Orthop** 193:57–63, 1985.
40. Ma GWC: Posterior lumbar interbody fusion with specialized instruments, in Lin PM, Gill K (eds): *Lumbar interbody fusion.* Rockville, MD, Aspen, 1989, pp 243–249.
41. Mardjetko: Spine.
42. Mercer W: Spondylolisthesis: With description of a new method of operative treatment and notes of 10 cases. **Edinburgh Med J** 43:545–572, 1936.
43. Mooney V: A randomized double-blind prospective study of the efficacy of pulsed electromagnetic fields for interbody lumbar fusions. **Spine** 15:708–712, 1990.
44. Nachemson A: Editorial comment: Lumbar discography—Where are we today? **Spine** 14:555–557, 1989.
45. Owens JM, Williams HG: Intervertebral spine fusion with removal of herniated intervertebral disk. **Am J Surg** 70:24–26, 1945.
46. Prolo DJ: Osteosynthesis in lumbar interbody fusion, in Lin PM, Gill K (eds): *Lumbar Interbody Fusions.* Rockville, MD, Aspen, 1989, pp 71–78.
47. Prolo DJ, Oklund SA, Butcher M: Toward uniformity in evaluating the results of lumbar spine operations. A paradigm applied to posterior lumbar interbody fusions. **Spine** 11:601–606, 1986.
48. Rish BL: A critique of posterior lumbar interbody fusion: 12 years experience with 250 patients. **Surg Neurol** 31:281–289, 1989.
49. Schlegel K, Pon A: The biomechanics of posterior lumbar interbody fusion in spondylolisthesis. **Clin Orthop** 193:115, 1985.

50. Simmons JW: Posterior lumbar interbody fusion with posterior elements as chip grafts. **Clin Orthop** 193:85–89.

51. Simmons JW: Posterior lumbar interbody fusion (PLIF), in Frymoyer JW *et al.* (eds): *The Adult Spine. Principles and Practices.* New York, Raven Press, 1991, pp 1961–1987.

52. Stambough JL: Indications for lumbar spine fusion in degenerative lumbar disease. **Contemp Neurosurg** 9:1–6, 1987.

53. Steffee AD: The variable screw placement system with posterior lumbar interbody fusion, in Lin PM, Gill K (eds): *Lumbar Interbody Fusion.* Rockville, MD, Aspen, 1989, pp 81–93.

54. Steffee AD, Sitkowski DJ: Posterior lumbar interbody fusion and plates. **Clin Orthop** 227:99–102, 1988.

55. Stender W, Meissner HJ, Thomas W: Ventral interbody spondylolisthesis using a new plug-shaped implant. **Neurosurg Rev** 13:25–34, 1990.

56. Stonecipher T, Wright S: Posterior lumbar interbody fusion with facet-screw fixation. **Spine** 14:468–471, 1989.

57. Tria: **Clin Orthop,** 1987.

58. Vaughan PA, Malcolm BW, Maistrelli GL: Results of 14-5 disc excision alone versus disc excision and fusion. **Spine** 13(6): 690–695, 1988.

59. Walker JL, Schulak D, Murtagh R: Midline disk herniation of the lumbar spine. **South Med J** 86:13–17, 1993.

60. Weinstein JN, Rydevik BL: The pain of spondylolisthesis. **Semin Spine Surg** 1:100–105, 1989.

61. Whitecloud TS, Davis JM, Olive PM.

62. Wiltberger BR: Intervertebral body fusion by the use of the posterior bone dowel. **Clin Orthop** 3S:69–79, 1964.

CHAPTER

19

Spinal Instrumentation for Degenerative Disease

RICHARD G. FESSLER, M.D., PH.D.

INTRODUCTION

Lumbar fusion, and in particular the use of lumbar instrumentation, for the treatment of degenerative disease of the lumbar spine is relatively controversial. Many surgeons argue that there are few or no indications for the use of lumbar instrumentation for the treatment of degenerative disease. Others are equally ardent in arguing that lumbar stabilization improves their results for surgery of the degenerative lumbar spine. Despite these strongly held opinions, relatively little prospective data exists on this topic.

To attempt to review data relating to this subject, it is important to be absolutely clear which aspect of the multiple "degenerative" disease processes one is considering. For our purposes, degenerative disease of the lumbar spine can be divided into 5 sub categories: (*a*) degenerative disc disease, (*b*) degenerative scoliosis, (*c*) degenerative spondylolisthesis, (*d*) lumbar stenosis, (*e*) postoperative instability. The following review will consider two distinct areas of degenerative disease of the lumbar spine. First a series of reports specifically addressing degenerative disc disease and the use of fusion and instrumentation for the treatment of disc disease will be considered. Second, a series of reports addressing more global issues of degenerative disease of the lumbar spine, including scoliosis, spondylolisthesis, and lumbar stenosis, will be reviewed. For each of these papers relative strengths, weaknesses, results, and conclusions will be evaluated. Finally, through this analysis we will attempt to answer the question, "does lumbar fusion and instrumentation improve the results of surgical treatment of degenerative disease of the lumbar spine?"

DEGENERATIVE DISC DISEASE/HERNIATED NUCLEUS PULPOSUS

Nachlas (3) compared the results of the treatment of herniated nucleus pulposus by excision with fusion and without fusion in nearly 400 patients with a 5-year follow-up. This analysis was retrospectively performed by the surgeon, and introduced a second possible selection bias by allowing follow-up of patients on a voluntary basis. Nachlas reported that patients undergoing fusion for herniated nucleus pulposus remained in the hospital nearly three times as long as non-fusion patients. In addition fusion patients had a higher incidence of shock and phlebothrombosis. Both groups has similar infection rates (Table 1). Fusion patients, however, had a slightly lower incidence of residual backache and radiculitis. There was approximately an equal incidence of patients in each group who complained of residual backache and radiculitis (Table 2). Nachlas defined an excellent clinical result as "freedom from symptoms and disabilities." A very good clinical result was the same as an excellent result except that the patient could have some sensory loss, atrophy, or loss of reflexes. A good result was one in which no disc recurrences, deformities, or disabilities occurred, but the patient had weakness or mild neurologic deficit. A fair result was one in which the patient experienced recurrences with disability and had a painful weak back. A poor result was one in which the patient's symptoms were not relieved. Based on these definitions Nachlas reported a slightly higher incidence of excellent and very good results in patients with fusions (Table 3). Despite slightly improved clinical results in his

TABLE 1

*Hospitalization and Complications in Fused and
Non-Fused Patients Undergoing Lumbar Discectomy*

	Non-Fusion	Fusion
Days in Hospital	15	58
Complications		
Shock	0.39%	2.54%
Infection	4.7%	5.1%
Phlebothrombosis	0.39%	2.54%

Nachlas, 1952.

TABLE 2

Residual Symptoms in Fused and Non-Fused Patients Undergoing Lumbar Discectomy

Residual Syptoms	Non-Fusion	Fusion
Backache only	21.5%	16.1%
Radiculitis	32.8%	29.7%
Both	13.7%	13.5%

Nachlas, 1952.

TABLE 3

End Results in Fused and Non-Fused Patients Undergoing Lumbar Discectomy

	Non-Fusion	Fusion
Excellent	2.3%	5.9%
Very good	12.9%	25.4%
Good	44.6%	38.1%
Fair	18.4%	13.6%
Poor	4.3%	1.7%
Re-operation	17.6%	15.3%

Nachlas, 1952.

fusion patients, Nachlas felt that the longer hospitalization stay, the longer delay in return to work, and the higher complication rate were of greater significance than his slightly improved clinical results. He therefore concluded that disc excision alone is the procedure of choice for the treatment of herniated nucleus pulposus.

White *et al.* (5) compared the use of lumbar laminectomy and discectomy alone versus discectomy with internal fixation and fusion in a prospective and controlled series of patients. Although there were relatively few subjects in this report, and among these few patients multiple lumbar levels were compared, White *et al.* reported that the success rate was equal between the groups. Fusion, however, led to longer recuperative time. Therefore, White *et al.* concluded that spinal fusion played no role in the management of simple herniated nucleus pulposus.

Vaughn (4) retrospectively compared patients undergoing L4/5 discectomy alone versus discectomy and fusion. Disease at only one level was analyzed in this report and patients had a mean follow-up of 7 years. Vaughn defined an excellent clinical result as a patient who had no pain and had returned to all previous activity. A good clinical result was that patient in whom occasional back pain occurred but in whom all activities were resumed. A fair clinical result was that patient who had persistent back pain requiring a brace and a poor clinical result was no relief of pain. Vaughn then categorized excellent and good results as "satisfactory," and fair and poor results as "unsatisfactory." Vaughn reported that 85% of his patients who had satisfactory results had successful fusion of L4/5. Patients who did not achieve successful fusion, or who were not fused, had only a 39% satisfactory rate (Table 4). This result was significant at $P < 0.001$. Causes of unsatisfactory results among patients with successful fusions were pseudoarthrosis (6%), pain at the graft site (6%), and progressive disc disease at L3/4 (3%). Unsatisfactory results in patients who did not achieve successful fusions or in whom fusion was not attempted resulted from progressive degenerative disc dis-

TABLE 4
End Results in Fused and Non-Fused Patients Undergoing Lumbar Discectomy

	Fusion	Non-Fusion
Satisfactory	85%	39%*
Unsatisfactory	15%	61%

Vaughn *et al.*, 1988.

ease (35%), recurrent disc (15%), foot drop (2%), infection (2%), and unknown etiology (4%). Vaughn concluded that the reoperative rate was higher in the non-fusion group, that fusion decreases the chance of recurrent disc herniation, and that overall satisfactory results were higher in the fusion group.

DEGENERATIVE DISC DISEASE-SCOLIOSIS, SPONDYLOLISTHESIS, STENOSIS

The clinical efficacy of spinal instrumentation in lumbar degenerative disc disease was reported by Zuckerman *et al.* (8). The main criterion for success in this study was relief of pain. To analyze the ability of spinal instrumentation to relieve pain, Zuckerman, *et al.* retrospectively matched groups who underwent fusion without instrumentation ($n = 30$), groups receiving fusion with Knodt rods ($n = 36$), patients receiving Harrington rods ($n = 30$), and patients receiving the Vermont spinal plate ($n = 30$). For inclusion in this study patients had to meet strict criteria and results were evaluated by individuals other than the operating surgeon. Rate of fusion was not evaluated in this study nor was fusion rate correlated with the pain results. As seen in Table 5, Zuckerman, *et al.* did not find significant differences in pain relief between any of these groups.

Lorenz *et al.* (2) compared single level fusion with and without instrumentation in a prospective randomized fashion. Although entrance criteria for this study were relatively strict, there were also relatively few patients entered into this study and the results were surgeon evaluated. Lorenz *et al.* reported that fusion rate improved from 42% in noninstrumented patients to 100% in instrumented patients (Table 6). Similarly a higher rate of pain relief and a more rapid return to work was reported in patients who received spinal instrumentation compared to those who did not. Lorenz *et al.* concluded that instrumentation was associated with a higher fusion rate and with improved pain and more rapid return to work.

Grubb and Lipscomb (1) prospectively evaluated the results of lumbosacral fusion for degenerative disc disease with and without instrumentation in a consecutive, nonrandomized, series of patients. These

TABLE 5
End Results in Fused Patients Lumbar Discectomy

Group	Excellent	Good	Fair	Poor
NIF (30)	50%	30%	16%	3%
KR (36)	53	22	22	3
HR (30)	53	13	7	27
VSP (30)	47	27	20	7

NIF, Non-instrumented fusions; KR, Knodt rod; HR, Harrington rod; VSP, Vermont spinal plate.
Zuckerman *et al.*, 1992.

TABLE 6
Fusion Rate, Pain Response and Return to Work Rate in Patients with Degenerative Disease of the Lumbar Spine Undergoing Fusion Without Instrumentation

	Non-Instrumented	Instrumented
Fusion rate	42%	100%
Improved pain	42%	77%
RTW	31%	72%

RTW, Return to Work.
Lorenz *et al.*, 1991.

patients had relatively uniform disease processes and 2- to 5-year follow-up. Similar to Lorenz *et al.*, Grubb and Lipscomb evaluated their results on the basis of fusion rate, decreased pain, and return to work and/or previous lifestyle.

Grubb and Lipscomb demonstrated that fusion rate increased from 15% in noninstrumented patients to 94% in instrumented patients. Postoperative pain rating in patients with successful fusion was scored at 4/10 versus 6/10 in patients with pseudoarthrosis. Return to full time employment was 67% in patients with successful fusion versus 31% in patients with pseudoarthrosis. Only 16% of patients with successful fusion were disabled versus 57% of patients with pseudoarthrosis. Despite their observation that fusion was associated with decreased pain and increased return to work, Grubb and Lipscomb concluded that beyond increasing fusion rate, instrumentation *per se* was of no benefit.

A prospective, randomized, evaluation of 124 patients was reported by Zdeblick (7). Follow-up was relatively short at 16 months and the results were evaluated by the surgeon. Zdeblick defined excellent clinical results as patients who were pain free and returned to work at their previous occupation. Good results were those patients with mild backache requiring only non-narcotic medication and who had returned to work. Fair results were those patients with continuing back pain which prevented return to work or required narcotic medication. Poor results were those patients whose condition was worse than previously or who required additional surgery at the same level. Patients were randomized between those receiving fusion without instrumentation, those receiving instrumentation of a "semi-rigid nature," and those receiving rigid pedicular fixation. Fusion rates varied between 65% in noninstrumented patients, to 77% in semirigid instrumented patients, to 95% in rigid instrumented patients. Excellent results were reported to improve from 49% in noninstrumented patients, to 60% in semirigid instrumented patients, and 70% in rigid instrumented patients. The highest percentage of fair to poor results were noted in noninstrumented patients (Table 7). Similar to Lorenz et al., Zdeblick concluded that rigid instrumentation improved fusion rate for degenerative disease of the lumbar spine and that solid fusion appeared to be associated with improved clinical results.

Finally, Wood et al. (6) compared fusion rates, pain reports, and return to work status, in a series of prospective, multi-institutional, patients who underwent independent evaluation, met strict criteria for study inclusion, and had a minimum 2-year follow-up. Wood et al. reported that fusion rates improved from 68% in noninstrumented patients to 100% in instrumented patients. Clinical improvement was 75% in instrumented patients with 25% receiving no improvement. Return to work status followed a similar pattern. Wood et al. used a literature review for matched control as comparison groups. Although instrumentation was reported to improve fusion rates, Wood et al. felt that beyond that instrumentation was of no benefit to the patient.

SUMMARY

In summary, the above nine clinical reports specifically evaluated fusion rates and clinical efficacy of lumbar fusion and instrumentation in the treatment of degenerative disease of the lumbar spine. Among

TABLE 7
End Results of Patient Undergoing Fusion With or Without Instrumentation for Degenerative Disease

	Non-Instrumented	Semi-rigid	Rigid
Excellent	49%	60%	70%
Good	22%	29%	24%
Fair/poor	29%	11%	5%

Zdeblick, 1993.

these, several reports dealt specifically with herniated nucleus pulposus, while the remainder dealt with more generalized degenerative changes including scoliosis, spondylolisthesis, and stenosis. Among these reports nearly all conclude that lumbar instrumentation improved fusion rates. However, four reports specifically conclude that improved clinical results are correlated with these improved fusion rates. Among these four reports, three are prospective and randomized. It should also be noted that among those reports that did not specifically conclude that instrumentation improved clinical results, the data of at least two does support improved clinical results.

It seems clear at this time that lumbar instrumentation unequivocally improves fusion rates in degenerative disease of the lumbar spine. It remains controversial, however, whether improved clinical results are in fact correlated with these improved fusion rates. Logically if the disease process causing pain is one of ongoing degenerative changes, then successful fusion could be beneficial. In that regard, one possibility is that the invasiveness and disruption of normal anatomy in current surgical technique are responsible for the less than satisfactory results often obtained. If that is the case, then the recent development of minimally invasive techniques for lumbar fusion could be the key to improved clinical results overall.

REFERENCES

1. Grubb SA, Lipscomb HJ: Results of lumbosacral fusion for degenerative disc disease with and without instrumentation. **Spine** 17:349–355, 1992.
2. Lorenz M, Zindirck M, Schwaegler P, *et al.*: A comparison of single-level fusions with and without hardware. **Spine** 16:s455–s458, 1991.
3. Nachlas, NE: End result study of treatment of herniated nucleus pulposus by excision with fusion and without fusion. **J Bone Joint Surg** 34A:901–908, 1952.
4. Vaughn R: Results of L4-L5 disc excision alone versus disc excision and fusion. **Spine** 13:690–695, 1988.
5. White AH, von Rogov P, Zucherman J, *et al.*: Lumbar laminectomy for herniated disc: a prospective controlled comparison with internal fixation fusion. **Spine** 12:305–307, 1987.
6. Wood GW, Boyd RJ, Carothers T, *et al.*: The effect of pedicle screw/plate fixation on lumbar/lumbosacral autogenous bone graft fusions in patients with degenerative disc disease. **Spine** 20:819–830, 1995.
7. Zdeblick TA: A prospective, randomized study of lumbar fusion. **Spine** 18:983–991, 1993.
8. Zucherman J, Hsu K, Picetti G, *et al.*: Clinical efficacy of spinal instrumentation in lumbar degenerative disc disease. **Spine** 17:834–837, 1992.

CHAPTER

20

Acquired Lumbar Spinal Stenosis

JOHN A. JANE, SR., M.D., PH.D., JOHN A. JANE, JR., M.D.,
GREGORY A. HELM, M.D., DAVID F. KALLMES, M.D.,
CHRISTOPHER I. SHAFFREY, M.D., JAMES B. CHADDUCK, M.D.,
AND CHARLES G. DiPIERRO, M.D.

INTRODUCTION

Through a complex series of events often involving all elements of the vertebrae, the lumbar spine is transformed in such a way that the neural elements contained within it are compressed (Fig. 1). The particular vertebral transformations that characterize lumbar stenosis are remarkably diverse. Inferior or superior facet hypertrophy, laminar or pedicle changes, ligamental hypertrophy, disc bulges or scoliosis, may be present in different combinations. But a narrow lumbar canal in and of itself is not always symptomatic. Apparently, some second factor must be present to produce either radiculopathy or claudication, the two principal symptoms. Surgical therapy must be directed toward the anatomic transformations and their relationship to the presenting symptoms.

PATHOGENESIS

Pertinent Anatomy (3, 16, 18, 25, 60, 78, 85)

Each lumbar vertebra is composed of a vertebral body and a neural arch that arises from the upper half of the vertebral body (Fig. 2). Adjacent vertebrae articulate via three joints, the intervertebral disc and the superior and inferior articular facets. These three joints share the spinal load and, depending on posture, the facets bear between 3 to 25% of the total load (85).

General Concepts (15, 21, 22, 25, 44, 45, 82, 86)

Kirkaldy-Willis *et al.,* (45, 86) studied the degenerative changes occurring in the spine and popularized the concept of the three-joint complex initially proposed by Farfan *et al.* (21, 22). Together they hypothesized that acquired spinal stenosis begins with the degeneration of the joints of the spinal canal: namely, the intervertebral disc and su-

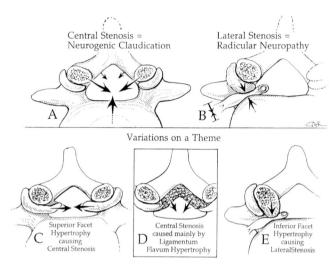

FIG.1 Spinal stenosis. Artist's diagrammatic representation of the various processes that result in spinal stenosis. (**A**) demonstrates the direction of movement of the lamina, inferior facet, and disc in narrowing the spinal canal. (**B**) shows compression of the nerve root in the lateral recess by a hypertrophied superior facet. (**C**) shows that occasionally superior facet hypertrophy may result in central stenosis. (**D**) shows the role of the hypertrophied ligamentum flavum narrowing the spinal canal. (**E**) shows that even inferior facet hypertrophy may compress the nerve root causing lateral stenosis.

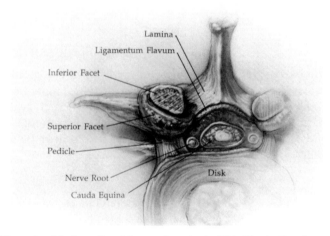

FIG.2 Normal axial view of vertebra and contents. This illustration demonstrates a normal axial view at a single lower lumbar vertebral level. Each of the bony and ligamentous elements captioned can be involved in spinal stenosis. Note the oblique orientation of the facet joints, placing this level in the lower lumbar region.

perior and inferior facets. These joints form a complex and as such are interdependent; degeneration of one joint ultimately affects the other two (45, 86).

When the intervertebral disc and posterior facets degenerate, the biomechanics of the spine are altered, causing microinstability. According to Wolf's Law, bone and soft tissues respond to this increased stress by hypertrophy. Ultimately, the pathological changes may include the following: (a) bulging of the disc; (b) hypertrophy of the ligamentum flavum and the superior and inferior facets; and (c) abnormal mobility including spondylolisthesis and descended pedicles. In our experience the most commonly affected levels are L4/5 and L3/4, followed by L2/3, L5/S1, and L1/2.

Although degenerative changes in the spine are almost universally apparent in individuals by the age of 60, morphometric analysis has revealed that only 6% of adult patients suffer from symptomatic lumbar stenosis (15). The National Center for Health Statistics' data revealed that lumbar surgical procedures for degenerative processes are performed in one of 1000 persons who were more than 65 years old (44). There may be certain predisposed individuals who develop spinal stenosis based on the shape of their canals, the orientation of their facet joints, or their particular endocrinologic and local inflammatory responses. Thus, while joint degeneration is universal, the consequences depend on other factors.

Bone and Soft Tissue Degeneration

THE DISC: PERTINENT ANATOMY (3)

The intervertebral disc has two main functions: it permits a ball-bearing motion in all planes and evenly dissipates concentrated mechanical loads. It is composed of the annulus fibrosis and the nucleus pulposus. The annulus is the outer shell of the disc and is composed of concentric layers, or lamellae, of type I collagen, which provides great tensile strength and surrounds the nucleus. The nucleus is composed of type II collagen, a more hydrated form of the protein, and proteoglycans that maintain the hydration of the disc. It is the fluid of the nucleus that permits the even redistribution of biomechanical loads.

THE DISC: PATHOGENESIS (3, 7, 17, 21, 22, 25, 45, 73, 78, 81, 86)

The major constituents of the intervertebral disc are collagen, proteoglycans, and water. However, these components are not static throughout one's lifetime. With increasing age the hydrated type II collagen decreases in proportion to type I and both are increasingly replaced by fibrous tissue. The proportion of proteoglycans in the entire disc also decreases, but especially in the nucleus; they become less aggregated and less able to maintain the hydration of the disc. As the absolute water content of the disc decreases, so does the disc's ability to evenly redistribute biomechanical loads.

Taken together these biochemical degenerative changes render the disc more prone to biomechanical damage. Without the even distribution of biomechanical forces, focal regions in the disc are subject to exceptional forces that finally lead to a circumferential tear in the annulus fibrosis. With repeated minor trauma, the tears coalesce producing a larger radical tear. This leads to internal disruption of the disc, loss of disc height, disc resorption, and microinstability. Secondarily, repetitive trauma and degeneration lead to bulging of the annulus into the canal (Fig. 3) and subperiosteal osteophyte formation where the annulus attaches to the vertebral body.

THE POSTERIOR FACETS: PERTINENT ANATOMY

The posterior facets bear a portion of the rotational forces of the spine. The upper lumbar facets are well-suited to do so because they are oriented in the sagittal plane. Unlike the upper lumbar vertebrae, the two lower lumbar facets are oriented in a more coronal plane (Fig. 2).

THE POSTERIOR FACETS: PATHOGENESIS (3, 7, 14, 17, 21, 22, 25, 45, 59, 73, 81, 86)

Whereas disc degeneration is mainly a function of biochemical changes related to aging, the posterior facets are primarily altered by biomechanical forces. The coronally oriented lower lumbar facets per-

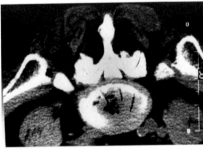
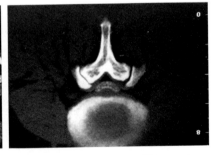

FIG.3 Disc bulge. (**A**) Diffuse intervertebral disc bulge: Axial contrast CT scan shows soft tissue bulging diffusely from the posterior aspect of the vertebral body. This bulging disk may narrow the central canal or lateral recess. (**B**) Central intervertebral disc bulge: Axial contrast CT scan shows a central soft tissue bulge from the posterior aspect of the vertebral body narrowing the central canal.

mit more rotational mobility and are more subject to injury in this plane. In addition to the rotational forces that normally are borne by the facets, disc degeneration transfers added axial load to the facets. The loss of disc space height alters the facets' alignment and reduces the cross-sectional area available to bear stress. Increased focal stresses across the facet joints produces focal cartilage destruction, causing the capsule to loosen. In response to this loosening and microinstability, the facets hypertrophy. Generally, superior facet hypertrophy narrows the intervertebral foramen and lateral recess, while inferior facet hypertrophy projects medially into the central canal (Fig. 4).

THE LIGAMENTUM FLAVUM: PERTINENT ANATOMY (3, 45, 50, 53, 59)

The ligamentum flavum supports the spine preventing hyperflexion of the spine. It has connections in both the central and lateral recesses attaching superiorly, to the central undersurface of the lamina above; inferiorly, to the superior edge of the laminae below; laterally, to the undersurface of the superior facet (Fig. 5); and medially, or centrally, to the interspinous ligament.

THE LIGAMENTUM FLAVUM; PATHOGENESIS (3, 25, 50, 53, 58, 59, 76, 78, 86, 87)

The effects of the degenerating three-joint complex are not limited to the joints. The ligamentum flavum also responds to the microinstability by hypertrophy (Fig. 5). There are three mechanisms for this hypertrophy: (a) proliferation of type II collagen, with relative depletion of the elastic fibers; (b) ossification, associated with proliferation of chondrocytes and hyalinization of collagen fibers; and (c) calcium crystal deposition, associated with granulomatous tissue proliferation. These changes typically occur at the insertion of the ligament on the facet joint.

Abnormal Mobility

PERTINENT ANATOMY (3, 10, 14, 18, 28)

In the normal spine, the facets bear up to 30% of the forces in the anteroposterior direction (10). These forces are borne well by the lower lumbar vertebrae because they are oriented oblique to the sagittal plane. However, there are individuals who have more sagittally oriented lower facets that do not adequately bear anteroposterior forces. Individuals with more sagittally oriented lower facets are more likely to experience stenosis and spondylolisthesis.

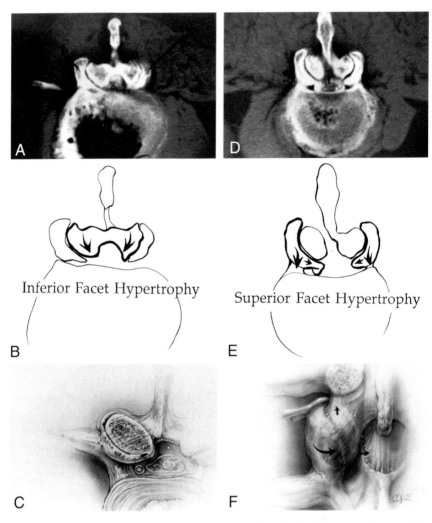

FIG. 4 Facet hypertrophy. Inferior facet hypertrophy: (**A**) Axial contrast CT scan, (**B**) its corresponding line drawing, and (**C**) another illustration at the level of the inferior articulating facet showing the medial projection of the hypertrophied facet and the resultant narrow central canal. Superior facet hypertrophy: (**D**) Axial contrast CT scan and (**E**) its corresponding line drawing at the level of the superior aspect of the superior articular facet demonstrating joint space loss and subarticular sclerosis typical of degenerated facet joints. The anteriorly directed osteophyte from the superior facet narrows the lateral recess (*large arrows*). (**F**) Drawing showing that with excessive hypertrophy, the superior facet will encroach medially into the central canal (*small arrows*).

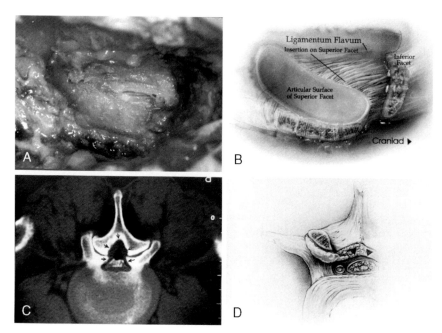

FIG.5 Ligamentum flavum. (**A**) Cadaveric dissection photograph and (**B**) its corresponding line drawing showing the lateral attachment of the ligamentum flavum. While most of the yellow fibers attach to the facet joint capsule, a smaller number of white fibers can be seen to attach to the undersurface of the superior articular facet. (**C**) Hypertrophy of the ligamentum flavum: Axial contrast CT shows convex bulge into the thecal sac resulting from degenerated and hypertrophied ligamentum flavum (*arrows*). Ossification is not uncommonly seen within the hypertrophied ligaments. (**D**) Artist's representation of the effects of ligamental hypertrophy.

PATHOGENESIS (1, 18, 20, 45)

Abnormal mobility occurs after the disc and facets have undergone degenerative change. With the loss of integrity of the supporting bone and ligamentous structures, the spine may become grossly unstable. Degenerative spondylolisthesis can narrow the central and lateral regions of the canal and occurs when the vertebral body above the degenerated disc moves anteriorly as the inferior facet subluxates anteriorly and superiorly (Fig. 6). The lateral recess may be narrowed when the intervertebral disc height narrows and the pedicle moves inferiorly pinching the spinal nerve (Fig. 7). Similarly, the pathological movements in scoliosis occurs when the pedicle on the convex side moves inferiorly and compresses the nerve root (Fig. 8).

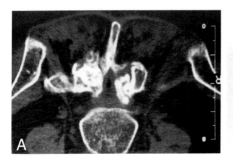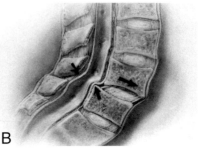

FIG.6 Spondylolisthesis. (A) Axial contrast CT scan demonstrates elongation of the central canal in the sagittal plane from anterolisthesis of the inferior vertebral body. Typically seen are degenerated facets, which have varying degrees of cartilaginous overgrowth. The apparent disc bulge actually represents an artifact of the axial scan technique; in lower images this soft tissue aligns with the posterior aspect of the inferior vertebral body. (B) Artist's rendering of spondylolisthesis in sagittal view.

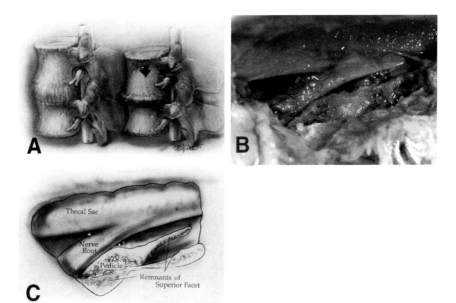

FIG.7 The pedicle. (A) This drawing demonstrates the impact of degenerative disc space narrowing on the pedicles. As the pedicle displaces inferiorly, its inferior border compresses the exiting nerve root adding to lateral recess stenosis. (B) A cadaveric dissection and (C) its illustration demonstrating nerve root compression by the pedicle.

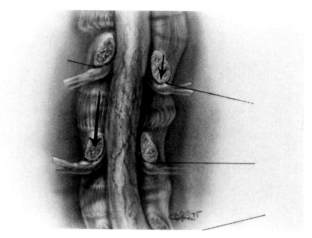

FIG.8 Scoliosis. Consequences of scoliosis: Scoliosis is not uncommonly a component of lumbar stenosis. This drawing depicts a scoliotic spine with the planes of angulation. The arrows depict the way in which the pedicle on the convex side impinges upon an exiting nerve root.

Congenitally Short Pedicles

While not properly considered as part of the pathogenesis of acquired spinal stenosis, congenitally short pedicles, a developmental disorder, may accompany and contribute to the narrowing of the canal. In this disorder, the narrow height of the pedicles causes stenosis of both the lateral recess and the central canal (Fig. 9).

PATHOLOGY

The particular manner in which these degenerative changes occur leads to two overlapping, but distinguishable, pathological and clinical entities: namely, central and lateral stenosis. It is unclear which predisposing factors lead to predominately central or lateral stenosis, but it is useful to discuss them separately.

Central Stenosis

PERTINENT ANATOMY (25)

The spinal canal is bordered anteriorly, by the vertebral body, intervertebral disc, and posterior longitudinal ligament; posteriorly, by the laminae, pars interarticularis, ligamentum flavum and the facet joints; and laterally, by the pedicles. Hypertrophy of any of these structures can narrow the central canal.

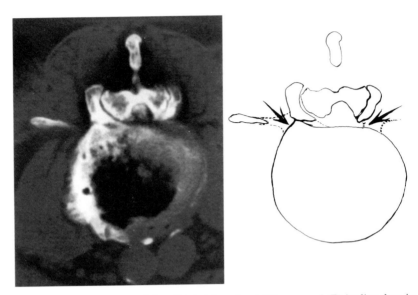

Fig.9 Congenital short pedicles. (**A**) Axial contrast CT scan and (**B**) its line drawing demonstrating the effects of congenitally short pedicles on the lateral recess and central canal. Although this is not a degenerative process, it is not uncommonly seen in concert with other elements of acquired lumbar stenosis.

PATHOLOGY (1, 7, 45, 50, 53, 59, 73, 78, 86)

The pathology of central stenosis most commonly involves the intervertebral disc, inferior facet, and ligamentum flavum (Fig. 1A). The central canal is narrowed anteriorly by central intervertebral disc bulge and vertebral body osteophytes; and posteriorly, by enlarged laminae, hypertrophy of the inferior facets (Fig. 4, **A** and **B**), which is often pronounced, and the ligamentum flavum, which is hypertrophied at the caudal edge of the laminae. Spondylolisthesis may cause further narrowing of the central canal. At times, marked superior facet hypertrophy can also narrow the central canal (Figs. 1, **C**, 4, **C** and **D**).

Lateral Stenosis

PERTINENT ANATOMY (14, 15, 25, 30, 45, 60)

The spinal nerves exit the spinal canal through the lateral recess, which is bounded anteriorly, by the vertebral bodies and disc; posteriorly, by the pars interarticularis of the superior vertebrae, the superior (located laterally) and inferior facets (located medially), and the ligamentum flavum; and superiorly and inferiorly, by the pedicles.

The shape of the central canal and lateral recess also has pathological significance. While most canals on transverse section appear dome-shaped, a variation in the normal anatomy is apparent in 14% of individuals who have what has been termed a "trefoil-shaped" canal (15). This trefoil configuration is characterized by a shorter sagittal diameter and a deep lateral recess in which the superior facet forms the roof and predisposes to lateral recess stenosis.

PATHOLOGY (1, 3, 7, 16, 17, 30, 45, 58, 76, 78, 86, 87)

The pathology of lateral stenosis most commonly involves the superior facet, ligamentum flavum, intervertebral disc, and pedicle (Fig. 1, **B, D,** and **E**). The lateral recess may be narrowed posteriorly by hypertrophy of the superior facet (Figs. 4, **C** and **D**) or ligamentum flavum; anteriorly by a laterally bulging disc (Fig. 3 **A**); or superiorly by a descending pedicle (Fig. 7). Significant inferior facet hypertrophy may also narrow the lateral recess (Fig. 1 **E**).

RADIOGRAPHIC MANIFESTATIONS OF SPINAL STENOSIS

The radiographic appearance of spinal stenosis is well described and can reveal the specific pathologic changes seen in the disease. This section contains a brief discussion of normal radiographic anatomy of the lumbar spine followed by separate consideration of the factors contributing to spinal stenosis.

Normal Anatomy

The normal appearance of the thecal sac in axial section is round to ovoid at L1 through L3, and is ovoid to triangular at L4 through S1. A trefoil shape secondary to prominent articular pillars is a normal variant at L5/S1, seen in 10 to 20% of patients. This should not be confused with the trefoil appearance of central causal stenosis from ligamentum flavum hypertrophy (13).

The exiting nerve root is surrounded by epidural fat at all levels. Obliteration of this fat should be considered evidence of nerve root compression. Researchers have offered multiple measurements of the normal dimensions of the thecal sac and lateral recess. Verbiest (74) reported that the normal midsagittal diameter of the lumbar thecal sac is 16 to 18 mm. A diameter between 10 and 12 mm is termed relative stenosis and less than 10 mm is absolute stenosis, since this latter measurement could lead to symptoms without other compressive factors (74). The lateral recess height, measured at the level of the superior aspect of the superior facet, should be greater than 5 mm in anterior to posterior dimension. Between 2 and 5 mm is suspicious for

stenosis, and less than 2 mm in width is usually pathological (61). However, because of individual variation, the diagnosis of spinal stenosis
should be based more on the appearance of the thecal sac and lateral
recess than on absolute measurements (13).

Although plain films and plain computerized tomography (CT) may
suggest the diagnosis of spinal stenosis, accurate depiction of both the
bones and soft tissues surrounding the thecal sac are necessary for the
evaluation of suspected spinal stenosis. This is best obtained using contrast myelography/CT or magnetic resonance (MR) imaging. Myelography allows a functional assessment of the degree of spinal block; CT
myelography provides an excellent depiction of bone anatomy. Magnetic resonance imaging is particularly useful for evaluating the
neural foramina because it enables direct sagittal imaging and provides outstanding contrast between the various soft-tissue elements in
the neural foramina, such as nerve roots, fat, and vessels (52).

Facet Hypertrophy

Degenerative change of the facet joints is manifested radiographically as narrowing of the joint space, subarticular sclerosis, and cyst
formation, and osteophyte formation (Fig. 4). The superior facet osteophytes tend to project anteriorly, while those of the inferior facet tend
to project anteromedially. Because the lateral recess is most narrow at
the level of the superior facet, anteriorly projected superior osteophytes often result in compromise of the lateral recess (51). Lateral recess stenosis is unusual in the upper lumbar spine given the relatively
short intraspinal segment of the nerve root sleeve at these levels (64).
Hypertrophy of the inferior facet, because of its anteromedial orientation, will usually contribute to central canal rather than lateral recess
stenosis. However, in some cases, inferior facet hypertrophy may also
lead to compromise of the lateral recess.

Hypertrophy of the Ligamentum Flavum

Thickening of the ligamentum flavum occurs as a manifestation of
degenerative change in the lumbar spine (Fig. 5). Various degrees of
ossification may also be present in thickened ligamentum flavum. The
thickened ligament produces a convex deformity on the posterior lateral aspect of the thecal sac, leading to the classic trefoil appearance
seen in central canal stenosis. Hypertrophy is most pronounced at the
interlaminar levels rather than at the level of the laminae.

Disc Bulge or Herniation

Bulging or herniation of the intervertebral disc may compound degenerative spinal stenosis (Fig. 3), compromising the central canal, lat-

eral recess, or intervertebral foramen; end-plate osteophytes may also affect these areas. On myelography, disc pathology typically results in ventral extradural defects and various degrees of nerve root cutoff. Axial contrast CT demonstrates soft tissue in the ventral extradural space with obliteration of epidural fat. Magnetic resonance imaging is most useful in the region of the neural foramina, where disc herniations initially obliterate fat in the inferior aspect of the neural foramen. Because the nerve root resides in the superior portion of the neural foramen, root compromise typically is not present until the fat in the neural foramen has been nearly completely obliterated.

Degenerative Spondylolisthesis

Degenerative spondylolisthesis rarely occurs in isolation, and is usually compounded by abundant bone overgrowth of the facet joints and thickening of the ligamentum flavum (Fig. 6). The intact posterior bone ring of the anteriorly subluxated vertebrae may produce central or lateral recess stenosis. Myelography is useful not only in demonstrating the malalignment of the lumbar spine, but also in assessing the location and degree of canal compromise. Axial images are useful in demonstrating the facet hypertrophy as well as the central canal and lateral recess stenosis. There is often a prominent band of soft tissue along the posterior aspect of the vertebral body, which may be mistaken for a bulging disc. However, the posterior margin of this apparent disc bulge is congruent with the posterior margin of the inferior vertebral body and represents an artifact of the axial scan technique (32).

CLINICAL PRESENTATION

The symptoms of lumbar stenosis are commonly either radiculopathy or neurogenic claudication. While radicular symptoms are most likely caused by lateral stenosis, neurogenic claudication is probably the result of narrowing of the central region of the spinal canal. Seventy-eight percent of our patients presenting with radiculopathy had pain that was worse in, or limited to, one leg. In a similar fashion, 75% of our patients with neurogenic claudication report that their pain is significantly worse on one side, although symptoms typically occur in both legs. This asymmetry permits us to choose the most appropriate side to fully decompress.

TREATMENT

Natural History

There are few reports of conservative treatment of symptomatic spinal stenosis. One recent study followed a group of 32 patients with myelogram-proven spinal stenosis. Seventy-five percent had neuro-genic claudication, 12.5% had radicular symptoms and another 12.5% had mixed symptoms. Following a mean time of observation of 49 months, pain was unchanged in 70%, worse in 15%, and improved in another 15%. Although no patients experienced neurologic deteriora-tion, the fact that 85% of these patients' pain was worse or unchanged at long-term follow-up makes surgery a reasonable option (43).

Current Surgical Therapy

A variety of surgical procedures are used to treat lumbar spinal stenosis. These procedures range from limited surgical decompression *via* laminotomy, laminaplasty, or limited laminectomy, to total laminectomy, wide foraminotomies, and instrumentation for fusion. Equally varied are the patient selection criteria and follow-up proto-cols used to determine the results of these procedures (2, 23–26, 29, 35–39, 41–44, 46, 54–56, 66, 67, 72, 75, 78, 79, 88).

Spinal Fusion

INDICATIONS

The only unequivocal indication for lumbar fusion is gross segmen-tal instability shown by flexion and extension films. Other relative in-dications include: significant preoperative segmental instability caused by either degenerative spondylolisthesis (>1 cm) or scoliosis; partial medial facetectomy and laminectomy with discectomy; and bi-lateral disruption of the posterior facets. Aside from these indications, the role of spinal fusion is both unclear and controversial.

AGAINST FUSION

A number of researchers have found that fusion either increases morbidity or adds no benefit to a standard decompression (12, 19, 27, 47, 63, 69, 70, 80, 89). Deyo *et al.* (11), reviewed 13,662 Medicare pa-tients treated for spinal stenosis of whom 6% received a fusion after to-tal laminectomy. These patients had 1.9 times higher complication rates, 5.8 times greater transfusion rates, 2.2 times greater chance of being placed, post hospitalization, in a nursing home, and 2.0 times greater chance of a 6-week postoperative mortality. They proposed that these complications resulted from the need for two incisions (as the il-iac crest was frequently used), increased operative time, increased area and extent of dissection, and use of instrumentation.

A recent randomized study of 45 patients with lumbar spinal steno-sis without instability compared three groups: decompression alone, decompression with arthrodesis of the most stenotic segment, and decompression with arthrodesis of all of the decompressed segments (27). There were no statistically significant differences in the relief of pain at an average follow-up of 28 months.

FOR FUSION

There are a number of theoretical advantages of adding fusion to laminectomy. As the disc degenerates with age, the posterior facets become more important to the structural stability of the spine. A wide laminectomy, especially if accompanied by facetectomy, compromises the integrity of the posterior elements and can cause both gross instability and microinstability, which is difficult to identify radiographically and may lead to recurrent stenosis at the operative site (6, 40). Stabilization at the decompressed level using bone grafts or instrumentation would greatly decrease the chance of re-stenosis resulting from either gross or microinstability. Whether the potential long-term improved outcomes are worth the added risk is not known.

Several researchers have reported results favorable to fusion. Although figures vary widely, most authors believe that following major lumbar decompressions, between 5 and 20% of individuals experience postoperative instability (5, 31, 40, 42, 43, 48, 49, 63, 65). Hopp and Tsou (40) demonstrated that degenerative disc disease, scoliosis, and total facetectomy were predictive indicators for postoperative instability. This postoperative instability is not without consequence. Chen *et al.* (6) found moderate or marked regrowth in 44% of cases with an average follow-up of 4.5 years. The authors reported that spinal instability accelerated bone regrowth at later follow-up and that spinal levels adjacent to fusion also showed more bone re-growth. Patients with moderate or marked bone regrowth had poorer clinical outcomes compared with those with mild or no regrowth.

Herkowitz and Kurz (34) studied 50 patients suffering from degenerative lumbar spondylolisthesis with spinal stenosis and compared the relief of pain in patients who received decompression alone to decompression with intertransverse fusion. The results were significantly better in patients receiving concomitant arthrodesis. Not only was their pain better relieved, only 28% of these patients had increased postoperative spondylolisthesis compared with 96% of patients who did not have arthrodesis.

The "Ipsi-Contra" Procedure (12)

The side to be decompressed is entered in the usual fashion. To verify position a number four Penfield is inserted in the epidural space and a cross-table lateral film is obtained. A hemilaminectomy is then performed in the standard fashion and extends to as many levels as is indicated clinically and radiographically.

Attention is then directed to enlarging the size of the canal. This is done with upbiting punches removing bone across to the contralateral side underneath the spinous process (Fig. 10). Using a cottonoid care is taken to dissect away the dura (Fig. 10C). The contralateral ligamentum flavum is also removed with the aid of a blunt nerve hook. This ligamentum is engaged and pulled toward the operator. The obliquely directed ligamentum is easily removed, but in addition, the more horizontal ligamentum flavum which inserts on the superior facet of the opposite side should also be removed (Figs. 5, **A** and **B**). With this maneuver it is usually possible to decompress the contralateral side enough so that the nerve roots are visualized. If the contralateral decompression still seems inadequate, a drill is carried through the facet capsule into the facet and spinal canal. Direct decompression of the nerve is then carried out (Fig. 11). Small pieces of fat are then placed into the facet.

The operator then directs his attention to the decompression of the ipsilateral lateral recess and this is best done from the opposite side of

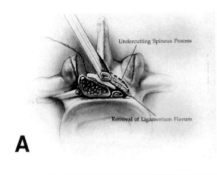

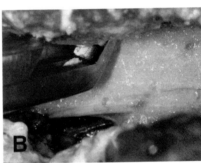

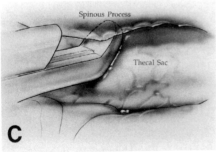

FIG.10 Undercutting of the spinous process. (**A**) Illustration showing an axial view undercutting the spinous process with removal of contralateral ligamentum flavum. (**B**) A cadaveric dissection and (**C**) its illustration depicting the undercutting permitting a good decompression of the central canal with a hemilaminectomy and does not disrupt the contralateral facet joint.

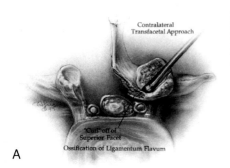 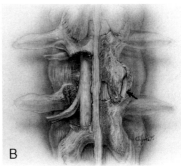

A   B

FIG.11 Contralateral transfacetal approach. (**A**) Illustration of the contralateral transfacetal approach in axial view. This approach may be used in patients with bilateral symptoms and permits a more adequate removal of the ligamentum flavum. (**B**) The ipsilateral decompression having been accomplished with arrows showing the transfacetal approach.

the table. The nerve roots are followed out into the lateral recess and whatever bone removal is necessary to decompress the nerve root is carried out. This often involves removing the inferior facet thereby exposing the surface of the superior facet. As much of the superior facet is removed as necessary and the nerve is followed out around the pedicle. Often it appears that the nerve root is tethered against the surface of the pedicle (Figs. 7, **B** and **C**). If this is the case, a drill is used to hollow-out the pedicle (Fig. 12) and then a curette breaks down the remaining shell. The decompressed nerve root often subsequently moves into the space previously occupied by the pedicle (Fig. 12**G**).

The contralateral bone is then decorticated, including the facet, lamina and spinous process. All of the bone which has been removed during the procedure is then added together and firmly packed into the contralateral space (Fig. 13). The muscle is approximated in the midline.

SPECIFIC SURGICAL CONSIDERATIONS

Our current approach to the treatment of lumbar stenosis tailors the surgical approach not only to the radiographic findings but also to the specific signs and symptoms of the patient.

Patients whose complaints are primarily of a unilateral radiculopathy with radiographic evidence of spinal stenosis are considered to suffer from lateral stenosis. This lateral stenosis is usually related to the superior facet but may often be due to inferior facet and ligamentum flavum hypertrophy, scoliosis, or pedicle impingement. For these individuals an extensive unilateral decompression is performed so that the

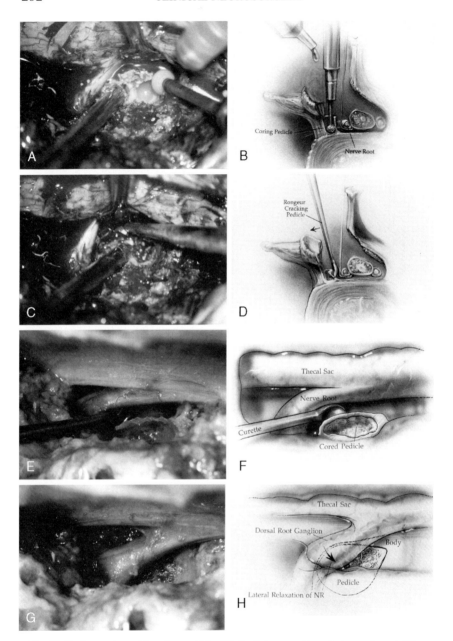

FIG.12 Coring and cracking the pedicle. (**A**) An intraoperative photograph and (**B**) an artist's rendering of the coring procedure (the head is to the right). (**C**) An intraoperative photo, (**D**) a drawing in axial view, (**E**) a cadaveric dissection and (**F**) its illustration of the cracking procedure of the cored pedicle. (**G**) A cadaveric dissection and (**H**) its drawing showing how the decompressed pedicle moves into the space previously occupied by the pedicle.

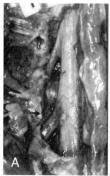
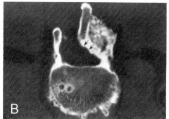
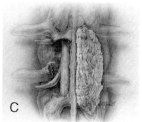

FIG.13 Postoperative views of the ipsi-contra procedure. (**A**) Cadaveric dissection. Note the radical lateral recess decompression (*arrow*) at multiple levels. (**B**) CT scan. Note the good central decompression achieved with hemilaminectomy, undercutting of the spinous process (*arrows*), as well as the large autologous contralateral fusion mass, and the shaved pedicle. (**C**) A drawing of the ipsi-contra procedure showing the ipsilateral decompression and the contralateral autologous bone fusion.

affected nerve root is completely decompressed. This commonly involves a unilateral hemilaminectomy, foraminotomy, pediculectomy, facetectomy, and occasionally, discectomy. The side with no symptoms is not attacked surgically except perhaps to remove the contralateral ligamentum flavum via the undercut spinous processes and laminae.

Patients who present with unilateral neurogenic intermittent claudication and with radiological confirmation of central stenosis receive an extensive unilateral decompression with hemilaminectomies. Enlargement of the contralateral spinal canal is achieved by extensive undercutting of the spinous processes and total removal of the contralateral ligamentum flavum. We believe that this approach can consistently enlarge both sides of the canal while maintaining the anatomical integrity of the spinous processes and contralateral lamina and facets.

In patients with bilateral neurogenic claudication, the side of decompression is determined by comparing the severity of pain in each leg. The more symptomatic side is chosen for the major decompression. In patients with claudication or radiculopathy whose pain is intolerable bilaterally and whose imaging studies demonstrate severe bilateral lateral stenosis, the side with the worst pain is decompressed extensively. In addition, however, the side that exhibits less pain is treated by removing the ligamentum flavum on that side and performing either limited foraminotomies or a transfacetal decompression to decompress the exiting nerve root. Again, this leaves the spinous processes, the majority of the laminae, and the facets mechanically intact.

Although we perform this procedure on most of our patients with spinal stenosis, we believe that a total laminectomy, facetectomy, and instrumented fusion may be indicated in many situations (Fig. 14).

Future Treatment

Although the general treatment of lumbar spinal stenosis has not dramatically changed in the last 2 decades, several potential improvements are on the horizon: spinal instrumentation and advances in the molecular approaches to improve bone deposition at the fusion site offer promise (83, 84). Advances in instrumentation and endoscopic techniques will make fusion more desirable and stereotactic-guided placement of pedicle screws will lower their complication rate.

Recent advances in molecular biology have made it possible to identify bone growth factors that can be used to promote bone fusion in the lumbar spine (8). It has been demonstrated in a canine that when bone morphogenic protein-2 (BMP-2) is added to an autologous bone graft, the amount of bone deposition at the fusion site as well as the rate of solid bone fusion is greatly enhanced (33). In addition, type I collagen gel added to the autologous bone graft provides an excellent matrix onto which osteoblasts may migrate, thereby improving bone deposition between the autologous bone chips (33, 71). Collagen may also be

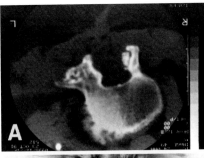
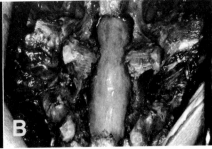
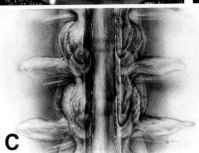

Fig.14 Standard total laminectomy. (A) Axial contrast CT scan at the level of the pedicles after a standard total laminectomy. (B) Cadaveric dissection and (C) an artist's illustration of a standard total laminectomy. Note the good central decompression as well as the fact that the lateral recesses have not been adequately decompressed. This procedure also disrupts the facet joints leaving them unstable.

an excellent carrier for osteogenic growth factors and may actually bind circulating growth factors that reach the fusion site (57).

SUMMARY

Based on the individual clinical presentation and radiographic findings, an operation that completely decompresses the neural elements in the spinal canal and neural foramina followed by posterior, posterolateral, or interbody fusion, with or without instrumentation should be the procedure of choice in the future. The introduction of pharmacological agents to decrease scarring around the decompressed nerve roots will also increase the number of successful procedures. It must be stressed, however, that any new operative technique must be tested in a rigorous fashion, ideally with a prospective randomized clinical trial.

REFERENCES

1. Alexander E, Kelly DL, Davis CH, *et al.:* Intact arch spondylolisthesis. **J Neurosurg** 63;840–844, 1985.
2. Aryanpur J, Ducker T: Multilevel lumbar laminotomies: An alternative to laminectomy in the treatment of lumbar stenosis. **Neurosurgery** 26:429–432, 1990.
3. Boden SD, Wiesel SW, Laws ER, Rothman RH: Anatomy of the spine and Pathophysiology of the aging spine, in Wickland E (ed): *The Aging Spine: Essentials of Pathophysiology, Diagnosis, and Treatment,* Philadelphia, W.B. Saunders Company, 1991, ed 1, pp 3–38.
4. Bohm H, Harms J, Dunk R, *et al.:* Correction and stabilization of angular kyphosis. **Clin Orthop Rel Res** 258:56–61, 1990.
5. Caputy AJ, Luessenhop AJ: Long-term evaluation of decompressive surgery for degenerative lumbar stenosis. **J Neurosurg** 77:669–676, 1992.
6 Chen Q, Baba H, Kamitani K, *et al.:* Postoperative bone regrowth in lumbar spinal stenosis. A multivariate analysis of 48 Patients. **Spine** 19(19):2144–9, 1994.
7 Ciricillo SF, Weinstein PR: Lumbar spinal stenosis. **West J Med** 158:171–177, 1993.
8. Cook SD, Dalton JE, Tan EH, *et al.:* In vivo evaluation of recombinant human osteogenic protein (rhOP-1) implants as a bone graft substitute for spinal fusion. **Spine** 19:1655–1663, 1994.
9. Cunningham BW, Sefter JC, Shono Y, *et al.:* Static and cyclical biomechanical analysis of pedicle screw spinal constructs. **Spine** 18(12):1677–88, 1993.
10. Cyron BM, Hutton WC: Articular tropism and stability of the lumbar spine. **Spine** 5(2):168–72, 1980.
11. Deyo RA, Ciol MA, Cherkin DC, *et al.:* Lumbar spinal fusion. A cohort study of complications, reoperations, and resource use in the medicare population. **Spine** 18(11):1463–70, 1993.
12. diPierro CG, Helm GA, Shaffrey CI, *et al.:* Treatment of lumbar stenosis by extensive unilateral decompression and contralateral autologous bone fusion: operative technique and results. **J Neurosurg** 84(2):166–173, 1996.
13. Dorward RH: Fundamentals of computed tomographic evaluation of lumbar disk disease, in Genant HK (ed): *Spine Update 1984.* San Francisco, Radiology Research and Education Foundation, 1983, pp 67–78.

14. Eisenstein S: The morphometry and pathological anatomy of the lumbar spine in South African negroes and caucasoids with specific reference to spinal stenosis. **J Bone Joint Surg** 59B:173–180, 1977.

15. Eisenstein S: The trefoil configuration of the lumbar vertebral canal. A study of South African skeletal material. **J Bone Joint Surg** 62B(1):73–77, 1980.

16. Epstein BS, Epstein JA, Lavine L: The effect of anatomic variation in the lumbar vertebrae and spinal canal on cauda equina and nerve root syndromes. **Am J Roentenol Rad Ther Nucl Med** 91:1055–1063, 1962.

17. Epstein JA, Epstein BS, Rosenthal AD, *et al.*: Sciatica caused by nerve root entrapment in the lateral recess: the superior facet syndrome. **J Neurosurg** 36:584–589, 1972.

18. Epstein JA, Epstein BS, Lavine LS, *et al.*: Degenerative lumbar spondylolisthesis with an intact neural arch (pseudospondylolisthesis). **J Neurosurg** 44:139–147, 1976.

19. Esses SI, Huler RH: Indications for lumbar spine fusion in the adult. **Clin Orthop Rel Res** 279:87–100, 1992.

20. Farfan HF: The pathological anatomy of degenerative spondylolisthesis. A cadaver study. **Spine** 5(5):412–418, 1980.

21. Farfan HF: Effects of torsion on the intervertebral joints. **Can J Surg** 12:336–341, 1969.

22. Farfan HF, Sullivan JB: The relation of facet orientation to intervertebral disc failure. **Can J Surg** 10:179–185, 1967.

23. Fast A, Robin CC, Floman Y: Surgical treatment of lumbar spinal stenosis in the elderly. **Arch Phys Med Rehab** 66:149–151, 1985.

24. Ganz JC: Lumbar spinal stenosis: postoperative results in terms of preoperative posture-related pain. **J Neurosurg** 72:71–74, 1990.

25. Garfin SR, Rydevik BL, Lipson SJ, *et al.*: Spinal Stenosis, in Rothman and Simeone (eds): *The Spine,* Philadelphia, WB Saunders Company, 1992, ed 3, pp 791–856.

26. Getty CJM: Lumbar spinal stenosis. The clinical spectrum and the results of operation. **J Bone Joint Surg** 62B:481–485, 1980.

27. Grob D, Humke T, Dvorak J: Degenerative lumbar spinal stenosis. Decompression with and without arthrodesis. **J Bone Joint Surg** 77A(7):1036–41, 1995.

28. Grobler LJ, Robertson PA, Novotny JE, *et al.*: Decompression for degenerative spondylolisthesis and spinal stenosis at L4-5: The effect on facet joint morphology. **Spine** 18:1475–1482, 1993.

29. Hall S, Bartels JD, Onofrio BM, *et al.*: Lumbar spinal stenosis. Clinical features, diagnostic procedures, and results of surgical treatment in 68 patients. **Ann Int Med** 103:271–275, 1985.

30. Hasegawa T, An HS, Haughton VM, *et al.*: Lumbar foraminal stenosis: Critical heights of the intervertebral discs and foramina. **J Bone Joint Surg** 77-A:32–38, 1995.

31. Hazlett JW, Kinnard P: Lumbar apophyseal process excision and spinal instability. **Spine** 7(2):171–6, 1982.

32. Heithoff KB, Ray CD: Principles of the computed tomographic assessment of lateral spinal stenosis, in Genant HK (ed): *Spine Update 1984,* San Francisco, Radiology Research and Education Foundation, 1983, pp 191–234.

33. Helm GA, Sheehan JM, Sheehan JP, *et al.*: The utilization of type I collagen gel, demineralized bone matrix and bone morphogenic protein-2 (rhBMP-2) to enhance autologous bone lumbar spinal fusion. **J Neurosurg** (In Press).

34. Herkowitz HN, Kurz LT: Degenerative lumbar spondylolisthesis with spinal stenosis. A prospective study comparing decompression with decompression and intertransverse process arthrodesis. **J Bone Joint Surg** 73A(6):802–8, 1991.

35. Herkowitz HN, Garfin SR: Decompressive surgery for spinal stenosis. **Semin Spine Surg** 1:163–167, 1989.
36. Herno A, Airaksinen O, Saari T: Long-term results of surgical treatment of lumbar stenosis. **Spine** 18:1471–1474, 1993.
37. Herron LD, Mangelsdorf C: Lumbar spinal stenosis: Results of surgical treatment. **J Spinal Disord** 4:26–33, 1991.
38. Herron LD, Trippi AC: L4-5 degenerative spondylolisthesis. The results of treatment by decompressive laminectomy without fusion. **Spine** 14:534–538, 1989.
39. Hood SA, Weigl K: Lumbar spinal stenosis: surgical intervention for the older person. **Israel J Med Sci** 19:169–172, 1983.
40. Hopp E, Tsou P: Postdecompression lumbar instability. **Clin Orthop Rel Res** 227:143–151, 1988.
41. Johnsson KE, Willner S, Johnsson K: Postoperative instability after decompression for lumbar spinal stenosis. **Spine** 11:107–110, 1986.
42. Johnsson KE, Redlund-Johnell I, Uden A, et al.: Preoperative and postoperative instability in lumbar spinal stenosis. **Spine** 14:591–593, 1989.
43. Johnsson KE, Rosen I, Uden A: The natural course of lumbar spinal stenosis. **Clin Orthop Rel Res** 279:82–6, 1992.
44. Katz JN, Lipson SJ, Larson MG, et al.: The outcome of decompressive laminectomy for degenerative lumbar stenosis. **J Bone Joint Surg** 73A(6):809–816, 1991.
45. Kirkaldy-Willis WH, Wedge JH, Yong-Hing K, et al.: Pathology and pathogenesis of lumbar spondylosis and stenosis. **Spine** 3:319–328, 1978.
46. Lassale B, Deburge A, Benoist M: Resultats a long terme du traitement chirurgical des stenoses lombaires operees. **Rev Rhum Mal Osteo-Artic** 52:27–33, 1985.
47. Laus M, Pignatti G, Alfonso C, et al.: Complications in the surgical treatment of lumbar stenosis. **Chir Degli Organi Mov** LXXVII:65–71, 1992.
48. Lee C: Lumbar spinal instability (olisthesis) after extensive posterior spinal decompression. **Spine** 8:429–433, 1983.
49. McPhee B: Spondylolisthesis and spondylosis, in Youmans JR (ed): *Neurological Surgery,* Philadelphia, W.B. Saunders Company, 1990, ed 3, pp 2749–2784.
50. Meredith JM, Lehman EP: Hypertrophy of the ligamentum flavum, **Surgery** 4:587–596, 1938.
51. Mikhael MA, Ciric I, Tarkingon JA, et al.: Neuroradiological evaluation of lateral recess syndrome. **Radiology,** 140:97–107, 1981.
52. Modic MT, Masaryk TJ, Ross JS: Degenerative diseases of the spine, in Modic MT (ed): *Magnetic Resonance Imaging of the Spine.* Chicago; Year Book Medical Publishers, 1989, pp 108–117.
53. Moiel RH, Ehni BE, Anderson MS: Nodule of the ligamentum flavum as a case of nerve root compression. **J Neurosurg** 27:456–458, 1967.
54. Nasca RJ: Rationale for spinal fusion in lumbar spinal stenosis. **Spine** 14:451–454, 1989.
55. Nasca RJ: Surgical management of lumbar spinal stenosis: **Spine** 12:809–816, 1987.
56. Pappas CTE, Harrington T, Sonntag VKH: Outcome analysis in 654 surgically treated lumbar disc herniations. **Neurosurgery** 30:862–866, 1992.
57. Paralkar VM, Nandedkar AK, Pointer R, et al.: Interaction of osteogenin, a heparin binding bone morphogenic protein, with type IV collagen. **J Biol Chem** 265:17281–17284, 1990.
58. Pennal BF, Schatzker J: Stenosis of the lumbar spinal canal. **Clin Neurosurg** 18:86–105, 1971.

59. Poletti C: Central lumbar stenosis caused by ligamentum flavum: Unilateral lamino-tomy for bilateral ligamentectomy: Preliminary report of two cases. **Neuro-surgery** 37:343–347, 1995.

60. Porter RW: Central spinal stenosis: Classification and pathogenesis. **Acta Orthop Scan** (Suppl 251) 64:64–66, 1993.

61. Prere J, Manelfe C, Salvolini U: Pathology of the neural arch, spinal stenosis, and spondylolisthesis, in Manelfe C (ed): *Imaging of the Spine and Spinal Cord,* New York; Raven Press, 1992, ed 1, pp 342–353.

62. Roberson GH, Llewellyn HJ, Taveras JM: The narrow lumbar spinal canal syn-drome. **Radiology** 107:89–97, 1973.

63. Selby DK, Gill K, Blumenthal SL, *et al.:* Fusion of the lumbar spine, in Youmans JR (ed): *Neurological Surgery,* Philadelphia: WB Saunders Company, 1990, ed 3, pp 2785–2804.

64. Shapiro R: The narrow spinal canal, in Shapiro R (ed): *Myelography,* Chicago; Year Book Medical Publishers, 1984, ed 4, pp 497–532.

65. Shenkin H, Hash C: Spondylolisthesis after multiple bilateral laminectomies and facetectomies for lumbar spondylosis. **J Neurosurg** 50:45–47, 1979.

66. Silvers HR, Lewis PJ, Asch HL: Decompressive lumbar laminectomy for spinal stenosis. **J Neurosurg** 78:695–701, 1993.

67. Spanu G, Messina AL, Assietti R, *et al.:* Lumbar canal stenosis: results in 40 patients surgically tested. **Acta Neurochirg (Wein)** 94:144–149, 1988.

68. Steinmann JC, Herkowitz HN, el-Kommos H, *et al.:* Spinal pedicle fixation. Confir-mation of an image-based technique for screw placement. **Spine** 18(13):1856–1881, 1993.

69. Stromqvist B: Postlaminectomy problems with reference to spinal fusion. **Acta Or-thop Scan** (Suppl) 251:87–89, 1993.

70. Summers BN, Eisenstein SM: Donor site pain from the ilium. **J Bone Joint Surg** 71B:677–680, 1989.

71. Sweeney TM, Opperman LA, Persing JA, *et al.:* Repair of critical size rat calvarial defects using extracellular matrix protein gels. **J Neurosurg** 83(4):710–715, 1995.

72. Surin V, Hedelin E, Smith L: Degenerative lumbar spinal stenosis. Results of oper-ative treatment. **Acta Orthop Scand** 53:79–85, 1982.

73. Teng P, Paptheodorou C: Lumbar spondylosis with compression of cauda equina. **Arch Neurol** 8:121–129, 1963.

74. Verbiest H: Stenosis of the bony lumbar vertebral canal, in Wackenheim A (ed): *The Narrow Lumbar Canal.* Berlin; Springer-Verlag, 1980, pp 115–145.

75. Verbiest H: Results of surgical treatment of idiopathic developmental stenosis of the lumbar vertebral canal. **J Bone Joint Surg** 59B:181–188, 1977.

76. Weinstein PR: Lumbar Stenosis in Hardy R (ed): *Lumbar Disc Disease,* New York; Raven Press, Ltd, 1993, ed.2, pp 241–254.

77. Weinstein JN, Scafuri RL, McNeill TW: The Rush-Presbyterian-St. Luke's lumbar spine analysis form: A prospective study of patients with "spinal stenosis." **Spine** 8:891–896, 1983.

78. Weinstein PR: The application of anatomy and pathophysiology in the management of lumbar spine disease. **Clin Neurosurg** 27:517–540, 1980.

79. Weir B, de Leo R: Lumbar stenosis: analysis of factors affecting outcome in 81 sur-gical cases. **Can J Neurol Sci** 8:295–298, 1981.

80. West JL, Olgilve JW, Bradford DS: Complications of the variable screw plate pedi-cle screw fixation. **Spine** 16:576–579, 1991.

81. Whiffen JR, Neuwirth MG: Spinal Stenosis, in Bridwell KH, DeWald RL (eds): *The Textbook of Spinal Surgery.* Philadelphia: J.B. Lippincott Company, 1991, ed 1, pp 637–656.
82. White AA, Punjabi MM: Clinical biomechanics of spine pain, in White AA, Punjabi MM (eds): *Clinical Biomechanics of the Spine,* Philadelphia: J.B. Lippincott Company, 1990, ed 2, pp 404.
83. Wozney JM: The bone morphogenic protein family and osteogenesis. **Mol Repro Dev** 32(2):160–167, 1992.
84. Wozney JM, Rosen V, Celest AJ, *et al.:* Novel regulators of bone formation: Molecular clones and activities. **Science** 242:1528–1534, 1988.
85. Yang KH, King AI: Mechanism of facet load transmission as a hypothesis for low-back pain. **Spine** 9(6):557–565, 1984.
86. Yong-Hing K, Kirkaldy-Willins WH: The pathophysiology of degenerative disease of the lumbar spine. **Orthop Clin North Am** 14:491–504, 1983.
87. Yoshida M, Shima K, Taniguchi Y, *et al.:* Hypertrophied ligamentum flavum in lumbar spinal canal stenosis. **Spine** 17:1353–1360, 1992.
88. Young S, Veerapen R, O'Laoire SA: Relief of lumbar canal stenosis using multilevel subarticular fenestrations as an alternative to wide laminectomy: Preliminary report. **Neurosurgery** 23:628–633, 1988.
89. Younger EM, Chapman MW: Morbidity at the donor graft site. **J Orthop Trauma** 3:192–195, 1989.

IV

General Scientific
Session IV—Innovations
in Minimalism

21

Innovation Through Minimalism: Assessing Emerging Technology in Neurosurgery

ISSAM A. AWAD, MD, MSC, FACS, MA (HON.)

Neurosurgical progress has been described as a "thorny road to minimally invasive techniques" (23). In effect, major neurosurgical advances in the 20th century have consistently aimed toward minimizing the invasiveness of neurosurgical intervention while enhancing the safety and effectiveness of surgical objectives. Preoperative and intraoperative localization techniques have strived toward improving the accuracy of the surgical approach so as to minimize damage to nonpathologic neural tissue (16, 19, 31). Surgical technology has evolved toward decreasing operative trauma and maximizing neural protection during the approach and handling of tissue (2, 7, 17, 18, 34). Major paradigm shifts in the past 25 years have included surgical microscopy, tomographic preoperative imaging, and computer assisted surgical planning and navigation (evolving from conventional stereotaxy toward frameless localizers), all aiming toward minimal invasiveness.

In this chapter, we review the forces urging minimalism in neurosurgery, and vulnerabilities and concerns introduced by these forces. We defined goals of minimalistic technology which are quantifiable and verifiable. Lastly, we propose scientific principles of technology assessment aimed toward the adoption of effective modalities, and discarding other concepts and techniques with false promise or potential harm.

FORCES URGING MINIMALISM

A "patient centered" philosophy has emerged as an essential neurosurgical value (3). Inherent to such philosophy is the attempt at minimizing harm and invasiveness to the person, while realizing maximum objectives of neurosurgical intervention. This has placed minimalism at the very core of "patient centered" neurosurgical philosophy.

Furthermore, minimalism has emerged as an integral component of "quality management." There is no disputing the concept that a less invasive approach achieving the same objectives and goals is necessarily of better quality. Minimalism harbors a unique conceptual appeal to patients, physicians, and third party adjudicators. It is especially appealing in an era of emphasis on "visible" versus "invisible" outcome, where parameters of surgical scar, cosmesis, length of hospitalization, and general patient comfort are greatly valued. A graphic example of such appeal is illustrated in highly colorful advertisements hailing the advantages of a "band aid" scar as opposed to the traditional surgical dressing. The "band aid" surgical scar has almost become an obsession in health care marketing to the general public. Avoiding hair shaving has also been pursued with an element of cosmetic appeal (33).

Other forces urging minimalism include the powerful socioeconomic currents shaping health care reform. Minimalism is thought to introduce powerful factors of shortened hospital stay, the potential attractiveness of decreased cost, and even the promise of more rapid convalescence, rehabilitation, and return to productive life. Of course, much of this appeal necessarily requires verification which has not always been forthcoming. In fact, there is nothing potentially more costly than an operation that achieves a visibly cosmetic result without treating the core of the pathologic problem effectively. Nevertheless, the visible outcome is often easier to quantify and justify than more invisible effectiveness parameters. Much of the appeal of minimalism in neurosurgery is inherently based on the promise of potential savings in treatment costs.

Lastly, perhaps the most powerful force urging minimalism in neurosurgery is the continuing explosion of technologic possibilities. While some minimalistic approaches have emerged from a genuine need to decrease invasiveness or to realize a difficult technical objective, many other approaches have become available, and have been adopted because of technologic evolution which made such approaches conceptually possible. In fact, evolving computer and robotic techniques promise to change the neurosurgical landscape through exploding possibilities which continuously challenging the neurosurgeons' imagination (1, 8, 20, 32).

VULNERABILITIES AND CAVEATS OF MINIMALISM

Bias and Myth

Despite the powerful forces urging continued evolution toward more minimally invasive techniques, neurosurgeons have begun to acknowledge unique vulnerabilities to bias and myth (3, 11, 12). Much of the neurosurgical observational database remains highly privileged and largely unverifiable. Observations on the ease of application of a technique, and to some extent its effectiveness, are generally contributed by the very champions of the technique. These individuals and teams are often "married" to such technology, through large personal and professional investments of infrastructure, resources and credibility. There is tremendous selection bias in cases subjected to various interventions, and a treatment bias when comparing conventional and innovative approaches. There is also a powerful outcome assessment bias, largely unblinded and uncontrolled, tending to exaggerate the promise and benefits of the technical approach being championed.

These powerful biases are further magnified through secondary gains that may potentially be realized by the very individuals promoting the new technique. In some instances, such secondary gains may be quite overt, with the individuals allegedly promoting the scientific merits of a tool or technology openly involved in financial or corporate schemes related to the technique. In other instances, they may receive percentage royalty from sales of tools or instruments, or at the very least, may witness substantial windfall to their clinical practices. While it is by no means wrong or unethical to realize fair financial return from innovative ideas or capital investment, it must be acknowledged that favorable financial incentive can at the very least introduce an unconscious bias, and worse yet the potential of misrepresentation of scientific facts. In other instances, secondary gains may be quite subtle, relating to academic credibility, stature within institutions or communities, and one's own reputation as having conceptualized or championed the technology. Regardless, such subtle potential gains can at the very least promote potential bias.

Conversely, the reputation and credibility of surgeons who have conceptualized or promoted a new technical tool may greatly impact on its acceptance and dissemination. Such weighted impact through credibility is particularly operative in the field of neurological surgery where allegiance and reverence to technical mentors and surgical heroes play a major role in career development. Timely consensus among a handful of key leaders in the field may promote the acceptance of a new surgical paradigm in an almost mystical fashion. Doubt and hypothesis driven questioning of the proposed technique would typically run against such strong currents.

The conceptual appeal of a technology, along with a timely key support by a few individuals may generate an insurmountable consensus despite the lack of objective scientific proof of any advantage of the technology. Acknowledging such vulnerability to bias and myth is not meant to discourage the adoption of innovative approaches, but rather to articulate and heighten awareness about potential false dissemination of ideas without sound scientific accreditation.

Limitations of Scientific Method in Technology Assessment

We have already addressed the issue of the credibility of proponents of technology, and how such credibility and reverence can generate an unscientific consensus. We also articulated problems of control and bias in patient selection, treatment, and outcome assessment. Other limitations of scientific method include the ever-changing state of evolving technology (3, 5, 11). It is nearly impossible to subject a technique or a tool to sound scientific accreditation when such technology is continuously evolving. On the one hand, newer versions of the technique promise to circumvent previous shortcomings. At the very least, newer versions of the technique provide its proponents with a powerful argument that any previous doubts may have been based on an earlier generation of the tool or technology. Similarly, the scientific question at the heart of assessing the effectiveness of emerging technology may also evolve during the process of assessments (5). Novel observations may raise new questions which had not been anticipated previously, or may trivialize other issues which had been thought to be more critical. At the same time, evolving understanding of the disease may change the cohort of patients being subjected to the technology, and also the relevant outcome parameters being measured. For example, as a technique becomes more disseminated, the types of patients being subjected to it may change dramatically, typically broadening the acceptance criteria, including cases with possibly less advanced stages of a disease. This may alter outcome assessment dramatically, or may require the introduction of additional more relevant outcome parameters.

There is also a wide complexity and variability of clinical scenarios where a technique is eventually applied. The preliminary feasibility studies on the use of a tool or a technology encourage its application in other clinical scenarios, and in broader patient cohorts. The potential of false generalization is ever present, as earlier favorable observations may be totally irrelevant when generalized to different clinical scenarios.

Caveats of Minimalistic Technology in Neurosurgery

Having acknowledged the vulnerability to bias and myth, and the definite limitations of classical scientific method in technology assessment, we must articulate a number of cardinal criteria aimed at enhancing the integrity of such assessment. First and foremost, minimalism should not be pursued "at any cost." It is extremely dangerous to champion a given technology to its utmost limits regardless of consequences. Clinical applications of any technology should therefore be aimed at defining specific goals of the technology, and the demonstration of equivalent or superior effectiveness in comparison to more traditional or conventional approaches (1). This should necessarily include demonstration of equivalent or superior durability of benefit in cases where long-term outcome may be critical. For example, a technique aimed at treating benign tumors or unruptured intracranial aneurysms cannot be validated through short-term results alone, but rather through its impact on the natural history of the disease over time (7, 14). Such data is excruciatingly difficult to gather, and requires very thorough and strict scientific methodology (see below). Yet, any shortcuts in this process, despite the powerful forces that may be urging them risk introducing serious scientific flaw. In such situations, there is no alternative to a thorough longitudinal integration of outcome assessment, as opposed to the assessment of morbidity of the intervention itself or a single episode of illness.

The integration of economic factors also requires longitudinal data collection. For example, a given technique may have strong conceptual appeal, a broad consensus of support, and may be applied with substantial cost savings in comparison to conventional approaches. Yet, such technology may be far more costly in the long run if it required frequent re-treatments, or if it incurred additional long-term costs due to lack of effectiveness. As an example, stereotactic radiosurgical treatment of vascular malformations may be associated with slightly lesser cost of initial hospitalization than microsurgical treatment of comparable lesions (20). Yet, cost savings may be eliminated or grossly exceeded by the necessity of continuing follow-up of the patient subjected to radiosurgery, management of radionecrosis in a substantial proportion of the cases, and the requirement of additional treatment of residual vascular malformation in another fraction of cases. Relative comparisons of cost of treatment are not valid unless they take in consideration such longitudinal integration of outcome and economic factors.

OBJECTIVES OF MINIMALISTIC TECHNOLOGY

The broad goal of minimalistic technology in neurosurgery is to improve management outcome. This must be assessed through clearly defined and relevant outcome parameters. These may include decease in perioperative or postoperative pain, discomfort, and anxiety. While highly subjective, these indicators greatly impact on patient satisfaction and represent powerful arguments for minimalistic technology, and they can be quantified through validated instruments controlling against placebo and treatment bias.

Other objectives of minimalistic technology include the facilitation of execution of surgical objectives (7, 16, 19, 31). A novel surgical localization or navigation strategy may greatly improve the ability to achieve tumor localization and maximize extent of resection. The use of intraoperative microscope in carotid endarterectomy may allow more precise removal of atherosclerotic plaque, and safer management of distal intimal flap. Yet, these conceptually appealing objectives can and must be validated through controlled observations aimed at quantifying the desired surgical objectives and testing the proposed hypothesis.

Other objectives which are easily subjected to quantification and verification include decreased operative time or hospital stay (including stay in critical care units, overall hospitalization, and length of rehabilitation) (15, 17). Time until return to premorbid activities or productive work may also be measured and quantified. Less invasive surgical approaches to lumbar disc disease have long been hailed as achieving such objectives. Yet, caution must be exercised against biases in outcome assessment or patient selection, and also against the lack of consideration of longer term outcome (11, 12, 24). For example, looser selection criteria might subject a broader cohort of patients to minimally invasive lumbar disc surgery who may otherwise not have been subjected to conventional surgical intervention (*i.e.*, failure of conservative therapy). Information on length of hospitalization and return to work in this cohort must be cautiously interpreted in comparison with data from conventional treatment strategies on what may be a different category of patients.

Lastly, cost of management may be an easily quantifiable variable accrediting a new technology. However, accounting principles and controls must be quite rigorous to avoid the attribution of cost savings to the technology itself at a time when length of stay and other health care costs may also be decreasing for other reasons. The use of hospital charges rather than costs may be quite unreliable for obvious reasons, while actual treatment costs are nearly impossible to obtain and validate at most institutions. Nevertheless, the acknowledgment of these limitations allows the introduction of rigorous controls when using management cost as an outcome variable. We have also eluded to the importance of longitudinal integration of economic factors whenever the disease is not totally cured by the intervention, and where costs of additional follow-up or further intervention may not be reflected in the initial cost of treatment. In this regard, "management cost" is a more accurate economic indicator than "treatment cost."

FALSE GENERALIZATION

The application of novel surgical technology requires generalization of observations from one set of patients and circumstances to a broader cohort of subjects. The threat of false generalization has long been recognized in scientific methodology. The French mathematician and scientific philosopher, Henri Poincare, expressed the threat as follows: "All generalization is an hypothesis. It ought always, as soon as possible, as often as possible, to be subjected to verification. If it does not stand this test, it ought to be abandoned without reserve. We do so with an ill humor. This ill humor is not justified" (26). No where is such ill humor evident as when proponents of a novel technology are asked to subject the technology to sound hypothesis testing before accepting its generalization!

Specific clinical scenarios can graphically illustrate the potential traps of false generalization. For example, preoperative embolization of brain arteriovenous malformations has been shown to be feasible, safe, and effective (10, 15). It has allowed the surgical excision of lesions, which were otherwise inoperable, and has been demonstrated to decrease operative time, blood transfusions, and postsurgical morbidity in these cases (15). The technique has been rapidly incorporated in the armamentarium of multidisciplinary teams managing brain vascular malformations, and has been increasingly applied to the treatment of all lesion types (10). However, the potential risk-benefit ratio of preoperative embolization in smaller, surgically accessible lesions has not been tested separately. In these cases, the potential morbidity of additional embolization may not be always justified, nor would the added cost which could easily exceed that of the surgical treatment of the lesion. This risk-benefit analysis may depend on numerous factors, including the lesion size, location in relation to eloquent brain regions, and preoperative patient condition. These considerations also depend, to a certain extent, on the practical capabilities and realistic outcomes of the endovascular and the surgical team at the particular institution (published rates of complications may not be generalizable to individual institutions). In these situations, as in all cases where generalization of observations may be required, a new hypothesis must be formulated and tested. For the specific example of embolization of arteriovenous malformations, prospective and controlled data collection stratified for relevant lesion and host factors must be undertaken, to justify the specific role of embolization in the various subgroups of cases (10).

Similarly, intraoperative angiography has recently been introduced into clinical practice. Several reports have emphasized its sensitivity, specificity and clinical usefulness (6, 21, 25). However, this information has largely emerged from specialized quaternary centers with high proportion of case complexity. Generalization of the use of intraoperative angiography would assume that the technique can be performed with comparable facility and morbidity at other centers, and that the case mix of more simple vascular procedures would also derive the same benefit from intraoperative angiographic findings. It is clear that both of these assumptions may not hold true, and that wide generalization of intraoperative angiography should require further hypothesis testing. Preliminary data from an ongoing prospective study at our center has suggested that this technique contributes useful information in giant and posterior circulation aneurysms, but not in smaller anterior circulation lesions (25). Its applicability following excision of thoroughly embolized arteriovenous malformations may also not be the same as following excision of non-embolized lesions.

Lastly, we wish to discuss the example of endosaccular aneurysm treatment with Guglielmi Detachable Coil as another potentially extreme case of false generalization. Preliminary safety and effectiveness studies for the purpose of approval of the device by the Food and Drug Administration limited it to the treatment of intracranial aneurysms where surgical morbidity would be expected to be prohibitive (due to lesion or host factors), or where surgical treatment may not be an option altogether (35). However, it soon became evident that numerous centers have experimented with the device in cases where surgical treatment of the lesion would have been possible without prohibitive morbidity (14). In fact, it has been suggested through uncontrolled observations in these cases, that the performance of the device (morbidity and effectiveness) may be far better in this latter subgroup of cases. This inconsistency in patient selection has significantly impacted on the reliability of outcome reporting of all cases treated with this device, with conclusions observed in a given cohort frequently implied as applicable to a broader group of patients. Pharmaceutical and device manufacturing companies have long used such an approach of accrediting a drug or device in a specific subgroup of cases, with the implication or full knowledge that clinicians would likely generalize those results to a wider "potential market." Surgeons should be aware of these and similar scenarios of false generalization, and potential pitfalls of scientific methodology that all but invalidate many of the initial outcome claims.

THE SCIENCE OF TECHNOLOGY ASSESSMENT

Evolution Through Hypothesis

Given the previously articulated concerns and caveats, neurosurgeons must articulate a credible scientific methodology applicable to the integration of novel technology. The experience of clinicians re-

mains the primary generator of doubts and concerns about the usefulness of any technology (26, 27). Favorable observations will thrust a
technology ahead, while carefully articulated concerns would create
need for further investigations. Similarly, novel technology may introduce conceptual solutions to old problems, hence thrusting ahead new
approaches and possibilities.

Whenever a novel technology is introduced in the setting of clinical
need or a promising new technical possibility, the first set of required information should document the feasibility and safety of the technology.
These two cardinal variables should be articulated using measurable
and relevant outcome parameters, in a suitable cohort of patients (13).

Following documentation of feasibility and safety, there should be an
attempt at quantification of the benefit and risk of the new technology.
This should be done in stages, aiming toward generalization of risk-
benefit considerations to broader cohorts of patients, and also to the
larger group of potential practitioners (beyond the initial expert proponents of the technique). It will become evident that some technologies will fail the test of generalization to either a wider cohort, or would
not be applicable with equal risk-benefit by all practitioners. In each
instance, information gathering should be driven by specific hypothesis, and all subsequent generalization should be executed through further hypothesis (26, 27).

The Scientific Method and Technology Assessment

Table 20.1 summarizes seven cardinal rules of scientific method that
must be at the heart of technology assessment in neurosurgery. First
and foremost, we have emphasized defining a specific hypothesis. Furthermore, there must be definition of the patient cohort, and the specific surgical objectives. These should be translated into relevant outcome parameters, preferably reflecting instruments which have been
validated for the particular disease, lesion, or intervention. As much as
possible, the technology being evaluated must be standardized, at least
for the purpose of initial evaluation. Further testing of more advanced
versions of the technology would be subjected to further hypothesis. It
may be advisable, in certain situations, to withhold large definitive
clinical trials until there is some consensus that the technology has stabilized. However, evolving technology cannot represent an excuse for
never performing thorough scientific evaluation of the modality.

As in all scientific undertakings, it is useful to acknowledge all potential biases, and construct a study design aimed at controlling such
biases (3, 5, 11, 12). The classical "double blinding" methodology of
pharmaceutical clinical trials may not always be applicable. However,

TABLE 1
Technology Assessment

A Cardinal Scientific Method in Neurosurgery

- Define the hypothesis (es)
- Define the patient cohort
- Define the surgical objectives
- Define relevant outcome parameters
- Standardize the technology being evaluated
- Acknowledge and control biases
- Third party adjudication of results

alternative methodologies of bias control must be rigorously introduced and adhered to, as appropriate within the constraints of ethical and practical considerations. The quality and reliability of the scientific results will always be proportional to the rigor of methodologic bias control. Whenever possible, results must be subjected to third party adjudication, and should never be left to the unverified observation by the very proponents of the technology. Third party adjudication may be the best alternative in situations when blinding of patients or clinicians may not be possible (3, 11).

An example of valid application of minimally invasive technology is the use of magnetic resonance angiography (MRA) as the preoperative diagnostic test before carotid endarterectomy. The increasing availability of MRA techniques, the continuing need for diagnostic tests without the risk of catheter angiography in elderly vasculopathic patients, and the potential cost savings have all urged the consideration of MRA as a sufficient diagnostic test prior to carotid endarterectomy. Before this concept could be accepted, specific studies were conducted documenting the sensitivity, specificity, and spacial fidelity of MRA diagnostic information in comparison with conventional catheter digital subtraction angiography (4, 22, 28, 29). Question driven clinical utility questions were addressed in large cohorts of cases with ischemic cerebrovascular disease (4). This experience not only demonstrated the potential validity of MRA, but also highlighted specific shortcomings. For example, the technique was not reliable in situations where the quality of the MRA exam was suboptimal, where there was discrepancy between MRA and doppler ultrasound testing, or where there was a question about occlusion or near-occlusion of the vessel. Also, a tendency by MRA to overestimate the degree of stenosis, and to distort the spatial geometry of the atherosclerotic plaque were clearly documented. Given these caveats, specific studies are currently being undertaken using MRA as the sole diagnostic test before carotid surgery in consecutive cases where the MRA study is a good quality, concordant with doppler ultrasound results, and where there is no question about possible occlusion of the artery or intracranial disease. Favorable results from these studies will allow cautious generalization of this technology, pending confirmation of such generalization among a broader spectrum of centers, surgeons, and patients, preferably in the setting of a controlled trial.

The concept of "Question-Driven Technology Assessment" as eloquently proposed by Caplan in 1991 remains the central theme of such graduated approach to technology evaluation and accreditation (9). The questions must be specific and relevant to the individual technology and applicable diseases, and should be assessed through clearly articulated hypothesis in the appropriate cohort of patients (3, 4, 9).

The range of scientific studies include carefully controlled consecutive observations in clearly defined cohorts of cases (23), registries with risk and lesion stratification (30), and clinical trials (5, 11). Each can contribute reliable scientific information, which validity and applicability are proportional to the rigors of scientific methodology and the statistical power of the cohort. Integration of information from a number of different studies is possible using sound statistical methods of meta-analysis, which can increase reliability of scientific consensus vis-a-vis smaller individual studies (3).

CONCLUSION

A neurosurgeon's practical dictum might be formulated as "never be the first to adopt a novel application, . . . and never be the last!" Such conventional wisdom reflects the potential quagmire surrounding a clinician's decision whether and when to adopt or discard a novel technology. Major forces have long shaped the field of neurological surgery toward increasingly minimalistic approaches to achieving surgical objectives. Exploding technological possibilities and socioeconomic forces have increased the power of this vector. However, the neurosurgeon must be aware of the vulnerability to bias and myth accompanying these forces, and major caveats of minimalistic technology. The limitations of scientific method in technology assessment should never be an excuse to bypass this methodology altogether. It has been said, and it remains so true for the foreseeable future, that the difficulties, complexities and costs of scientific assessment of surgical technique can only be exceeded by the costs and damage of integrating useless or harmful paradigms (5).

Acknowledgment and control of potential sources of bias can enhance the validity of any scientific observation, whether in an isolated clinical setting or in complex multi-institutional trials. Defining the question and the cohort is another essential requirement, while constantly bewaring of the threat of false generalization. Lastly, neurosurgeons should openly acknowledge the importance of third party adjudication in study design, data collection, and interpretation. This may be the only practical and valid alternative to blinded methodology (which is not often possible in surgical settings) and as an effective deterrent to the ever prevalent potential of secondary gains by the proponents of novel technology.

The future of neurological surgery carries the promise of an incredible journey into technical possibilities scarcely imagined today (8, 32). As numerous modalities are being proposed, the neurosurgeon is advised to consider four cardinal questions as recently proposed by the American College of Surgeons (1):

1. Has the new technology been adequately tested for safety and efficacy?
2. Is the new technology at least as safe and effective as existing, proven techniques?
3. Is the individual proposing to perform the new procedure fully qualified to do so?
4. Is the new technology cost-effective?

The answers to these questions often require thorough scientific testing, and will likely as often discredit as endorse novel techniques and minimally invasive modalities.

REFERENCES

1. American College of Surgeons: Statement on issues to be considered before new surgical technology is applied to the care of patients. **Bull Am Coll Surg** 80(9): 46–47, 1995.
2. Akabane A, Saito S, Suzuki Y, Shibuya M, Sugita K: Monitoring of visual evoked potentials during retraction of the canine optic nerve: protective effect of unroofing the opting canal. **J Neurosurg** 82:284–287, 1995.
3. Awad IA: Neurological surgery and clinical science, in Awad IA (ed): *Philosophy of Neurological Surgery,* American Association of Neurological Surgeons, Park Ridge, Illinois, 1995; pp 117–124.
4. Awad IA, McKenzie R, Magdinec M, Masaryk T: Application of magnetic resonance angiography to neurosurgical practice: A Critical Review of 150 Cases. **Neurolog Res** 14:360–368, 1992.
5. Awad IA, Spetzler RF: Extracranial-Intracranial bypass surgery: A critical analysis in light of the International Cooperative Study. **Neurosurgery** 19:655–664, 1996.
6. Barrow DL, Boyar KL, Joseph GJ: Intraoperative angiography in the management of neurovascular disorders. **Neurosurgery** 30:153–159, 1992.
7. Braun V, Richter HP: Preservation of hearing and facial nerve function in surgery for acoustic neuroma: Effect on tumor recurrence in 74 cases (German). **Laringo-Rhino-Otologie** 70:663–669, 1991.

8. Bucholz RD: Introduction to Journal of Image Guided Surgery. **J Image Guided Surg** 1(1):1–3, 1995.
9. Caplan LR: Question-Driven Technology Assessment: SPECT as an example. **Neurology** 41:187–191, 1991.
10. Frizzel RT, Fisher WS: Cure, morbidity, and mortality associated with embolization of brain arteriovenous malformations: A review of 1246 patients in 32 series over a 35 year period. **Neurosurgery** 37:1031–1040, 1995.
11. Haines SJ: Randomized clinical trials in the evaluation of surgical innovation. **J Neurosurg** 51:5–11, 1979.
12. Haines SJ: The art and science of evaluating neurosurgical treatment. **Clin Neurosurg** 35:451–458, 1989.
13. Hawkins C, Sorgi M, Eds: *Research: How to Plan, Speak, and Write About It,* Springer-Verlag, New York, 1985.
14. Hopkins, LN, Guterman LR, Livingston K, Gibbons KJ, Ahuja A: Endovascular treatment of aneurysms and cerebral vasospasm, in Awad IA (ed): *Current Management of Cerebral Aneurysms,* American Association of Neurological Surgeons, Park Ridge, Illinois 1993, pp 219–242.
15. Jafar JJ, Davis AJ, Berenstein A, Choi IS, Kupersmith MJ: The effect of embolization with N-butyl cyanoacrylate prior to surgical resection of cerebral arteriovenous malformations. **J Neurosurg** 78:60–69, 1993.
16. Jani AB, Cychra JJ: MR image classification algorithms for neurosurgical and stereotactic radiosurgery trajectory planning and volumetric analysis. **Neurolog Res** 17:17–23, 1995.
17. Jones RF, Kwok DC, Stening WA, Vonau M: The current status of endoscopic third ventrisculostomy in the management of non-communicating hydrocephalous. **Minimally Invasive Neurosurg** 37:28–36, 1994.
18. Kageyama Y, Fukuda K, Kobayashi S, Odaki M, Nakamura H, Satoh A, Watanabe Y: cerebral vein disorders and postoperative brain damage associated with pterional approach in aneurysm surgery. **Neurologia Medico-Chirurgica** 32:733–738, 1992.
19. Kunz U, Goldmann A, Bader C, Oldenkott P. Stereotactic and ultrasound guided minimal invasive surgery of subcortical cavernomas. **Minimally Invasive Neurosurg** 37:17–20, 1994.
20. Lindquist C, Kihlstrom L, Hellstrand E: Functional Neurosurgery: A future for the Gamma Knife? **J Stereotactic Functional Neurosurg** 57:72–81, 1981.
21. Martin NA, Bentson J, Vinuela F, Hieshima G, Reicher M, Black K, Dion J, Becker D: Intraoperative digital subtraction angiography and the surgical treatment of intracranial aneurysms and vascular malformations. **J Neurosurg** 73:526–533, 1990.
22. Masaryk AM, Ross JS, DiCello MC, Modic MT, Paranandi L, Masaryk TJ: 3DFT MR Angiography of the carotid bifurcation: Potential and limitations as a screening examination. **Radiology** 179:797–804, 1991.
23. Moses LE: The series of consecutive cases as a device for assessing outcomes of intervention. **N Engl J Med** 311:705–710, 1984.
24. Pasztor E: The thorny road to minimally invasive techniques in neurosurgery. **Minimally Invasive Techniques Neurosurg** 37:64–69, 1994.
25. Perl J, Masaryk TJ, Awad IA: Imaging of cerebral aneurysms, in Awad IA (ed): *Current Management of Cerebral Aneurysms,* American Association of Neurological Surgeons, Park Ridge, Illinois 1993, pp 43–70.
26. Poincare H: *La Science et L'Hypothese,* Flammarion Publishers, Paris, France, 1906.

27. Popper KR: *The Logic of Scientific Discovery,* Basic Books, New York, 1959.
28. Riles TS, Eidelman EM, Litt AW, Pinto RS, Oldford F: Thoe Schwartzenbert GWS. Comparison of magnetic resonance angiography, conventional angiography, and duplex scanning. **Stroke** 23:341–346, 1992.
29. Ross JS, Masaryk TJ, Ruggeri PM. Magnetic resonance angiography of the carotid bifurcation. **Top Magn Reson Imaging** 3:12–22, 1991.
30. Rosati RA, Lee KL, Califf RM, Pryor DB, Harrel FE: Problems and advantages of an observational database approach to evaluating the effect of therapy on outcome. **Circulation** 65(suppl 1):27–32, 1982.
31. Sandeman DR, Patel N, Chandler C, Nelson RJ, Coakham HB, Griffith HB: Advances in image-directed neurosurgery: Preliminary experience with the ISG viewing wand compared with the leksell G frame. **Br J Neurosurg** 8:529–544, 1994.
32. Satava RM: Virtual reality, telesurgery, and the new world order of medicine. **J Image Guided Surgery** 1:12–16, 1995.
33. Scherpercel B: No hair shaving (French). **Neurochirurgie** 39:374–375, 1993.
34. Slosarek J, Bajko J, Kojder I, Kaczor R: Effects of classical and microsurgical methods of exclusion of cerebral aneurysms on the structural and functional changes near the operation site. **Neurologia I Neurochirurgia Polska** 26:201–207, 1992.
35. Target Therapeutics. Product Information Summary. Guglielmi Detachable Coil (GDC). US Patent 5, 122, 136 and foreign patents pending. Customer Service, Target Therapeutics, Fremont, California, 1995:1–8.

22

Minimalism Through Stereotactic Technique

DONALD A. ROSS, M.D.

I. HISTORY

Below is an outline covering some of the important events in the development of stereotactically guided craniotomy. The number of papers published in the last 10 years has increased exponentially; therefore, no attempt has been made to include every reference from this time period. The contributions of Dr. Patrick Kelly deserve special mention as being undeservedly minimized by this approach, and no attempt has been made to deal with the expanding field of "frameless" stereotactic surgery.

Guiot et al. (11) has been credited with first proposing that stereotactic guidance could be usefully applied during open craniotomy, and Reichert and Mundinger (27) reported in 1964 on the utility of this technique for locating the feeding vessels to deep vascular lesions. It was not until 1980, however, that reports of more widespread application of existing stereotactic frames to open surgery began to appear. Jacques et al. (17) and Shelden et al. (30) reported in 1980 on the development of unique instruments specifically designed for stereotactic craniotomy. In 1981, Kelly and Alker (18) described the use of the Todd-Wells frame and laser for stereotactically guided tumor resection, one of many subsequent papers on this subject. In 1985, Hitchcock began using the term "open stereotactic neurosurgery."

In 1989, a report by Moore et al. (21) noted that the use of the open stereotactic technique could allow the use of local anesthesia, shortened operating time, decreased morbidity, and shortened hospitalization, thus suggesting that this technique could contribute to minimalism in neurosurgery. By 1990, Kelly (19) had reported on the results of 374 stereotactically guided craniotomies, firmly establishing the technique. Reports by Zamorano (32) and Cosgrove (6) also mention local anesthesia, decreased morbidity, and shortened hospitalization as advantages of this technique.

A. Pre-CT Era

Guiot *et al.* 1960 (11)—Proposed stereotactic guidance for operations on deep-seated vascular lesions

Riechert and Mundinger 1964 (27)—Described stereotactic localization of the feeding vessels of deep AVMs

B. Post-CT Era

Zamskaya *et al.* 1976 (33)—Described the combined use of stereotactic localization and open craniotomy for epilepsy surgery

Garcia de Sola 1980 (9)—Described a single case of a deep seated AVM resected with stereotactic guidance using the Talairach frame (see Carillo 1986 (4))

Jacques *et al.* 1980 (17)—Described the use of the Reichert-Mundinger frame and a unique stereotactic retractor for the resection of small intracranial lesions

Nguyen *et al.* 1980 (23)—Described a transformation from CT to plain films to localize lesions intraoperatively

Shelden *et al.* 1980 (30)—Described stereotactic craniotomy using CT localization and a number of novel instruments including a tulip retractor and endoscope

Kelly and Alker, 1981 (18)—First description of combined stereotactic localization with the Todd-Wells frame and carbon dioxide laser for guided resection of neoplasms

Heilbrun *et al.* 1983 (13)—Described seven open procedures with stereotactic guidance using the BRW frame

Boethius and Ribbe 1984 (3)—Described a modified stereotactic frame specially designed for use during open microsurgery with a large range of available trajectories and intraoperative localization using x-ray film

Hitchcock 1985—Used the term "open stereotactic surgery" at Toronto 9th Meeting of WSSFN

Carillo *et al.* 1986 (4)—Described the use of the Talairach frame to localize deep AVMs

Hariz and Fodstad 1987 (12)—Described the use of the Laitinen stereoadapter for guided craniotomy

Patil 1987 (25)—Described the use of a stereotactic probe guided retraction system

Sedan *et al.* 1988—Described localization of superficial lesions by superimposition of CT onto stereotactic plain films and deep lesions by stereotactic guide placement prior to craniotomy

Moore *et al.* 1989 (21)—Described the use of the BRW frame for guided craniotomy. Noted the use of local anesthesia, shortened operating time, decreased morbidity, and shortened hospitalization.

Chan *et al.* 1989 (5)—Described small craniotomies centered on the site of a skin mark placed in the CT scanner using the laser marker light to localize the slice of interest

Hirsch *et al.* 1989 (14)—Described the use of the BRW frame with CT or MR imaging in combination with open craniotomy for small or deep lesions

Hitchcock *et al.* 1989 (15)—Described 14 CT guided stereotactic craniotomies, some using a cylindrical retractor (resectoscope)

Kelly 1990 (19)—Results of 374 stereotactic craniotomies

Sabin and Whittle 1990—Described the use of the BRW frame with CT or MR imaging in combination with open craniotomy for small or deep lesions

Zamorano *et al.* 1990 (32)—Image guided stereotactic resection with mention of local anesthesia, decreased morbidity, and shortened hospitalization as advantages

Cosgrove and Steiner 1993 (6)—Stereotactic craniotomy with the Leksell system. Average length of hospital stay 2.8 days. Indications are for benign lesions and metastases less than 3.5 cm, but not malignant gliomas

II. IMPORTANT FEATURES OF STEREOTACTICALLY GUIDED CRANIOTOMY

Standard, frame-based stereotactically guided craniotomy has a number of desirable features. It is widely available in the neurosurgical community; it is relatively inexpensive when compared with the cost of the frameless systems currently available; it provides rigid head fixation during the operative procedure; and it provides precise target localization. Stereotactic guidance allows the surgeon to make a small skin incision, small craniotomy, and small cortical incision in the preselected gyrus or sulcus of the surgeon's choice. The decreased size of the opening in turn allows a switch to local anesthesia, decreased operating time, a shortened hospitalization and recovery time, and decreased cost of care.

III. CURRENT APPLICATIONS

Stereotactic craniotomy may be indicated in the following scenarios. Small lesions are especially amenable to this technique. Small metastases, primary brain tumors, and vascular malformations are good examples of lesions that can be removed by stereotactically guided craniotomy. Small cortical lesions may be removed through a single burhole if the opening is placed precisely over the lesion with stereotactic guidance. These cases are routinely done under local anesthesia with a 1-day hospitalization and in selected cases, no intensive care unit stay.

Deep lesions are also good candidates for stereotactically guided craniotomy. Metastatic tumors, primary brain tumors, and colloid cysts are examples of pathologies for which this technique is useful. Stereotactic guidance allows the selection of the cortical entry point and precise lesion localization through a small craniotomy. A cylindrical retractor such as that used by Dr. Kelly or which we have described (28) is useful in these cases.

Some large lesions may be appropriate for stereotactically guided craniotomy. In particular, some more extensive gliomas can be resected through relatively small craniotomies if the incision can be precisely located based on stereotactic coordinates. This in turn makes the use of local anesthesia better tolerated which allows for intraoperative neurologic examination.

We have substantiated the utility of the use of stereotactically guided craniotomy in a retrospective study at the University of Michigan Hospital. Twenty-nine patients undergoing stereotactic craniotomies were compared with 12 patients who underwent standard craniotomy and whose lesions were judged to have been suitable for a stereotactically guided procedure. The first difference noted was in the use of local anesthesia. While all 15 of the standard craniotomy patients had a general anesthetic, 14 of the stereotactically guided cases had a local anesthetic, and the trend was toward decreasing use of general anesthesia over time. The switch to local anesthesia improved the safety of the procedure by allowing intraoperative neurologic examination and decreased the cost of the procedure substantially (see below). In addition, stereotactically guided local anesthetic cases used an average 90 minutes of operating room time versus 106 minutes for stereotactically guided cases with a general anesthetic and 176 minutes for the conventional cases.

The use of stereotactic technique shortened the hospital stay. The average length of hospitalization for the standard craniotomies was 4.9 days versus 2.1 for the stereotactically guided procedures. Average ICU stay for the standard procedures was 1.8 days versus 0.9 for the stereotactic procedures.

Despite the increased cost of imaging incurred by using the stereotactic technique, there was an overall cost savings in the stereotactically guided craniotomy patients versus the conventional craniotomy group. We compared total cost of hospitalization, including operating room, hospital room, medications, radiology, and professional fees between the two study groups. We emphasize that these are not the charges for goods and services because charges are set arbitrarily, but the actual cost to hospital for caring for these patients. The conventional craniotomy group incurred a total average cost of $11,176 per case versus $8,645 for the stereotactically guided group, a decrease of 25%. When the stereotactic group was further subdivided into those receiving a general anesthetic versus those operated under local anesthesia, the total costs were $9,531 and $7,886, respectively. These data include that stereotactically guided craniotomy can save considerable cost by reducing anesthesia and operating room cost, intensive care unit stay, and length of hospitalization.

IV. FUTURE DIRECTIONS

The future of stereotactically guided craniotomy will no doubt include the widespread application of "frameless" or image-guided techniques. Other speakers have covered this emerging technology in detail.

The future is likely to hold an expanded array of stereotactic imaging techniques for preoperative planning. Stereotactic SPECT (2), PET, and functional MRI are already available in some centers and their utility is being evaluated.

Another area which may emerge from dormancy is the use of intraoperative dyes to aid in the resection of tumors. Fluorescein was used successfully for the localization of brain tumors 50 years ago (20) but has only rarely been used in recent years (22), probably because of the emergence of intraoperative ultrasound, computed tomography, and stereotactic guidance. Fluorescein crosses the blood-brain barrier in a manner analogous to radiologic contrast media and can be used to visualize a contrast-enhancing mass in the operating room. We have used fluorescein in combination with light source and eyepiece filters for the operating microscope to enhance the excitatory and fluorescent wavelengths, respectively. This allows intraoperative visualization of the contrast-enhancing portions of the mass with minimal disruption in standard neurosurgical procedure. More specific tumor markers based on laser fluorescence (26) or perhaps on immunologic reagents may improve the sensitivity and specificity of this technique.

Finally, the question of outpatient craniotomy no longer seems ridiculous as stereotactically guided procedures become minimally invasive and safety continues to improve.

REFERENCES

1. Alesch F, Ostertag CB, Koos WT: Combined stereotactic and microsurgical approach to cerebral lesions. **Acta Neurochir** (suppl)53:19–22, 1991.
2. Alexander E III, Loeffler JS, Schwartz RB, Johnson KA, Carvalho PA, Garada BM, Zimmerman RE, Holman BL: Thallium-201 technetium-99m HMPAO single-photon emission computed tomography (SPECT) imaging for guiding stereotactic

craniotomies in heavily irradiated malignant glioma patients. **Acta Neurochir** 122:215–217, 1993.

3. Boethius J, Ribbe T: A new stereotactic instrument which can be used in conjunction with open surgery. **Acta Neurochir** (Suppl) 33:559–565, 1984.

4. Carillo R, Garcia de Sola R, Gonzalez-Ojellon M, Garcia-Uria J, Bravo G: Stereotactic localization and open microsurgical approach in the treatment of some intracranial deep arteriovenous malformations. **Surg Neurol** 25:535–539, 1986.

5. Chan K-H, Mann KS, Ngan H: Computed tomography guided preoperative localization of small intracranial lesions. Short report. **Br J Neurosurg** 3:127–130, 1989.

6. Cosgrove GR, Steiner L: Stereotactic microsurgical resection of cerebral lesions. **Stereotact Funct Neurosurg** 61:182–194, 1993.

7. David DH, Kelly PJ: Stereotactic resections of occult vascular malformations. **J Neurosurg** 72:698–702, 1990.

8. Esposito V, Oppido PA, Delfini R, Cantore G: A simple method for stereotactic microsurgical excision of small, deep-seated cavernous angiomas. **Neurosurgery** 34:515–519, 1994.

9. Garcia de Sola R, Cabezudo J, Areitio E, Bravo G: Combined approach (stereotactic-microsurgical) to a paraventricular arteriovenous malformation. Case report. **Acta Neurochir** (suppl) 30:413–416, 1980.

10. Garcia de Sola R, Pulido P, Kusak E: Trans-fissural or trans-sulcal approach versus combined stereotactic-microsurgical approach. **Acta Neurochir** (suppl) 52:22–25, 1991.

11. Guiot G, Rougerie J, Sachs M, Hertzog E, Molina P: Reperage stereotaxique de malformations vasculaires profondes intra-cerebrales. **Sem Hop Paris** 36:1134–1143, 1960.

12. Hariz MI, Fodstad H: Stereotactic localization of small subcortical brain tumors for open surgery. **Surg Neurol** 28:345–350, 1987.

13. Heilbrun MP, Roberts TS, Apuzzo MLJ, Wells TH Jr, Sabshin JK: Preliminary experience with the Brown-Roberts-Wells (BRW) computerized stereotaxic guidance system. **J Neurosurg** 59:217–222, 1983.

14. Hirsch JF, Sainte Rose C, Pierre-Kahn A, Renier D, Hoppe-Hirsch D: Stereotaxic technics with an open skull in the treatment of space-occupying brain lesions. **Neurochirurgie** 35:164–168, 1989.

15. Hitchcock ER, Issa AMA, Sotelo MG: Stereotactic excision of deeply seated intracranial mass lesions. **Br J Neurosurg** 3:313–320, 1989.

16. Hitchcock ER: Open stereotactic surgery. **Acta Neurochir** (suppl) 52:9–12, 1991.

17. Jacques S, Shelden CH, McCann GD, Freshwater DB, Rand R: Computerized three-dimensional stereotaxic removal of small central nervous system lesions in patients. **J Neurosurg** 53:816–820, 1980.

18. Kelly PJ, Alker GJ: A open stereotactic approach to deep-seated central nervous system neoplasms using the carbon dioxide laser. **Surg Neurol** 15:331–334, 1981.

19. Kelly PJ: Stereotactic craniotomy. **Neurosurgery Clin North America** 1:781–799, 1990.

20. Moore GE, Peyton WT, French LA, Walker WW: The clinical use of fluorescein in neurosurgery: The localization of brain tumors. **J Neurosurg** 5:392–398, 1948.

21. Moore MR, Black PM, Ellenbogen R, Gall CM, Eldredge E: Stereotactic craniotomy: Methods and results using the Brown-Roberts-Wells stereotactic frame. **Neurosurgery** 25:572–578,1989.

22. Murray KJ: Improved surgical resection of human brain tumors: Part 1. A preliminary study. **Surg Neurol** 17:316–319,1982.

23. Nguyen JP, Van Effentere R, Fohanno D, Robert G, Sichez JP, Gardeur D: Practical method for the preoperative spatial localization of small intracranial neoplasms from scanner data. **Neurochirurgie** 26:333–339, 1980.

24. Patil AA, Woosley RE: Scalp marking of intracranial lesions using computed tomography (CT) images. A technical note. **Acta Neurochir** 80:62–64, 1986.

25. Patil AA: Stereotactic excision of deep brain lesions using probe guided brain retractor. **Acta Neurochir** (Wien) 50:152–1987.

26. Poon WS, Schomacker KT, Deutsch TF, Martuza RL: Laser-induced fluorescence: experimental intraoperative delineation of tumor resection margins. **J Neurosurg** 76:679–686, 1992.

27. Riechert T, Mundinger F: Combined stereotaxic operation for treatment of deep-seated angiomas and aneurysms. **J Neurosurg** 21:358–363, 1964.

28. Ross DA: A simple stereotactic retractor for use with the Leksell stereotactic apparatus. **Neurosurgery** 32:475–476,1993.

29. Sedan R, Peragut JC, Farnarier P, Derome P, Fabrizi A: Guidage stereotaxique de certaines interventions a crane ouvert **Neurochirurgie** 34:97–101, 1988.

30. Shelden CH, McCann G, Jacque S,Lutes HR, Frazier RE, Katz R, Kuki R: Development of a computerized microstereotaxic method for localization and removal of minute CNS lesions under direct 3-D vision. **J Neurosurg** 52:21–27, 1980.

31. Sisti MB, Solomon RA, Stein BM: Stereotactic craniotomy in the resection of small arteriovenous malformations. **J Neurosurg** 75:40–44, 1991.

32. Zamorano L, Dujovny M, Chavantes C, Malik G, Ausman J: Image-guided stereotactic centered craniotomy and laser resection of solid intracranial lesions. **Stereotactic and Functional Neurosurg** 54–55:398–403, 1990.

33. Zamskaya AG, Garmeshor JA, Ryabukha NP: Application with classical craniotomy in the treatment of focal epilepsy. **Acta Neurochir** (Wien)(suppl) 23:147–151, 1976.

CHAPTER

23

Minimalism Through Intraoperative Functional Mapping

MITCHEL S. BERGER, M.D.

Intraoperative functional mapping has evolved over the past several years as a form of surgical methodology used during tumor and epilepsy surgery to lessen the operative morbidity, improve the quality of life, and prolong survival by enhancing the extent of tumor resection. Notwithstanding, these collective techniques often require extra time in the operating room. On average, asleep motor mapping requires an additional 10 to 15 minutes following dural opening to stimulate the cortex and evoke site specific contralateral motor responses. During the tumor or epileptic focus removal it is often necessary to restimulate as the resection encroaches upon functional tissue, especially when infiltrating tumor tissue is removed within descending subcortial motor pathways. This is usually combined with somatosensory mapping when the patient is awake and the area to be removed involves the Rolandic cortex. When cortical and subcortical sites are resected within the dominant cerebral hemisphere, stimulation mapping of language pathways for speech, reading, and naming often requires several steps that may prolong the procedure by 30 to 45 minutes. This involves number counting to localize Broca's area contiguous to the face motor cortex, reading, and common object naming. The latter two tasks require at least three rounds of slide viewing and cortical stimulation to identify sites that are significantly essential to this aspect of language. This is first preceded with electrocorticography to determine the current necessary to stimulate the cortex without evoking after-discharge potentials as documented with simultaneous electroencephalographic recordings. For seizure mapping, electrocorticography is used before resecting a seizure focus and subsequently recording again the cortical region found initially to be epileptogenic. Postresection electrocorticography is an integral component of the mapping procedure when the patient presents with intractable seizures. Each recording may last 15 minutes when the patient is awake or twice as long if the patient is asleep due to the anesthetic condition of the cortex.

The cost of the local anesthetic is nearly identical to that of the asleep procedure due to the need for the prolonged administration of intravenous Propofol (Diprivan). Equipment costs range between $4,000 and $5,000 and include the cortical stimulation unit along with strip and cortical electrodes. A horseshoe skull-mounted holder is also needed to secure the recording electrodes to the surface during the procedure. The surgeon must work with an electroencephalographer and a skilled technician well versed in the process of language mapping. This latter individual is also responsible for recording the accuracy of each slide that is named to ensure that stimulation induced errors are correctly documented (Table 1).

Although the mapping procedure intraoperatively requires special technical adjuncts and trained personnel, the potential benefits both in the short and long term make this surgical approach minimalistic in several ways. Before the routine use of intraoperative functional mapping the morbidity was excessive and resulted in prolonged hospital stays, including several days to weeks on the physical rehabilitation ward. The incidence of postoperative paresis has been greatly diminished and a permanent paresis or plegia occurs in less than 5% of all cases having resections within or directly adjacent to the Rolandic cortex. Likewise, permanent expressive or receptive aphasia is avoided if the resection distance is greater than 10 mm from a mapping verified essential language site (1). Thus, the current hospital stay has been reduced to a mean of 3 to 5 days. Use of rehabilitation hospitalization has been reduced by nearly 80%; the usual length of stay on this service is now typically less than 1 week. Patients return to work much sooner when functional mapping is used to avert motor and language deficits. Nearly 75% of patients return to work in their original capacity if

TABLE 1

MAXIMAL ASPECTS OF FUNCTIONAL MAPPING

Additional Operative Time:
  Asleep Sensori-motor Mapping—10 to 15 minutes
  Awake Language Mapping—30 to 45 minutes
    (includes electrocorticography for afterdischarge potentials)
  Electrocorticography for Seizure Mapping—15 minutes per recording session

Equipment Costs:
  Stimulation Unit, Stimulating, and Recording Electrodes,
    Horseshoe Electrode Holder—$4,000 to $5,000

Personnel:
  Electroencephalographer
  Electroencephalography Technician

employed preoperatively, while 20% of patients continue to work at a reduced or different schedule. Less than 5% of patients become incapable of working in some capacity due to morbidity inflicted as a result of surgery.

Patients with intractable seizures are often rendered seizure free as a result of the electrocorticography guided surgery. In the tumor patient population, nearly 85% of adults will be seizure free with more than half of these individuals on no or greatly reduced doses of antiepileptic drugs (2). Children and adolescents who have intractable seizures nearly always, *i.e.,* 85% to 90%, are able to discontinue their seizure medication and remain seizure free when the epilepsy is associated with a structural lesion (3). An aggressive tumor resection with the aid of intraoperative mapping results in a significantly lower incidence of time to tumor progression and an increase in survival for both low and high grade glial neoplasms (4, 5). In addition, with mass effect relieved as a result of a radical tumor resection, it is more likely to taper and eventually discontinue the use of corticosteroids, which are often required for long periods of time to alleviate the swelling associated with incompletely resected gliomas.

The indications for intraoperative stimulation mapping revolve around the concept of resecting cortical and subcortical areas within or adjacent to functional sites for language, movement, and sensation. Examples include dominant hemisphere perisylvian regions, rolandic cortex, and subcortical motor and sensory pathways. Electrocorticography is used to guide the resection of seizure foci and when coupled with functional mapping, become highly useful surgical methods to safely work within critical areas. Examples of circumstances where functional mapping is beneficial will be described in this chapter, thus emphasizing the role of minimalism, in the long term, for this surgical methodology.

PREPARATION FOR INTRAOPERATIVE MAPPING

A retrospective analysis of magnetic resonance (MR) imaging studies in comparison to intraoperatively derived functional brain maps has yielded a consistent set of sulcal landmarks on the imaging studies, allowing for preoperative localization of the motor and somatosensory gyri. When examining the rostral T-1 or T-2 axial images, a mirror image sulcal landmark is apparent, indicating the Central sulcus (Fig. 1). This sulcus is nearly perpendicular to the falx and while it may be displaced by a mass lesion it is always delineated (6, 7). The Rolandic cortex may also be found on the mid-sagittal image by identifying the cingulate sulcus and following this posteriorly as it

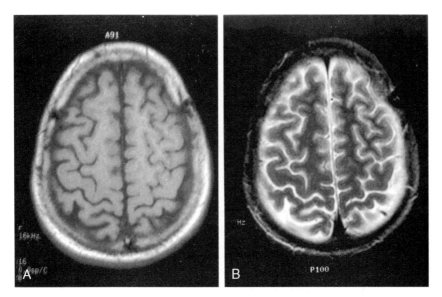

FIG. 1 T-1 weighted (**A**) and T-2 (**B**) rostral axial image, demonstrating a mirror image sulcus on the left and right, indicative of the central sulcus. The motor cortex is found directly anterior to the sulcus.

terminates in the marginal sulcus. The gyri in front of this sulcus collectively comprise the sensori-motor region in either hemisphere. If a far lateral sagittal image is used to preoperatively identify the Rolandic cortex, the insular triangle is noted and a perpendicular line drawn superiorly from its back margin will usually bisect the motor and sensory cortex. While functional MR imaging and magnetoencephalography are becoming clinical tools to identify the motor cortex preoperatively, the use of standard MR scans will yield accurate localization of this critical pathway in all cases if these important landmarks are recognized.

The patient must be tested for functional integrity on a volitional basis prior to entering the operating room. Individuals with a dense hemiparesis will be difficult to map while asleep and may require an awake operation to enhance stimulation mapping. No patient who is plegic preoperatively will be a functional mapping candidate. Children may often have an electrically inexcitable cortex due to their age, thus requiring somatosensory evoked potentials to identify the central sulcus as opposed to stimulation mapping (8, 9), although exceptions to this rule do apply under certain circumstances (10). Direct stimulation mapping is certainly less time-consuming than using evoked potentials, thus supporting the minimalistic approach. Additionally, subcortical mapping may be accomplished only with the former method leaving the use of evoked potentials to those few circumstances, *e.g.,* pediatric population, where it may be preferable (11, 12). When language deficits are prominent preoperatively, these difficulties will often be exacerbated during surgery. Thus, if a patient is tested for object naming and misses the correct name more than 25% of the time, language mapping for naming and reading will not be effective for avoiding further deficits and should not be attempted. Likewise, if a patient cannot count numbers out loud, Broca's area will be difficult, if not impossible, to accurately identify.

To enhance the ability to document epileptic foci during the surgical procedure, it is prudent to discontinue antiepileptic medication a day or 2 before the procedure. This is particularly helpful when the patient will be mapped asleep. The electrocorticography recordings will yield more useful information for planning the resection when the patient is operated upon while awake. Occasionally, subclinical epileptogenic activity may be recorded from the cortex if a bolus injection of Brevital is given (13). This may be helpful if the intraoperative recordings do not localize a seizure focus.

TECHNICAL ASPECTS OF MAPPING

Positioning, Exposure, and Equipment

Once in the operating room, the patient is positioned on his right side for a dominant hemisphere exposure. A Foley catheter is inserted, and the scalp is injected with a local anesthetic mixture of 0.5% lidocaine and 0.25% marcaine together with epinephrine. The injection should surround whatever skin incision is planned. This is done while the patient is sedated with propofol (Diprivan). This suffices to induce a deep sedative-hypnotic state while the scalp is opened and the bone is removed. The surgeon and anesthetist should avoid using small doses of barbiturates or narcotics for anxiety as these will affect the condition of the patient when they are awake and potentially reduce the reliability of the mapping. Once the bone is removed, the skull clamp that will hold the electrode array is attached to the skull and the dura around the middle meningeal articel is infiltrated with the same anesthetic mixture using a 30 gauge needle. This blocks the painful sensation experienced by patients when they are awake and the dura is manipulated. The propofol is discontinued and it usually takes between 10 and 30 minutes for the patient to awaken. In the author's experience, it appears that patients will rouse faster if they have less body fat and get a restful sleep the night before surgery. Once the patient is awake, the dura is opened. This step should not be done before having the patient wake up because of the potential deleterious effects, *e.g.*, swelling, coughing, and struggling, while emerging from the propofol sedation. It is generally advisable to expose more than less of the cortex to provide an adequate surface area to stimulate. Although motor mapping may be reliably accomplished with the patient asleep, it is preferable to perform this while the patient is awake if he or she has a preoperative deficit or if the tumor or epileptic focus involves the Rolandic cortex. A more detailed map of the motor homunculus may be obtained with the patient awake.

Stimulation mapping is achieved using a constant current generator that produces a train of biphasic square wave pulses with a frequency of 60 Hz and a single phase duration of 1.25 msec. The current is delivered via a bipolar stimulator with the tips spread 5 mm apart. The total current will usually vary between 2 mA and 16 mA. It typically takes less current to evoke motor or sensory responses and interrupt language function when the patient is awake. The current is adjusted in 1 to 2 mA increments until the desired response is elicited. If the patient is asleep it is imperative that all paralytic agents are discontinued and a train of four peripheral muscle twitches are obtained. At times the bone exposure may be on either side of the Rolandic cortex, thus making it difficult to find the motor or sensory cortex. In this setting, placing a strip electrode under the dura and stimulating through the electrode contacts will readily localize the hidden functional cortex. Likewise, if the leg and foot motor cortex need to be identified, a strip electrode may be placed alongside the falx to elicit the desired responses. All essential cortical regions should be marked with sterile numbered tickets and left in place until the procedure has been completed.

Motor and Somatosensory Pathways

Once the cortical surface is exposed, the bipolar stimulator is gently pressed onto the surface and held in place while saying, "on, off" (Fig. 2). The technician or anesthetist indicates if any movement occurs and documents what the response is. If stimulation evokes a brief focal motor seizure no intervention should be undertaken. However, if the seizure lasts 10 or more seconds or spreads to adjacent muscle groups, the cortex can be gently irrigated with cool saline where the stimulation occurred and this usually stops the neuronal hyperactivity. If this is not effective, then 0.5 to 1.0 mg of ativan is administered. There is no difference in technique whether the motor or sensory cortex is stimulated. Following mapping of the cortex, the subcortical pathways may

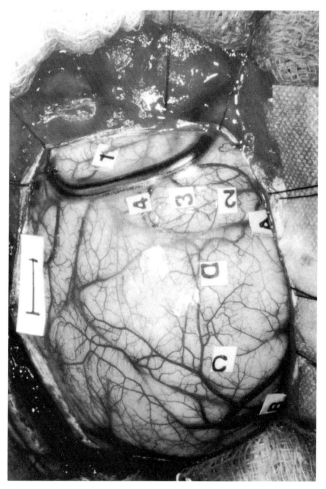

FIG. 2 Intraoperative photograph of motor cortex depicted by numbers *1, 2, 3,* and *4,* all representing stimulation induced contraction of the contralateral upper extremity. The tumor expands the somatosensory cortex as delineated by the letters **A, B, C, D.**

be identified by using the same current and stimulus duration as was used for the cortical response. The descending motor and sensory tracts may be followed throughout the resection in any part of the brain, brainstem, or spinal cord (Fig. 3). During the course of resecting an intramedullary tumor, small currents in the range of 0.5 to 2.0 mA will result in depolarization of anterior motor horn cells or corticospinal tract axons. This technique will be particularly helpful in avoiding damage to nearby motor pathways infiltrated by tumor.

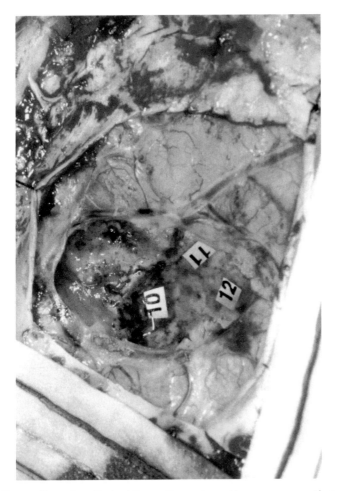

FIG. 3 Descending subcortical white matter motor pathways, representing the contralateral upper extremity, depicted by numbers *10, 11* and *12*.

Electrocorticography

Before language zones are mapped, the corticography and strip electrodes are placed over the surface and under the temporal lobe in accordance with scalp electroencephalographic recordings done preoperatively for localizing seizure foci. Interictal activity is readily identified (Fig. 4) and resected in a tailored fashion. For temporal lobe epileptic regions it is often necessary to place several strip electrodes under the temporal lobe to record off mesial structures. The temporal horn of the ventricle should be entered and direct recordings performed from the

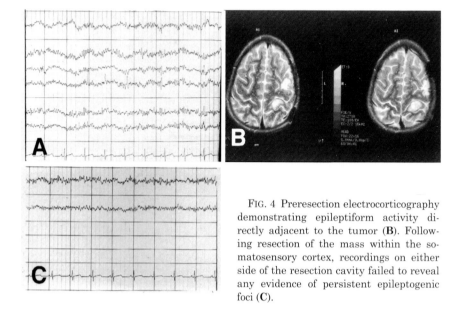

FIG. 4 Preresection electrocorticography demonstrating epileptiform activity directly adjacent to the tumor (**B**). Following resection of the mass within the somatosensory cortex, recordings on either side of the resection cavity failed to reveal any evidence of persistent epileptogenic foci (**C**).

hippocampus. Postresection recordings should always be done in those patients with intractable seizures to ensure that an adequate resection has been accomplished (14). When a structural lesion such as a glioma is present it is typical, rather than the exception, for the seizure focus or foci to originate from the brain adjacent to the tumor. This has been linked to compressed normal brain having fewer somatostatin and GABA immunoreactive neurons resulting in focal areas of hyperexcitability (15).

After the initial set of surface recordings have been completed, and before any resection, the cortical area under the electrodes is stimulated with escalating currents starting at 2 mA to attempt evoking afterdischarge potentials. When this is achieved the current should be lowered by 1 mA not to elicit seizure activity during the language recordings. Once this step is completed, it is now possible to begin the most complex aspect of the intraoperative functional mapping, namely, language localization.

Language Mapping

In most individuals, essential cortical zones for language will be confined to an area of 2 cm^2 or less (16). Although language sites predominate within the confines of the perisylvian region in the dominant hemisphere, language localization for reading and naming are variable and not predictable from any preoperative test or particular appearance of the cortex (Fig. 5). While the area, *i.e.*, Broca's, subserving motor speech is virtually always contiguous with the face motor cortex, sites essential for naming and reading vary and may not even be present in the temporal lobe in 16% to 18% of the population (1). Additionally, language is not present in the anterior temporal lobe (pre-Rolandic) in as much as 14% of the population. Most individuals will have two or more language sites, usually in the inferior frontal region and temporoparietal area. Because of this variability in language site localization, as it pertains to naming and reading, it becomes imperative to map language during any dominant hemisphere resection for tumor or intractable seizures when working within the perisylvian area.

Once the ideal current is chosen, which does not evoke afterdischarge potentials, language mapping begins by first identifying Broca's area in the inferior, posterior frontal lobe. This is done by having the patient count to 50 while the cortex is stimulated every 5 mm. Broca's area is defined by counting arrest without any oral facial movements. With the electrodes in place recording surface activity, the cortex is stimulated every one centimeter while the patient is reading the slides and naming the object that appears. Stimulation occurs as every other slide is shown to the patient. Each cortical site is tested three separate times without testing the same site more than once consecutively.

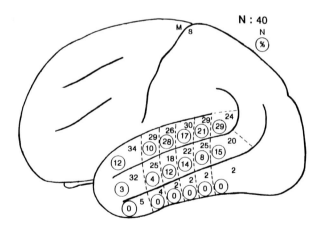

FIG. 5 Language localization in 40 patients with temporal lobe gliomas. In the upper right hand corner is the number of patients who had testing done at a particular site. The number within the circle represents the percentage of those patients who had stimulation induced language deficits for naming. (Printed with permission, **Neurosurgery** 34 (4), 1994).

TABLE 2

Minimalism Associated With Mapping

Average postoperative length of stay reduced (including in-hospital rehabilitation)

Significantly reduced incidence of permanent postoperative paresis, plegia, or expressive or receptive aphasia

Return to original work capacity expected

Electrocorticography for seizure control often obviates the use of long-term antiepileptic drugs

Mapping–enhanced radical tumor resection reduces mass effect, thus reducing the need for long-term steroid use

Radical tumor resection prolongs time to tumor progression and lengthens survival

Anomia is the sine qua non of an essential language site, and two out of three incorrect naming attempts implies significance. Repetitive dysnomia should also be respected and the corresponding cortex not violated. Hesitation in naming is not enough evidence to prevent resection of that site. It is usually necessary to test, on average, 20 or more

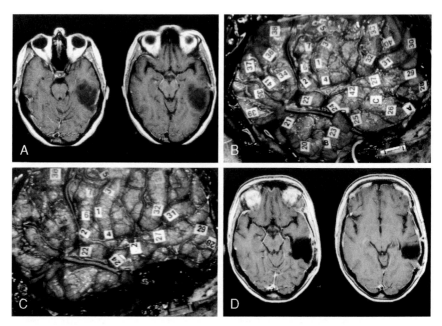

FIG. 6 Preoperative T-1 weighted axial image (**A**) of a noncontrast enhancing low grade glioma. Intraoperative map (**B**) demonstrating sites specific for anomia as 41 and 37. No language representation was found in the temporal lobe. Postresection intraoperative map (**C**) and postresection MRI scan (**D**) showing complete resection of the tumor.

cortical sites within the operative field (Fig. 6). When naming an adequate predictor of language localization is known (17), repetitive errors will indicate that the site tested must not be violated. Our experience with temporal lobe language indicates that resecting contiguous cortex closer than 7 mm from the stimulating electrode will result in permanent language deficits in up to 40% of cases (1). Thus, a 1-cm rule is invoked which indicates that the resection should not come within 10 mm of an essential language site (Fig. 7).

SUMMARY

Intraoperative stimulation mapping may be used to avoid unnecessary risk to functional regions subserving language and sensori-motor pathways. Based on the data presented here, language localization is variable in the entire population, with only certainty existing for the inferior frontal region responsible for motor speech. Anatomical landmarks such as the anterior temporal tip for temporal lobe language sites and the posterior aspect of the lateral sphenoid wing for the frontal lobe language zones are unreliable in avoiding postoperative aphasias. Thus, individual mapping to identify essential language sites has the greatest likelihood of avoiding permanent deficits in naming, reading, and motor speech. In a similar approach, motor and sensory pathways from the cortex and underlying white matter may be reliably stimulated and mapped in both awake and asleep patients.

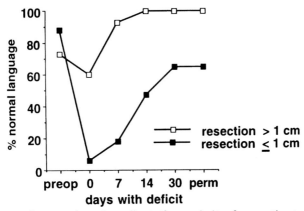

FIG. 7 One-centimeter rule, as it applies to the proximity of a resection to an essential language site. Resection of cortex greater than 1 cm away from an essential language site does not result in any permanent deficits, as opposed to a resection less than 10 millimeters from an essential language site (Printed with permission, **Neurosurgery** 34 (4), 1994.)

Although these techniques require an additional operative time and equipment nominally priced, the result is often gratifying, as postoperative morbidity has been greatly reduced in the process of incorporating these surgical strategies. The patient's quality of life is improved in terms of seizure control, with or without antiepileptic drugs. This avoids having to perform a second costly operative procedure, which is routinely done when extraoperative stimulation and recording is done via subdural grids. In addition, an aggressive tumor resection at the initial operation lengthens the time to tumor recurrence and often obviates the need for a subsequent reoperation. Thus, intraoperative functional mapping may be best alluded to as a surgical technique that results in "minimalism in the long term."

ACKNOWLEDGMENTS

This work was supported by the American Cancer Society Professor of Clinical Oncology Grant #071, NIH-NINCDS T32 NS07289, the American Cancer Society Grant #EDT-53 and the American Cancer Society's Rex and Arlene Garrison Summer Fellowship Program.

REFERENCES

1. Haglund MM, Berger MS, Shamseldin M, Lettich E, Ojemann GA. Cortical localization of temporal lobe language sites in patients with gliomas. **Neurosurgery** 34(4):567–576, 1994.
2. Berger MS, Ghatan S, Haglund MM, Dobbins J, Ojemann GA. Low grade gliomas associated with intractable epilepsy: seizure outcome utilizing electrocorticography during tumor resection. **J Neurosurg** 79:62–69, 1993.
3. Berger MS, Ghatan S, Geyer JR, Keles GE, Ojemann GA. Seizure outcome in children with hemispheric tumors and associated intractable epilepsy: the role of tumor removal combined with seizure foci resection. **Pediatr Neurosurg** 17:185–191, 1992.
4. Berger MS. Malignant astrocytomas: surgical aspects: In: *Seminars in Oncology.* Jaeckel K, M.D. and Aiken R, M.D. (eds): W.B. Saunders Co. Publishers, Vol. 21(2), pp. 172–185, 1994.
5. Berger MS, Keles GE, Ojemann GA, Ghatan S, Deliganis A. Extent of resection affects recurrence patterns in patients with low grade gliomas. **Cancer** 74:1784–1791, 1994.
6. Berger MS, Cohen W, Ojemann GA. Correlation of motor cortex using intraoperative brain mapping data with preoperative magnetic resonance imaging anatomy. **J Neurosurg** 72:383–387, 1990.
7. Berger MS. Preoperative magnetic resonance imaging localization of the primary motor cortex. **Perspect Neurol Surg** 2:23–32, 1991.
8. Berger MS, Kincaid J, Ojemann GA, Lettich E. Brain mapping techniques to maximize resection, safety and seizure control in children with brain tumors. **Neurosurgery** 25:786–792, 1989.
9. Goldring S, Gregorie EM. Surgical management of epilepsy using epidural recordings to localize the seizure focus. **J Neurosurg** 60:457–466, 1984.

10. JayaRai P. Physiological principles of electrical stimulation. **Adv Neurol** 63:17–27, 1993.
11. Gregorie EM, Goldring S. Localization of function in the excision of lesions from the sensorimotor region. **J Neurosurg** 61:1047–1054, 1984.
12. Luders H, Leser RP, Morris HH. Chronic intracranial recording and stimulation with subdural electrodes. In: Engel JP (ed): *Surgical Management of the Epilepsies.* New York: Raven Press; 1987:297–321.
13. Berger MS, Ojemann GA, Lettich E. Neurophysiological monitoring to facilitate resection during astrocytoma surgery. In: *Neurosurgery Clinics of America.* Vol. 1, No. 1, pp. 65–80, 1990.
14. Berger MS, Ojemann GA. Intraoperative brain mapping techniques in neuro-oncology. **Stereotact Funct Neurosurg** 58:153–161, 1992.
15. Haglund MM, Berger MS, Kunkel DD, Franck JE, Ghatan S, Ojemann GA. Changes in GABA and somatostatin in epileptic cortex associated with low grade gliomas.
16. Ojemann GA, Ojemann J, Lettich E, Berger MS. Cortical language localization in left, dominant hemisphere. An electrical stimulation mapping investigation in 117 patients. **J Neurosurg** 71:316–326, 1989.
17. Ojemann GA. Some brain mechanisms for reading. In: Euler C, Lundberg I, Lennerstrand G (eds): *Brain and Reading.* New York, MacMillan; pp. 47–59, 1989.

CHAPTER

24

Innovations in Minimalism: Intraoperative MRI

EBEN ALEXANDER, III, M.D., THOMAS M. MORIARTY, M.D., PH.D.,
RON KIKINIS, M.D., AND FERENC A. JOLESZ, M.D.

The application of imaging techniques to neurosurgical planning and procedures has been a major component in the growth of neurosurgery in this century. In fact, the major developments in neurosurgery have been rooted in advances in imaging: ventriculography in the 1920s, angiography in the 1930s, the operating microscope in the 1960s, computerized tomographic (CT) imaging in the 1970s, and magnetic resonance (MR) imaging in the 1980s. All of these developments enabled significant advances in the performance of neurosurgical procedures and treatments.

The linkage of imaging data to the physical space of the operating environment began with the advent of stereotactic frames, which came into clinical use in the late 1940s. They enabled precise localization of intracranial targets based on plain skull x-rays, pneumoencephalograms, or arteriograms. The development of CT and MR has provided a tremendous increase in the utilization of imaging information in the stereotactic operating environment (1, 2) wherein preoperatively acquired images are registered to the operative field in some way to guide surgical procedures. These modern imaging modalities have enhanced not only the ability to guide procedures with stereotactic frames (3, 4, 5, 6) but have also ushered in the use of frameless mechanical, optical, and acoustic arms and wands (7, 8). Similarly, they have enabled development of video displays that link to microscopes and show the region from imaging space correlating with the field in the focus of the microscope. These latter devices (arms, wands, and microscope-associated displays) all use high-speed graphic computer workstations and involve multiple point-to-point linkage of the 3-dimensional image reconstruction and the physical operating environment (9, 10, 11, 12).

One major problem inherent in the use of stereotactic frames and the frameless arms, wands, and guided microscopic systems popular today is the shift of intracranial soft tissue during the performance of operative resection. This results in significant shifts of important anatomical structures away from their position mapped from preoperative imaging data. This may result in inadequate treatment (resection, thermocoagulation, etc.) of a lesion or of unanticipated damage to the nervous system resulting in postoperative neurologic deficits.

The intraoperative MR project (MRT, or Magnetic Resonance Therapy) has been a joint effort of the Brigham & Women's Hospital (BWH) and Harvard Medical School Departments of Radiology and Surgery (Neurosurgery) with the Medical Imaging Division of the General Electric (GE) Corporation (Milwaukee, WI) to develop an "open" magnet, with sufficient room for the surgeon and an assistant to operate within the MR during imaging (13, 14). This radical new design effort began at GE in 1987, involved significant collaborative work beginning with the BWH team beginning in 1990, and progressed to the installation of a working large bore open MR system at the BWH in January 1994.

THE OPEN MR SYSTEM

The system allows a surgeon and assistant to perform procedures on a patient while imaging the region of interest (15). The field strength of 0.5 T is higher than has been achieved with other interventional MR units and, with the various surface coils available, provides high resolution images of the progress of the operation. The other major advantage of the GE design over that of other interventional MR designs is that the two MR tori are standing on end next to each other (Fig. 1), allowing the surgeon and an assistant to stand between them, on either side of the patient couch (Fig. 2), which slides through the axis of the two tori (doughnuts). The option of bringing the patient couch in to the assistant's position, perpendicular to the more standard configuration, is available. However, this omits the possibility of an assistant to the surgeon.

The prototype intraoperative MR facility opened at the Brigham & Women's Hospital in Boston, MA is composed of: 1) a novel open-configuration, cryogenless 0.5 T superconducting magnet, 2)a standard GE MR user interface {including standard Signa console, electronics and software for image acquisition (GE Medical Systems, Milwaukee, WI)}, 3) integrated optical digitizer 3-D tracking system (Integrated Technologies, Inc., Boulder, CO) with specialized image guidance software implemented on a window-driven interactive SUN 4/670 workstation (Sun Microsystems, Mountain View, CA), 4) standard RF and gradient coils as well as novel open-configuration transmit/receive (T/R) coils, 5) MR compatible essential OR tools, including the anesthesia machine (XL10 MRI Compatible Anesthesia Station; Ohmeda,

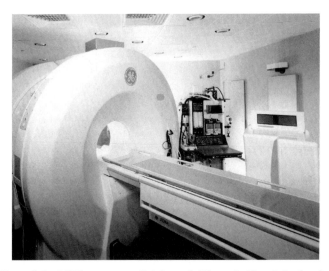

FIG.1 View of the MRT system at Brigham & Women's Hospital, showing patient couch entry into torus axis (inside diameter 55 cm). The MR compatible anesthesia machine and monitoring equipment stand to the right, behind the patient couch.

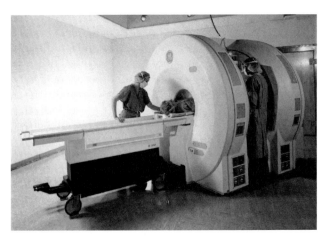

FIG.2 Patient being inserted feet first into the axis of the MRT system, with surgeon in place between the tori.

Madison, WI), electrophysiological monitors (MagLife ODAM; Bruker, Wissembourg, France), modified liquid crystal display video monitors (model LQ6NC01; Sharp Electronics, Rahwah, NJ), 2-way audiovisual communications, bipolar cautery (Force II, Valleylab, Boulder, CO), and various surgical instruments (Fig. 3).

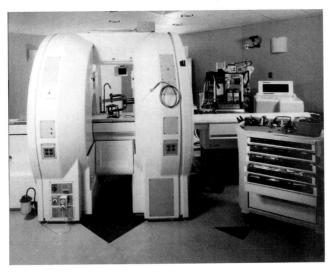

FIG.3 View into the surgeon's area between the tori. The Bookwalter flexible "snake" arm is attached on the left aspect of the operative field between the tori. The 3-point head holder projects in from the right. A flexible head coil is lying on the patient couch where the patient's head would be, in the middle between the tori. Note the liquid crystal display screen suspended from the overhead support, directly above the head holder. The optical digitizer tracker is hanging beside its coiled cable on the outer aspect of the right magnet torus. Outlets for electricity, oxygen, nitrous oxide, suction, laser, etc. are located on the lower outer aspects of the two tori. Other channels from the control areas and computer room are available in the same base area.

The superconducting magnet is composed of two sets of niobium tin coils housed in separate but communicating cryostats (16). A two-stage cryocooler assembly (Kelcool UC130; Balzers, Hudson, NH) is used to maintain a shield temperature of 10° K, and liquid cryogens are not necessary. The superconducting transition temperature of 18.1° K for niobium tin (as opposed to the more commonly used niobium titanium, transition temperature 10.1° K) allows coil operation without the use of a liquid helium bath. This enables much improved patient access by reducing space between the superconducting coils and cryostat walls (15).

The magnet and software environment are optimized to routinely operate at a field strength of 0.5 T. The system is a fully functional, multiplanar, high-resolution, wholebody imaging system that maintains a stable spherical imaging volume 30 cm in diameter at the center of the imager's axis. There is a 56-cm gap at the center of the magnet to allow the surgeon and assistant full vertical access to the patient during operative procedures.

Computer modeling was used to define the optimal configuration and number of coils, based on the standard Helmholtz pair, to optimize access between the innermost coils and the volume of the highly homogeneous magnetic field. This required sufficient space between the cryostats such that a surgeon and assistant could stand (or sit) between the coils and still have a system that generated a high-quality image. Because liquid cryogens are not used and their obligatory bulky cooling baths are not necessary, the width of each cryostat/coil unit is significantly smaller than conventional MR systems. In the prototype at the Brigham & Women's Hospital, the vertical access (*i.e.,* the space between the coils) is 56 cm, which is sufficiently wide to permit one surgeon to stand on either side of a patient at the center of the imaging volume.

Patient positioning within the magnet is accomplished in several ways, three of which are currently in use at the prototype facility. The first uses a standard MR couch docked at the front of the magnet such that the patient is passed through the bore of the coils into the imaging volume (inner diameter 56 cm). Alternatively, the MR couch is docked perpendicular to the magnet (head-first) with the patient passed between the coils, obviating space for the assistant. The 45° diagonal orientation of the main MR axis relative to the room axes facilitates couch approaches along both directions within limited operating room space. The third configuration uses a removable chair that can be adjusted to center various anatomical regions of interest in a seated or semireclining patient in the imaging volume. This arrangement is particularly well adapted for dynamic imaging of the spine, genitourinary system, or various joints (hip, knee, wrist, or ankle).

The Intraoperative MR system is located in a specially modified operative suite that combines the essential features of an MR imaging suite with a fully functional operating room (OR). The room is magnetically shielded, and the floor is reinforced to support the imager. The Signa console and SUN workstation are located directly outside the main room in the control area. Several video monitors and a two-way audiovisual system keep the members of the Intraoperative MR team, both inside and outside the room, in constant contact. The room meets the institutional requirements for airflow, cleanliness, and sterility set for the main OR. An MR compatible anesthesia machine (XL10 MRI Compatible Anesthesia Station; Ohmeda, Madison, WI) and patient monitoring device (MagLife ODAM; Bruker, Wissembourg, France) are located next to the magnet. A tunnel beneath the floor carries lines for air, suction, gases, fiberoptic laser, electrocautery, ultrasonic aspiration, etc. into the jacket of the magnet for use intraoperatively. The non-MR compatible components of the latter three devices are thus safely located outside of the strong MR field, with an approximate conduit distance of 7.4 m from the computer or control rooms into the central operating field. Adjacent to the Intraoperative MR room is a special sub-sterile zone where the scrub sinks and instrument handling rooms are located. An autoclave is located nearby. A three bed post anesthesia care unit (PACU) is located within the Intraoperative MR suite.

The position of various instruments, platforms, and supports (such as a head-holding fixation device) may all be mapped and monitored in the operative field using three charge-coupled device (CCD) video cameras mounted in the overhead support truncheon that track various light emitting diodes (LEDs) on the devices. This system of multicamera infrared source mapping has been used in other frameless stereotactic systems. This tracking system can alternatively be used as a pointer by the operating surgeon to rapidly define the MR view plane required at any given time in the procedure.

The current version of the software allows for the optical digitizer "virtual-probe" to define a vector in space. The MR image plane can then be defined as the axial, coronal, or sagittal view through a point a given distance (say, 15 cm) along the vector beneath the probe. It may also be defined as a less conventional view plane perpendicular to the defined vector, or in some orientation parallel and along the vector ("in-plane 90°" or "in-plane 0°")

Conventional radio-frequency and gradient coils typically surround the patient and preclude access to the region of interest in a diagnostic MR scanner. With the Intraoperative MR system, a variety of flexible transmit/receive surface coils were designed to take full advantage of its open patient access. These pliable devices, which can be wrapped in a sterile fashion, are applied to the body surface to surround the operative region, while only minimally obstructing the operative approach. They operate in both transmit and receive modes. Various sizes and shapes have been implemented to accommodate the body part of interest, keeping in mind that the coil must have access sufficient to encompass the operative site (17). For neurosurgery, for example, the cranial coil is a 1-inch wide strip shaped into a pair of 8-inch squares that lie on either side of the head. For the cervical spine, the surface coil is incorporated into a modified Philadelphia collar.

The current user interface is based on the standard SIGNA console, electronics, and software, with several additional modules for interactive image-guided procedures. The basic software, implemented by a technologist located outside the MR room on a push-button plasma screen, is the equivalent to that available on the commercial 0.5 T Signa Advantage system. Scan orientation, acquisition modes, and the basic pulse sequences are the same. A number of pulse sequence enhancements are included for MRT. Development of more robust 3-dimensional software in conjunction with the Surgical Planning Laboratory at the Brigham & Women's Hospital is the subject of significant effort.

With the use of identical phantoms, the MRT system has been shown to possess imaging capabilities comparable, or even slightly superior (by 10%), to a conventional 0.5 T MR scanner (15). This assessment is based on signal-to-noise (S/N) of the MRT system in comparison with a second 0.5 T MR imager with similar receiver electronics (Signa Advantage; GE Medical Systems, Milwaukee, WI). Absence of a body coil in the open imager and lack of associated noise coupling in the head coil attribute, in part, to this improvement.

The surgeon and assistant working in the magnet with the patient communicate with the control room technologist via a two-way audiovisual connection. Two modified liquid crystal display screens are mounted on the magnet housing for the surgeon to monitor the images during procedures. Different views may be presented to the two viewing screens, for instance MRT planes in one and endoscopic views in the other.

REGISTRATION OF IMAGING AND PHYSICAL SPACE

A three-dimensional optical digitizer system (Integrated Technologies, Inc., Boulder, CO) is integrated into the system to allow prescription of interactive image-plane acquisition, and to allow the system to be used as a stereotactic device. Three high resolution linear charge-coupled-device (CCD) video cameras are rigidly fixed to the upper support beam of the magnet over the operative field. These cameras can visualize the position of multiple small light emitting diodes (LEDs) in the imaging space, each with a different firing frequency. A number of instruments, termed "trackers", have been modified to include two or more LEDs. A software routine compares the location and firing pattern of the various LEDs mounted on these tracks and can determine the location and pointing direction of the tracker or the location of a tool mounted in the tracker, in three dimensional space.

The trackers are used for both determination of position and orientation for image acquisition and for tracking any manipulations of tools in the operative field. Along with the standard orthogonal, multislice image acquisitions run under Signa, the tracker can be used analogously to an ultrasound handpiece to prescribe image location and orientation. Software provides the location and vector of a probe or needle mounted in the tracker. Image planes can be selected in three standard orthogonal planes through a point defined by the tracker (for example, a point 15 cm along the biopsy needle from its connection at the tracker), or 3 orthogonal planes linked to the direction vector of the needle (in-plane zero, in-plane 90°, or perpendicular plane at a fixed distance along the needle vector). This can be followed in the imaging volume or a predicted pathway to a particular location can be projected onto the images based on current needle position.

Evaluation of the linearity, accuracy, and precision of the tracking system within the imaging space is of paramount importance. Before the use of the system for stereotactic neurosurgical procedures, it was critical to verify that spatial fidelity of imaged structures and instruments was preserved within certain tolerances. Schenk et al. have recently performed the fundamental assessment of imaging linearity, homogeneity, and performance (15). A formal, quantitative protocol is used to evaluate magnetic susceptibility artifacts in all instruments and equipment used in the MRT system at the Brigham & Women's Hospital. Our assessment of the integrated system for neurosurgical applications, including the reliability of the optical tracking system, registration of the tracking system to image acquisition and the performance of the various trackers in the system, is currently being analyzed. In general, the system is linear to within 1% throughout the 30 cm imaging volume. Tracking the tip of an instrument in the imaging volume can be accomplished with milimetric accuracy.

Rapid, facile navigation through imaging space is achieved using a hand-held pointer under control of the optical digitizer tracker. With the use of software to define the length of a virtual probe relative to the tracker, it is possible to use it to identify an intracranial point, such as the border of a tumor or other anatomic structure. Through software, it is trivial to switch between standard orthogonal planes (coronal, sagittal, and axial) around the point of interest to gather anatomical reference information in near real time. The scan time, image contrast, and resolution may be changed to alter image definition. In the current software version of planar image presentation, this index (pointer) function of image acquisition is used to guide surgery or other interventional procedures.

The tracker can be used to place an actual probe (*e.g.*, a biopsy needle) into the brain. A modified Mayfield clamp (Ohio Medical Instruments, Cincinnati, OH) is used to limit movement of the patient's head. A flexible T/R surface coil is positioned for imaging. A number of tracker-prescribed volumetric images are utilized to plan the biopsy. After prepping and draping in the magnet, a skin, bone, and dural incision is made.

Then, with the use of only MR images acquired intraoperatively, a modified Sudan side-biting brain biopsy needle (Elekta Instruments, Inc., Atlanta, GA) is advanced to the lesion with the window positioned across the border of the lesion. The projected needle path is easily displayed on the in-plane images to assist in safe needle passage. A biopsy is obtained. While waiting for the neuropathologists to evaluate the biopsy specimen, one obtains a number of imaging sequences to watch for the possibility of hemorrhage. The incision is then closed. The time for the entire procedure, from image acquisition for biopsy planning, through the biopsy itself and the postbiopsy imaging was less than two hours in preliminary cases.

THREE-DIMENSIONAL GRAPHIC SOFTWARE DEVELOPMENT

Much of the potential for development in the MRT project will depend on work done in various 3-dimensional medical imaging laboratories, such as the Surgical Planning Laboratory (SPL) at the Brigham & Women's Hospital (8, 14, 19, 20, 15). To fully appreciate the impact that the MRT system will have on surgical procedures, one needs to appreciate the revolution occurring in the world of advanced data acquisition and 3-dimensional image fusion and reconstruction.

Much work so far consists of 3-dimensional reconstructions of MR derived data, using segmentation and registration algorithms to define normal and abnormal anatomic structures that are then presented to the surgeon as a 3-dimensional view. This computer model of the region of interest (for example, the head and brain) may be viewed in a variety of ways, with various structures (e.g., scalp region, part of the skull) removed to simulate a surgical approach. The entry pathway for various probes or electrodes may be easily projected, evaluated, and adjusted. Vascular structures can be visualized and protected by adjusting the surgical trajectory appropriately.

The ability to enhance and view various anatomic structures has tremendous appeal for surgeons operating anywhere in the body. Otolaryngologists and general surgeons have already used the planar views of MRT to enhance their ability to navigate within the body. For neurosurgeons, there is an entirely new level of critical operative information that may be incorporated into the surgeon's realm. The various neural functions of many structures in the central nervous system may be identified and mapped into the computer model for presentation to the surgeon.

For example, preoperative use of transcranial magnetic stimulation to define a cortical map of motor or speech cortical structure may be fused onto the 3-dimensional preoperative MR computer model of the brain, labeling gray and white matter regions with their specific anatomic and functional correlates. Likewise, preoperatively acquired somatosensory evoked response mapping (vector evoked response) or electrocorticographic information may be projected into the reconstructed 3-dimensional MR model for use by the surgeon during the planning and actual performance of the procedure. Other standard image data sets, such as those defined using positron emission tomography (PET), single photon emission computed tomography (SPECT), magnetic source imaging (MSI), or specialized MR {magnetic resonance angiography MRA, MR spectroscopy, "flash" MRI with rapid temporal analysis of gadolinium enhancement patterns, or MR sequences that use paramagnetic analysis of the oxyhemoglobin levels to monitor metabolism in various cortical regions during specific task activation} may all be blended into a preoperative computer model.

This information-rich model can then be presented in various ways to the operating surgeon preoperatively as well as during the procedure to assist in more safely and effectively removing a tumor or vascular anomaly or in making a functional pathway lesion. The MRT system offers a very sophisticated real-time monitoring technique to adjust the spatial distribution of this computer model during the performance of the operation. Soft tissue shifts present a significant challenge to stereotactic neurosurgeons who use preoperative data without any means of updating the anatomic representation to account for these shifts that occur during a procedure. Ultrasound has been proposed as a real-time imaging technique to provide this soft-tissue shift ability (2), but MR provides a much richer dataset on which to base analysis of anatomic shifts.

INSTRUMENT ISSUES

A significant number of instruments and tools used in the standard operating room have required modifications for this project. The main consideration is the avoidance of ferromagnetic materials within the MRT operating room that might become airborne and fly into the magnet at high speed, damaging the system and injuring or killing personnel or patients. In addition, many materials distort the magnetic field and may lead to imaging artifacts. The artifacts created by each instrument must be considered in terms of their proximity to the imaging space at specific points in the procedure, as to their interference with the resolution and spatial fidelity of the image.

Major equipment that has been modified and currently operational in the MRT suite include a general anesthesia apparatus, a bipolar cautery unit, and a high speed gas drill with multiple handpieces and drill bits (Midas Rex, Fort Worth, TX). Various other pieces of equipment have been modified such that they can drive capabilities within the operating environment through conduits from the computer or control areas of the suite, even though the main "box" must be outside of the MRT Operating Room. These include a Neodymium/YAG and KTP fiberoptic laser system (Laserscope, Santa Clara, CA) that powers a laser in the operative field. A piezoelectric ultrasonic aspirator is in advanced stages of development for use in the MRT environment (Elekta, Inc., Stockholm, Sweden). Many of the microinstruments commonly used in neurosurgical procedures are made from titanium and are thus compatible with the MRT environment. Note that titanium does cause local image artifact, and this must be considered for instruments that are used during critical imaging phases of the procedure.

MINIMALLY INVASIVE MRT PROCEDURES

The intraoperative MR system will serve as a revolutionary platform for standard neurosurgical procedures, but the uncharted future for the MRT system will likely incorporate novel technologies and approaches. The ability to image and see beyond the visible operative field will give rise to clever adaptations of minimally invasive procedures. One example is the coupling of the strengths of cranial endoscopy with intraoperative MR imaging. The tunnel vision limitations of endoscopy will be augmented by the global imaging and visualization provided by Intraoperative MR. Conversely, the moderate resolution view of MR will be augmented by the local illumination and magnification of the endoscope. The limited range of lesions currently treated endoscopically will likely increase, and the morbidity and mortality will decrease. The field of skull base surgery, too, which has evolved around radical tissue manipulation to visualize critical structures, may take full advantage of the MR's view to see around and behind critical structures and the extent and morbidity of these procedures should decrease.

Another major advantage of MR is the ability to generate images showing temperature contrast, enabling assessment of the temperature changes during thermal surgery (*e.g.*, with cryoprobe, radiofrequency electrode, or fiberoptic laser). This capability offers a new world of percutaneous therapeutic intervention in the form of thermal destruction of tumors or vascular targets, as well as the possible creation of functional neural lesions. MR has the potential to monitor temperature changes in tissues with resolution in the range of 1 to 3°C, such that the signal change is seen before the tissue is irreversibly damaged (22, 23, 24, 16). The ability to monitor tissue temperature changes during procedures may revive the clinical interest in thermal therapies for various deep seated tumors. Heat deposition via laser can kill tumor cells and may be an effective therapy for cancer (25, 26, 27, 28, 29, 30, 31, 32, 33). However, the inability to monitor temperature deposition during the procedure and monitor the progress of therapy has previously limited the therapeutic use of lasers (34). MRT may facilitate the intraoperative monitoring of interstitial laser therapy. Other interstitial thermal therapies, such as cryotherapy, will also play a role in the future of intraoperative MRI.

One of the most exciting new modes of thermal generation in creating these lesions is with focused ultrasound (27, 28, 31). The recent progress with phased array focused ultrasound allows for transmission of ultrasound energy through a small cranial opening on the order of 2.0 cm across, much smaller than with standard focused ultrasound. This technique enables the visualization of a small region of minimal temperature increase above ambient temperature, which can be steered around within the MR image until it is centered at the desired point within the target. The energy input and local temperature may then be increased to create the lesion under direct thermal visualization, with accurate mapping of the temperature across the anatomic MR image. This technique may prove to be a superior mechanism for making fully image-guided functional lesions within the nervous system (for the treatment of pain, movement and behavioral disorders).

CLINICAL CASES

As of November 1995, more than 85 cases have been performed in the prototype MRT facility at the Brigham & Women's Hospital in Boston. These include 65 general surgical biopsies (percutaneous needle biopsies of liver, pancreas, adrenal, psoas muscle, groin, retroperitoneal area, lymph nodes, etc.). There have been 9 otolaryngological endoscopic sinus cases, 2 biopsies of neck masses, 1 nephrosotomy tube placement, and 3 breast tumor wire localizations. Neurosurgical cases include catheter drainage of 2 chronic subdural hematomas and 4 deep brain tumor biopsies. MRT imaging capabilities have also been used to assess dynamic loading effects on spine and joint imaging, as well as dynamic MRI of pelvic floor continence.

The MRT system has worked very well to provide real-time imaging during the four brain biopsies performed thus far. It is particularly well suited for the biopsy of cystic lesions or those intimately associated with the ventricular system, because standard stereotactic biopsies in these settings may be frustrated by the corruption of preoperatively acquired imaging data if significant fluid is released during the biopsy. It has also been very useful in assessing exactly where in the tumor a biopsy is obtained, especially in low grade lesions where the neuropathologist has difficulty assessing the grade or reporting one is "near" the tumor (as opposed to many millimeters inside of it).

The most significant obstruction to progress has been the exhaustive process of obtaining MR compatible instruments and equipment. The acquisition of a suitable brain biopsy needle alone took 18 months. Most of the equipment is now in place for performing neurosurgical resections, which should provide some exciting developments in the near future. Ongoing progress in more exotic fields such as laser ablation, cryoprobe lesioning, phased array focused ultrasound, endoscopic control, etc. should offer additional therapeutic advantages over the longer term.

FUTURE DIRECTIONS

Intraoperative MR is in its infancy. Many physicians and surgeons have expressed an interest in this potentially revolutionary technology, but the increasing concern about the cost of high technology in the medical sector has quenched some of the enthusiasm. To prove itself as a vital contribution to the practice of medicine and surgery, interventional MR must provide improved outcomes for various diseases, with high treatment safety and efficacy, AND efficient throughput of cases so as to justify its expense.

The situation is very similar to that of the early 1960s with the operating microscope. A revolutionary technique of assisted visual guidance for the surgeon is available. Entire new capabilities for dealing with various diseases will be offered. It is likely that this powerful new technology will provide treatment of disorders that we can not even visualize today, creating entirely new subspecialties of clinical management, just as we saw happen with the operating microscope 30 years ago. As happened then, our patients stand to benefit substantially from our endeavors in Intraoperative MR.

ACKNOWLEDGMENTS

The authors acknowledge the many collaborators from both the Brigham & Women's Hospital and the General Electric Corporation, including but not limited to the following: S. Morry Blumenfeld, Ph.D., Robert W. Newman, M.S., John F. Schenck, M.D., Ph.D., Kirby G. Vosburgh, Ph.D., Peter B. Roemer, Ph.D., Harvey E. Cline, Ph.D., William E. Lorenson, M.S., Steven G. Hushek, Ph.D., Robert V. Mulkern, Ph.D., Holly G. Isbister, R.T.(R), Catherine E. Holley, R.N., Maureen D. Ainslie, B.S., R.T., Douglas P. Dietz, M.D., Michael R. Figueira, M.S., Kenneth W. Rohling, P. Langham Gleason M.D., Stuart G. Silverman, M.D., Marvin P. Fried, M.D., Peter McL. Black, M.D., Ph.D., and Robert B. Lufkin, M.D.

REFERENCES

1. Lunsford L, Martinez A, Latchaw R: Stereotaxic surgery with a magnetic resonance and computerized tomography-compatible system. **J Neurosurgery** 1986;64: 872–878.

2. Maroon J, Bank W, Drayer B, Rosenbaum A: Intracranial biopsy assisted by computerized tomography. **J Neurosurgery** 1977; 46:572.

3. Brown R: A stereotactic head frame for use with CT body scanners. **Invest Radiol** 1979;14:300–304.

4. Horsley V, Clark R: The structure and functions of the cerebellum examined by a new method. **Brain** 1908;31:45–124.

5. Leksell L: The stereotaxic method and radiosurgery of the brain. **Acta Chir Scand** 1951;102:316–319.

6. Lunsford L: *Modern Stereotactic Neurosurgery.* Boston, MA: Martinus Nijhoff, 1988.

7. Barnett G, Kormos D, Steiner C, Weisenberger J: Intraoperative localization using an armless, frameless stereotactic wand. **J Neurosurg** 1993;78:510–514.

8. Galloway R, Maciunas R: Stereotactic neurosurgery. **CRC Crit Rev Biomed Eng** 1990;18:181–205.

9. Olivier A, Germano I, Cukiert A, Peters T: Frameless stereotaxy for surgery of the epilepsies: preliminary experience. **J Neurosurg** 1994;81:629–633.

10. Olivier A, Peters T, Bertrand G: Stereotactic system and apparatus for use with magnetic resonance imaging, computerized tomography and digital subtraction imaging. **Appl Neurophysiol** 1985;48:94–96.

11. Roberts D, Strohbehn J, Hatch J, Murray W, Kettenberger H: A frameless stereotaxic integration of computerized tomographic imaging and the operating microscope. **J Neurosurg** 1986;65:545–549.

12. Shelden C, McCann G, Jacques S, *et al.*: Development of a computerized microstereotaxic method for localization and removal of minute CHS lesions under direct 3-D vision: technical report. **J Neurosurgery** 1980;52:21–27.

13. Alexander E, III, Kooy HM, Van Herk M, *et al.*: Magnetic resonance image-directed stereotactic neurosurgery: use of image fusion with computerized tomography to enhance spatial accuracy. **J Neurosurg** 1995;83:271–276.

14. Alexander E III, Kikinis R, Jolesz F: Intraoperative Magnetic Resonance Imaging, In: Barnett GH, Roberts D, Guthrie B, (eds): *Image-Guided Neurosurgery: Clinical Applications of Interactive Surgical Navigation,* McGraw-Hill, Inc., New York, (in press, 1995).

15. Schenck J, Jolesz F, Roemer P, *et al.*: Superconducting open-configuration MR imaging system for image-guided therapy. **Radiology** 1995;195:805–814.

16. Kelly P, Kall B, Goerss S, Earnest F: Computer assisted stereotaxic laser resection of intra-axial brain neoplasms. **Journal of Neurosurgery** 1986;64.

17. Schenck JF, Hart HR Jr, Foster TH, Edelstein WA, Hussain MA: High resolution magnetic resonance imaging using surface coils. In: Kressel HY (ed). *Magnetic Resonance Annual.* New York, NY, Raven, 123–160, 1986.

18. Alexander E III, Loeffler JS, Lunsford LD: *Stereotactic Radiosurgery.* New York: McGraw-Hill, 1993.

19. Jolesz F, Bleier A, Jakab P, Ruenzel P, Huttl K, Jako G: MR imaging of laser-tissue interactions. **Radiology** 1988; 168:249–253.

20. Moriarty TM, Kikinis R, Jolesz FA, Alexander E III: Magnetic resonance-imaging therapy (MRT): Intraoperative MRI, In: Maciunas R (ed): *Clinical Frontiers of Frameless Stereotaxis. Neurosurgical Clinics of North America,* W.B. Saunders Co., Philadelphia (in press, 1995).

21. Berger M: Ultrasound-guided stereotaxic biopsy using a new apparatus. **J Neurosurg** 1986;50:550–554.
22. Bleier A, Higuchi N, Panych L, Jakab P, Hrovat F, Jolesz F: Magnetic resonance imaging of interstitial laser photocoagulation. **Proc SPIE** 1990;1202:188–195.
23. Bleier A, Jolesz F, Cohen M, *et al.*: Realtime magnetic resonance imaging of laser heat deposition in tissue. **Magn Reson Med.** 1991;21:132–137.
24. Jolesz F, Moore G, Mulkern R, *et al.*: Response to and control of destructive energy by magnetic resonance. **Invest Radiol** 1989;24:1024–1027.
25. Bettag M, Ulrich F, Kahn T, Seitz R: Local interstitial hyperthermia in malignant brain tumors using a low power Nd:YAG laser. **Proc SPIE** 1991;1525:409–411.
26. Castro D, Lufkin R, Saxton R, *et al.*: Metastatic head and neck malignancy treated using MRI guided interstitial laser phototherapy: an initial case report. **Laryngoscope** 1992;102:26–32.
27. Cline H, Schenck J, Hynynen K, Watkins R, Souza S, Jolesz F: Magnetic resonance guided focused ultrasound surgery. **Radiology.**
28. Cline H, Schenck J, Watkins R, Hynyen K, Jolesz F: Magnetic resonance guided thermal surgery. **Magn Res in Med** (submitted).
29. Dowlatshahi K, Babich D, Bangert J, Kluiber R: Histologic evaluation of rat mammary tumor necrosis by interstitial Nd:YAG laser hyperthermia. **Lasers Surg Med.** 1992;12:159–164.
30. Fan M, Ascher PW, Schrottner O, *et al.*: Interstitial 1.06 Nd:YAG laser thermotherapy in malignant gliomas under real-time monitoring of MRI: experimental studies and phase I clinical trial. **J Clin Laser Med Surg** 10:355–361, 1992.
31. Masters A, Steger A, Bown S: Role of interstitial therapy in the treatment of liver cancer. **Br J Surg** 1991;78:518–523.
32. Matsumoto R, Oshio K, Jolesz F: T1-weighted MR monitoring for interstitial laser- and freezing-induced ablation in the liver. **JMRI** 1992;2:555–562.
33. Matthewson K, Barr H, Tralau , Bown S: Low power interstitial Nd:YAG laser photocoagulation: studies in a transplantable fibrosarcoma. **Br J Surg** 1989;76: 378–381.
34. Wyman D, Wilson B, Malone D: Medical Imaging Systems for Feedback Control of Interstitial Laser Photocoagulation. **Proc IEEE** 1992;80:890–902.

25

Intraoperative Cranial Navigation

ROBERT J. MACIUNAS, M.D.

"Less is more."

Mies Van Der Rohe

Human beings are inveterate map makers. Many of our earliest, and arguably some of our most compelling, images are scaled representations of the world around us. It was partly our love of maps that led us to complete them at their edges, leading us to new continents and conquests. Because the maps possessed by early seafarers were at best inexact and fanciful expressions of reality, their translation into practical information required an individual who was both experienced in traversing that region and familiar with the conventions used by the map makers. These navigators of seafaring ships constituted a highly trained, skilled, and experienced group of professionals, passing on their expertise only to those under them who were committed to long and often arduous apprenticeships.

We, who practice the surgical arts, have turned inward this very human bent for map making as we explore and conquer the new medical frontiers to be found within our patients' bodies. Every neurosurgeon develops and maintains a richly detailed and carefully cross-indexed three-dimensional model for the practical understanding of intracranial anatomy. This personal atlas must reliably serve us in the face of complex anatomic relationships distorted by individual variations, the impact of disease, and the sequelae of prior therapeutic efforts. The development of this personal navigational sense has been one of the key missions programmed into the core of every neurosurgical residency training program structure. Grounded in prior analyses codified into textbooks, explored in anatomic dissections, reinforced by the systematic querying of faculty members and more senior residents, and put to use in the surgical theater, this sense of place is a precious legacy that is imparted to each of us. We maintain and refine it with expanding clinical experience throughout our careers.

This art of surgical navigation, involving the use of anatomic maps as illustrative pictures, has traditionally taught us to use specific landmarks as touchstones during our operations, and to "hug the shore" of the inner skull surface as we orient ourselves, while approaching our targets. If we must venture deeper into subcortical parenchyma, we place a heavy emphasis upon skill, judgment, experience, apprenticeship, and lore as we use methods of reckoning little changed over the history of neurosurgery. We are very much like the ancient navigators in this aspect of our profession.

The ancient navigators are no longer with us, aboard seafaring vessels. Precise and accurate localization techniques, quantitatively registered to exact maps, have replaced lore with LORAN. The captain of a vessel now knows with certainty its position and trajectory and can use that information effectively and decisively to maximum advantage. We must become like these modern captains in this utilization of modern technology in order to assure a dynamic future for our profession of neurosurgery.

NAVIGATIONAL TECHNOLOGY

A variety of techniques currently assist physicians in localizing the pathology relevant to a given disease process and its treatment. The recent revolution in digital tomographic imaging has fundamentally altered the practice of medicine by giving us exquisite pictures of compelling detail for each individual patient. Although these images use a coordinate system, internal to the scanner machinery, to organize the acquisition of information, that coordinate system is jettisoned once the patient leaves the scanner itself. For these pictures to become true maps that serve the purposes of surgical navigation, these image data within their coordinate systems must be mapped, or registered, to the physical space in which the patient exists. When the addresses of points in one image volume are mapped onto the points of another image volume, or onto physical space itself, then these volumes are said to have been registered with one another. When image spaces are registered with one another and with physical space, medical images become true, point-to-point maps capable of precise surgical guidance.

The first example of this in our profession was the introduction of stereotactic methodology to benefit selected neurosurgical procedures. These frame systems have been modified to accommodate the advances of digital imaging, but they remain fundamentally the same devices first seen nearly a century ago (1, 2).

The major benefits of stereotactic systems include a rigid coordinate frame providing a stable and redundant frame of reference, an aiming arc assembly that is mechanically stable as it holds the probe in position along a trajectory, and preoperative planning methods allowing surgical simulation. Unfortunately, these also produce the greatest limitations on stereotactic systems as seen in Table 1. The rigid frame is a

TABLE 1
Benefits and Limitations of Stereotactic Frames

Benefits of Stereotactic Frames
- Rigid coordinate frame provides a stable and redundant frame of reference
- Aiming arc is mechanically stable, holding the probe in position along a trajectory
- Planning allows preoperative simulation of operation

Limitations of Stereotactic Frames
- Rigid frame is a restrictive head holder; also must be a temporary frame of reference
- Aiming arc is mechanically complex, bulky, limited to one target/trajectory at a time
- Planning is computationally limited, nonintuitive, and not updated in real time

restrictive head holder that can interfere with surgical positioning and approaches, and it is only a very temporary frame of reference; the aiming arc assembly is mechanically complex, bulky, and limited to dealing with only one target/trajectory coupling at a time; the preoperative planning is often computationally limited, nonintuitive, and not updated in real time. These limitations have precluded the application of the stereotactic discipline to all intraoperative cranial navigation.

Several investigators have pursued novel technologies of interactive image-guided neurosurgery to provide accurate intraoperative cranial navigation without the constraints imposed by the design limitations inherent to stereotactic frame systems. These systems consist of five fundamental elements, detailed in Table 2.

REGISTRATION TECHNIQUES

A variety of registration techniques offer alternative methods for achieving the mapping of images to each other and to physical space. As seen in Table 3, they may be classified into several types: (1) point methods, including stereotactic frame systems, (2) curve and surface methods, (3) moment and principal axes methods, (4) correlation methods, (5) interactive methods, and (6) atlas methods.

Point-based registration methods define corresponding points in different images and physical space, determine their spatial coordinates, and calculate a geometric transformation between the volumes. These points may be intrinsic and are based upon patient-specific anatomic landmarks (7). While this allows registration to be fully retrospective, the selection and definition of anatomic landmarks have proven to be labor-intensive processes that are subject to significant inaccuracies.

TABLE 2
Interactive Image-Guided Neurosurgery

- Registration of image and physical space
- Interactive localization device
- Computer and interface
- Integration of real-time data
- Robotics

TABLE 3
Registration Techniques

- Interactive
- Correlation
- Moment and principal axes
- Atlas
- Curve and surface
- Point
  - Intrinsic
  - Extrinsic
    - Nonrigid
      - Fiducials
    - Rigid
      - Fiducials
      - Stereotactic frames

Extrinsic point-based registration methods, requiring artificially applied markers such as stereotactic frames or fiducial markers, do not allow for retrospective registration of images. However, several significant advantages accrue with this technique (Table 4). Any and all imaging modalities and physical space can be registered as long as a detectable marker can be constructed (Fig. 1). The markers may be designed for optimal automatic or semiautomatic detection, allowing for straightforward extraction of their positions from medical images. The advantages of point-based registration methods have led to their widespread use throughout a variety of surgical guidance systems (5, 6, 7, 8, 9, 4, 10, 11, 12, 13, 14).

Two types of fiducial markers have been used for extrinsic point-based registration: (1) mobile markers that are taped or otherwise affixed to soft tissue such as the scalp and skin, and (2) rigidly affixed markers that anchor to the skull or other bone. Mobile markers are easily affixed to soft tissues but are associated with inconsistent registration accuracy.

TABLE 4
Advantages of Fiducial Markers

- Most accurate method of registration
- Can inform the physician of a precisely determined measure of accuracy
- Do not require special scanning protocols or intensive user interfaces to achieve proper registration

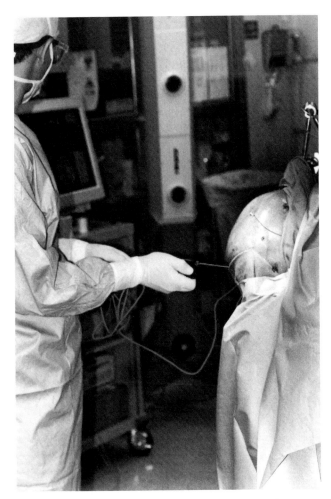

FIG. 1 Registration of image space to physical space by means of an interactive localization device, which is used to touch each of four implanted fiducial markers, providing spatial coordinates for the intraoperative computer to perform an appropriate transformation matrix calculation.

Rigidly affixed markers require a minor surgical intervention for their application (Figs. 2 and 3), but this disadvantage is offset by the dramatically increased level of registration accuracy afforded by this rigid fixation. Additionally, rigid fixation of markers provides a unique advantage: unlike any other form of registration, this method produces a known geometric relationship between the fiducial markers, thereby precisely defining for each individual patient what the registration accuracy will be for that particular surgical intervention (Table 4).

Surface-based registration systems fit sets of points extracted from contours in one image set to surface models extracted from contours in other images or physical coordinates of the patient's cranium. This is the only registration technique able to be both fully retrospective and to register image-to-physical space. The accuracy, however, is currently less than when employing point-based registration methods (15, 7, 16).

Other registration techniques, of limited value to neurosurgeons, include those based upon principal axes, correlation, and interactive means. None of these techniques can register images to physical space, therefore precluding their surgical use. They are primarily used by radiologists as retrospective methods for registering sets of medical images one to another.

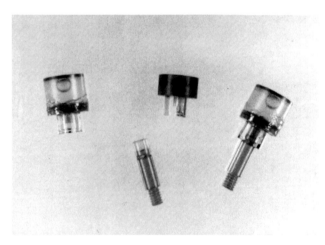

FIG. 2 Implantable fiducial markers. Pictured are the imaging fiducial marker, the implanted marker base, the intraoperative localization cap, and the assembly of the imaging fiducial marker/implanted marker base. Reproduced with permission from Maciunas RJ, Fitzpatrick JM, Galloway RL, Allen GS. Beyond stereotaxy: Extreme levels of application accuracy are provided by implantable fiducial markers for interactive image-guided neurosurgery. *In* Maciunas RJ (ed). *Interactive Image-Guided Neurosurgery.* Park Ridge, IL, American Association of Neurological Surgeons, 1993, pp 259–270.

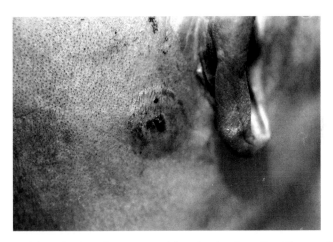

FIG. 3 Fiducial marker base in proper position after implantation. The specific cranial location is chosen on the basis of an individual patient's clinical requirements.

Anatomic atlases of intracranial landmarks have been long available. Unfortunately, it has proven difficult to adequately define the warping necessary to map such atlas coordinates onto an individual brain distorted by pathologic processes and mass lesions. Nonetheless, it is probable that atlas methods will continue to be combined with methods using extrinsic point registration to amplify their utility for diagnosis and surgical planning.

INTERACTIVE LOCALIZATION DEVICES

To register image-to-physical space, it is necessary that a physical pointer be used to identify the points or surfaces to be registered. These interactive localization devices (ILD) are the second fundamental part of any system of intraoperative cranial navigation. These devices may be classified into two categories: linked or nonlinked, depending upon whether or not they require an unbroken physical connection between the device and the patient. They are listed in Table 5.

Linked systems began with stereotactic frame-mounted aiming arc assemblies, have included active robotic and passive articulated localizing arms (Fig. 4), and now include intraoperative tomography with CT and MR imaging (because the scanner itself provides the only coordinate system for the patient's images (15, 8, 17, 10, 11, 12, 14).

Nonlinked ILDs began with techniques of sonic triangulation on spark-gap emitters (Figs. 5 and 6) (5, 13) and have substituted infrared light for sound in the infrared emitting diode (IRED) devices triangulated upon by linear charge-coupled device (LCCD) three-camera arrays

TABLE 5
Interactive Localization Devices

Linked
- Stereotactic aiming arcs
- Active robotic arms
- Passive articulated arms
- Intraoperative MR and CT

Nonlinked
- Sonic triangulation
- IRED optic triangulation
- Machine vision - passive video
- Magnetic field deflection
- Gyroscopes, gravitometers, and inertial guidance
- Real-time ultrasound

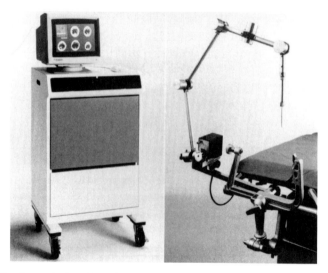

FIG. 4 Passive articulated localization arm, with computer video display of intraoperative end-point position on preoperative images. Reproduced with permission from Watanabe E. The Neuronavigator: a potentiometer-based localization arm system. *In* Maciunas RJ (ed). *Interactive Image-Guided Neurosurgery*. Park Ridge, IL, American Association of Neurological Surgeons, 1993, 135–148.

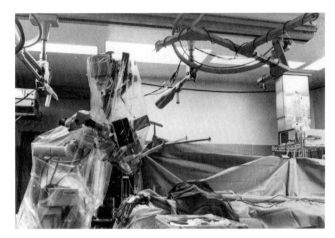

FIG. 5 Sonic localizing operating microscope fitted with spark-gap emitters. Sound detectors mounted about the operating room. Reproduced with permission from Roberts DW, Friets EM, Strohbehn JW, Nakajima T. The sonic digitizing microscope. *In* Maciunas RJ (ed). *Interactive Image-Guided Neurosurgery.* Park Ridge, IL, American Association of Neurological Surgeons, 1993, pp 105–112.

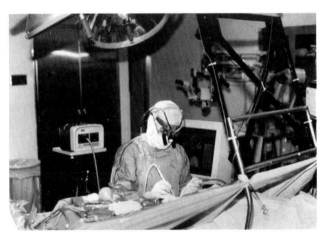

FIG. 6 Sonic localizing handheld intraoperative localization device. Sound detectors mounted in a plate on the operating table. Reproduced with permission from Barnett GH, Kormos DW, Steiner CP, *et al.* Frameless stereotaxy using a sonic digitizing wand: Development and adaptation to the Picker Vistar medical imaging system. *In* Maciunas RJ (ed). *Interactive Image-Guided Neurosurgery.* Park Ridge, IL, American Association of Neurological Surgeons, 1993, pp 113–120.

(Fig. 7) (18, 4, 19). Although more expensive than sonic systems, these light-based systems are immune to the interference from sonic echoes off echogenic operating room environments and from the spatial uncertainty introduced by the speed of sound changing approximately 6% per degree of temperature fluctuation (7). Passive object recognition techniques, using two video cameras at two different viewpoints trained

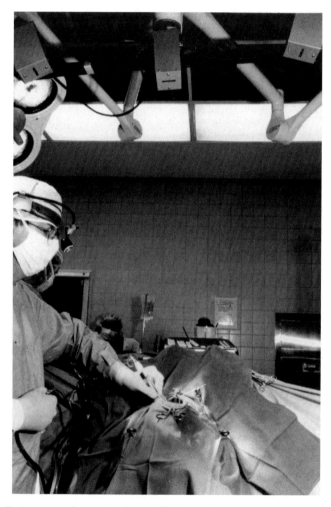

FIG. 7 Optic triangulation by three LCCDs tracking a surgical instrument with IREDs. Reproduced with permission from Bucholz RD, Smith KR: A comparison of sonic digitizers versus light emitting diode-based localization. *In* Maciunas RJ (ed). *Interactive Image-Guided Neurosurgery.* Park Ridge, IL, American Association of Neurological Surgeons, 1993, pp 179–200.

upon marked objects within the operating field, are showing promise as the computing capabilities improve for object recognition software (Fig. 8) (9, 20). Magnetic field deflection has been exploited in compact and inexpensive devices for spatial localization (Fig. 9), although use of this technique continues to be plagued by the unpredictable and variable degrees of field distortion caused by random metal objects and radio

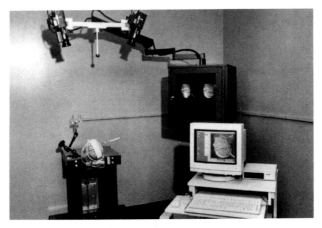

FIG. 8 Machine vision localization. Reproduced with permission from Heilbrun MP, Koehler S, McDonald P, et al. Implementation of a machine vision method for stereotactic localization and guidance. *In* Maciunas RJ (ed). *Interactive Image-Guided Neurosurgery.* Park Ridge, IL, American Association of Neurological Surgeons, 1993, pp 179–200.

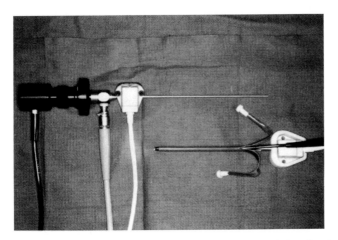

FIG. 9 An endoscope and shunt catheter stylet fitted for magnetic localization. Reproduced with permission from Manwaring KH. Intraoperative microendoscopy. *In* Maciunas RJ (ed). *Interactive Image-Guided Neurosurgery.* Park Ridge, IL, American Association of Neurological Surgeons, 1993, pp 217–232.

frequency fields in the operating theater environment (21). Gyroscopes, gravitometers, and other methods of inertial guidance offer theoretical promise as localization devices, although significant problems of miniaturization and reliability remain unsolved. Taken as a whole, ILDs have progressed from pointing machines that physically dominated the operating room to surgical instruments that can also impart localization information.

COMPUTER AND INTERFACE

The rapid evolution of computer hardware and software is one of the main engines driving development of surgical navigational systems. Collaborative teams of neurosurgical end users, basic scientists, and engineers working together have provided the model for platform development in this field. While a cladistic explosion of alternative treatment planning and display solutions was initially in evidence, a striking coalescence has resulted in an emerging dominant standard of rapidly refreshed multiplanar slice images combined with visually straightforward and computationally simple rendered images (Fig. 10). As the price of hardware and software plummets, rapidly refreshed rendered displays will likely become more popular. A considerable amount of experimentation continues with "heads up" displays, although no totally satisfactory solution has been found to balance the competing threats of loss of information and confusion due to visual overload (Fig. 11). The interface between contemporary digital imaging scanners and these systems remains a major source of inconsistency and failure. With increasing standardization of image data formats, this should become less of a problem.

REAL-TIME INTRAOPERATIVE FEEDBACK

Once reliable methods of spatial localization have been established, they may be augmented by incorporating real-time feedback from the surgical work space (Table 6). Preoperative digital imaging data, even when registered to physical space, remain historical information in essence and are subject to becoming obsolete in the operating room as surgical manipulation of the tissues changes the landscape being viewed. By integrating real-time feedback from the surgical work space, the feedback loop of intraoperative cranial navigation can be completed as this new information is used to refresh and update the registered image data being used for guidance. A number of intraoperative visualization and data gathering techniques can be digitized in the form of digital video images, which then may be registered to the preoperative images. These databases are derived from the output

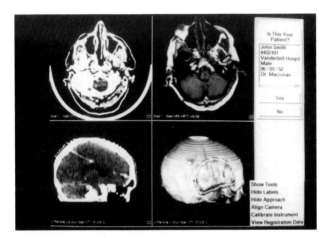

FIG. 10 An intraoperative multimodality display of image slices and shaded surface renderings. Reproduced with permission from Maciunas RJ. Surgical aspects and general management of ganglion cell tumors. *In* Apuzzo MLJ (ed). *Benign Cerebral Gliomas: Neurosurgical Topics* Book 22, vol II. American Association of Neurological Surgeons, Park Ridge, IL, 1995, pp 427–444.

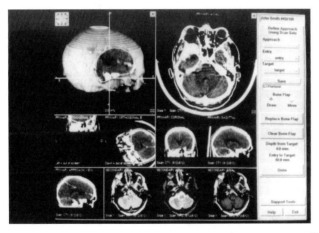

FIG. 11 A preoperative surgical treatment planning software program. Reproduced with permission from Maciunas RJ. Surgical aspects and general management of ganglion cell tumors. *In* Apuzzo MLJ (ed). *Benign Cerebral Gliomas: Neurosurgical Topics* Book 22, vol II. American Association of Neurological Surgeons, Park Ridge, IL, 1995, pp 427–444.

TABLE 6
Integration of Real-Time Data

- Electrophysiology
  - Intraoperative stimulation mapping
  - electrocorticography
  - Microelectrode recording
- Microscopy and endoscopy
- Ultrasonography
- Tomography
  - CT
  - MR

---

of intraoperative stimulation mapping and electrocorticography; endoscopy and microscopy; ultrasonography; and tomography. Preliminary steps are being taken to accomplish this integration (18).

In our experience, spatially registered intraoperative electrophysiologic recordings have proven to be extremely useful in guiding the resection of deep-seated primary brain tumors in and around functionally eloquent cortical pathways (Fig. 12).

Although the in-plane pixel resolution of video LCCD cameras and monitors does not yet equal that of the finest optical surgical microscopes, the digital video display of endoscopic images has proven quite adequate for surgical visualization. Spatially registered endoscopy is technologically straightforward and clinically inevitable, especially when the added benefit of having routine three-dimensional localization on preoperative images is considered (6). Spatially registered transcranial Doppler information has been used, to some advantage, by several groups.

Ultrasonography, a digital real-time imaging modality, is theoretically an ideal choice for spatial integration. The image resolution of ultrasonography, however, is at times suboptimal for precise surgical navigation. Also under investigation is the question of whether the imaging distortions inherent to ultrasonography can be overcome, so that it may be used intraoperatively to re-register or warp outdated preoperative tomographic images (18, 12).

The apotheosis of the principle of real-time feedback would appear to be performing the entire surgery within an MR imaging scanner, with fresh imaging data continuously available on command. Significant corporate investment in this field has guaranteed that it will provide an attractive, albeit expensive, technologically intensive adjunct to navigational systems in the decade to come. On a somewhat expanded time

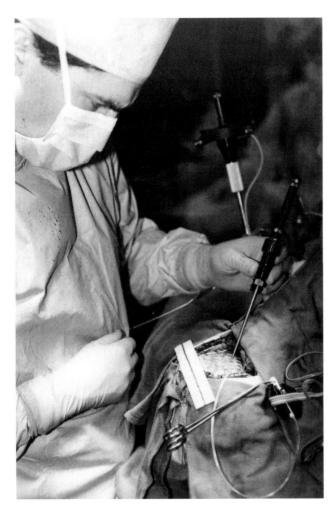

FIG. 12 Spatially registered intraoperative grid electrocorticography to define senso-rimotor cortex before resection of pediatric ganglion cell tumor.

scale, it is quite possible that flatbed MR imaging scanners with low-field magnets and miniaturized radio frequency field coils may be improved sufficiently to allow routine intraoperative scanning capabilities.

NONRIGID BODY REGISTRATION

The analysis of real-time imaging data demonstrates that many bio-logical tissues are in a state of dynamic flux. To date, however, all reg-istration techniques for surgical navigation have made the presumption

that the object they registered was solid and nondeforming. Thus, these
are termed "rigid body" registration techniques. This basic assumption
fails when the tissue being registered is not rigid. Examples of this include when the brain shifts intraoperatively after release of cerebrospinal fluid or removal of tissue, when pliable soft tissue such as surrounds peripheral nerves is registered but then moves during surgical
manipulation, when articulated bone moves segmentally as in the
spine, and when respiration or other disturbances complicate extracranial navigation. No universal solution to these situations exists; a partial listing of particular solutions to individual cases appears in Table
7. In every case, the neurosurgeon is called upon to continually exercise
judgment and maintain an appropriate level of skepticism towards navigational devices as is done with all other instruments in the armamentarium.

Several stereotactic surgeons, including Dr. Patrick J. Kelly, have
suggested that certain constraints be applied to surgical technique to
minimize the potential for intracranial shifts, including the avoidance
of osmotic diuretics, the positioning of the head such that the craniotomy is at its uppermost aspect and the trajectory to the lesion is directed straight down, the performance of small cranial openings, and
the use of a cylindrical retractor to restrain brain movement when exposing the lesion. These techniques are best suited to the surgical attack of relatively small, deep-seated, and well-circumscribed tumors.

If such constraints are deemed unacceptable (Fig. 13), the progress
of the operation can be modified and redirected by providing spatially
registered real-time feedback to the operating surgeon, using ultrasonography, endoscopy, electrophysiology, and even tomography with
CT or MR imaging.

TABLE 7
Non-Rigid Body Registration

Brain shift, soft tissue, articulated bone, respiration, extracranial navigation
- Exercise surgical judgment
- Constrain operative technique
- Add data: ultrasound, endoscopy, electrophysiology
- Piezoelectric tactile feedback
- Refresh, update registration
- Warp preoperative images to new registration
- Reacquire intraoperative image data
- Dynamic, weighted data integration

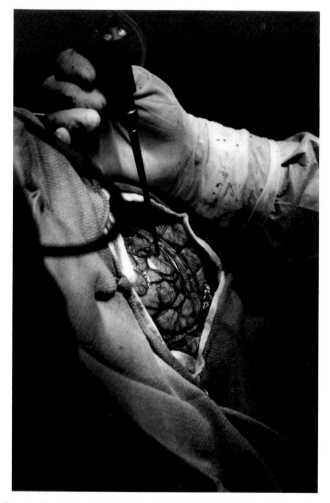

FIG. 13 Interactive image-guided delineation of resection margins for an extensive left frontal grade 2 mixed oligodendroglioma/astrocytoma.

It is possible that some or all of these additional sources of intraoperative data will be used to refresh the original registration or to warp the preoperative images to reflect the changing intraoperative anatomy; reacquiring intraoperative tomographic image data will provide the most detailed matrix by which to refresh registration. The dynamically computed integration of these information sources in a practical manner for clinical use will require considerable work before becoming a reality.

ROBOTICS

Advances in micromachine technology are sufficiently rapid that within a decade we can expect to see server control mechanisms capable of scaling down human hand movements to allow micromanipulation capabilities for industrial production, which can then be translated to equipment for surgical purposes (15, 8, 17). U.S. Defense Department efforts, such as that termed ARPA, are enthusiastic in their advocacy of telesurgery using virtual reality technologies. Piezoelectric tactile feedback sensors being developed for "smart" components of bridges and other stress elements in construction may find themselves applied to virtual reality gloves in the entertainment industry and, by translation, to the surgical control of micromachinery end effectors. The European Union has supported medical robotics through direct and indirect grant support (6).

PRESENT BENEFITS

At this time, the state of the art for interactive image-guided neurosurgery is that at least one system based on implantable fiducial markers and active optical IRED triangulation has shown itself to be as accurate as stereotactic frames (4); other techniques are somewhat less accurate, although they clearly furnish clinically valuable information to the neurosurgeon. Individual investigators have consistently perceived certain benefits to the use of such systems (Table 8), including less invasive surgery and a shortened operating time due to increased surgeon confidence, because of better lesion definition and spatial orientation as well as a greater degree of lesion resection associated with less collateral dissection injury, leading to improved clinical outcomes and a shorter hospital stay. The practical utility of these systems of intraoperative cranial navigation may be highlighted by several examples (Table 9).

TABLE 8
Surgeons' Perceptions

- Less invasive surgery
- Shortened operative time
- Better lesion definition
- Increased confidence
- Less collateral dissection injury
- Shortened hospitalization
- Improved clinical outcomes

TABLE 9
Practical Utility of Intraoperative Cranial Navigation

- Planning the operation
- Placement of the scalp incision
- Designing and executing the craniotomy flap
- Directing/defining the approach
- Working around and within the lesion
- Integrating real-time data in the operating room
- Confirming the execution of surgery

Because these systems are not limited to the clinical indications previously associated with stereotactic frame solutions, the benefits of preoperative computer treatment planning now can be extended to all of cranial neurosurgery. The extent of preoperative "scripting" of an operation can be tailored to suit the complexity of anatomic relationships involved and tempered by the requirements for surgical flexibility to appropriately reassess plans when faced with additional intraoperative information. A broad spectrum of preoperative imaging modalities potentially can be queried in order to create the optimal, anatomically correct map of functionally critical structures surrounding the target lesion. Preoperatively defining the location of the periRolandic cortex in relation to a frontoparietal ganglioglioma (by anatomic criteria applied to spin echo T1- and T2-weighted MR images, and functional activation observed in echoplanar MR imaging scans, MSI, or activation positron emission tomography [PET] adds considerably to the neurosurgeon's reassurance that motor cortex is not violated in a child, where intraoperative stimulation mapping may prove inconsistent or equivocal and techniques of awake craniotomy may not be tolerated by the patient.

The proper placement of a scalp incision and craniotomy flap are mundane but relevant capabilities of all navigational systems, especially appreciated in the case of a high parietal metastasis or a parasagittal meningioma near the junction of the middle and posterior thirds of the superior sagittal sinus (Fig. 14). Often, the greater confidence in directing placement of such flaps allows them to be made no more extensive than truly necessary, while avoiding the need for a second bone flap or suboptimal intraoperative redraping of an expanding surgical field.

Directing and defining the approach to the lesion may be elegantly precise and subtle or simply straightforward. The benefit that can accrue to transphenoidal surgery for a sellar tumor obviously includes the

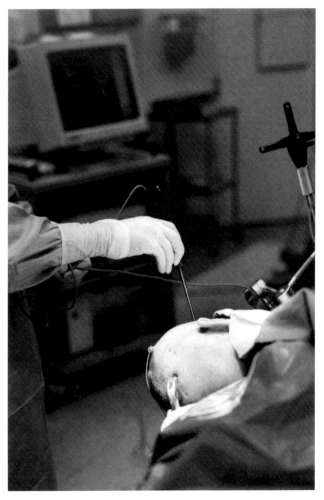

FIG. 14 Defining the scalp incision by reference to the underlying location of a sub-cortical tumor.

ability to confirm the surgeon's anterior-to-posterior (AP) location during exposure, eliminating the need for the bulk of the intraoperative C-arm radiographic unit (Fig. 15). Additionally, this AP information is displayed simultaneously with right-to-left lateralizing information: this can provide useful cautionary information when dealing with a deviated midline septum in an acromegalic, when exposing the lateral pituitary gland adjacent to the cavernous sinus and underlying internal carotid artery during resection of an ACTH-secreting microadenoma, or when resecting a nonsecreting macroadenoma with sphenoid sinus extension

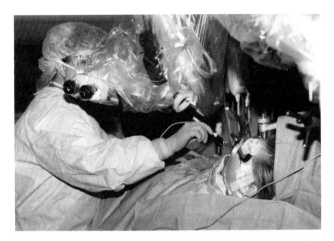

FIG. 15 Defining parasellar anatomic relationships during transphenoidal resection of a microadenoma, using an IRED-based ILD probe.

destroying the cranial base landmarks (Fig. 16). When approaching deep-seated subcortical metastatic tumors, a minimal and precisely directed corticotomy might lessen the opportunity for perioperative neurologic morbidity (Fig. 17). Although the approach to an intracranial aneurysm is conceptually straightforward, the additional reassurance provided by continuous spatial feedback during exposure of a middle cerebral artery aneurysm can reduce operative time and unnecessary dissectional trauma to perforating arteries in the Sylvian fissure. In the case of a patient with bilateral middle cerebral artery trifurcation aneurysms and a P1-region posterior cerebral artery aneurysm, navigational assistance may help to minimize the length of surgery and the extent of dissection needed to properly expose the aneurysms.

Working around and within the lesion is greatly enhanced by spatial feedback. The intracapsular debulking of a fibrous cerebellopontine angle meningioma approached retrosigmoidally, or of a clival chordoma approached transorally, can proceed more rapidly when the surgeon's orientation is preserved by reinforcing imaging-based knowledge of the tumor's relation to key neurovascular structures. Even when dissecting along the surface of the capsular plane, the ability to "see around the corner" is beneficial to anticipate potential hazardous structures or disorientingly projecting tumor lobules (Fig. 18). The irregular contours of the solid tumor tissue components of most glial neoplasms, which lend themselves to spatial disorientation and are therefore often incompletely resected, are better defined and tracked using these systems.

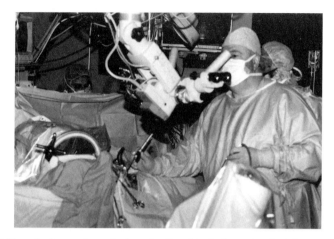

FIG. 16 Use of advanced surgical navigational techniques to identify anatomic relationships adjacent to the cavernous sinus during transphenoidal resection of an extensively eroding pituitary macroadenoma.

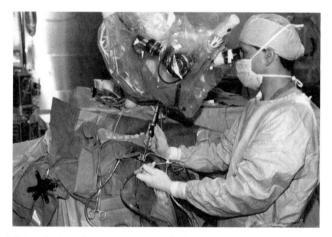

FIG. 17 Minimally invasive craniotomy technique to approach a 4-cm diameter tumor; adenocarcinoma metastatic to the left parietal lobe.

Low-grade gliomas, especially those that are intimately related to functionally eloquent cortex and its subcortical pathways, present an excellent opportunity for improving surgical outcome by incorporating the anatomic and functional feedback from spatially registered intraoperative stimulation mapping (Fig. 19). Use of cavitating ultrasonic aspiration under microscopic illumination can help to reduce sur-

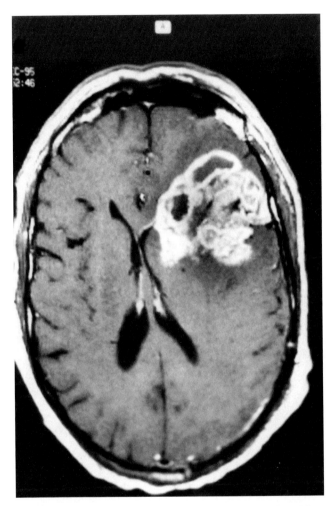

FIG. 18 Irregularly contoured solid tumor tissue component of glioblastoma multi-forme, which was able to be resected up to the contrast-enhanced T1-weighted imaging margins without incurring a neurologic deficit.

geon fatigue and undue tissue manipulation during resection of these ill-marginated, often rubbery, infiltrating tumors. The optimal surgi-cal treatment for both cytoreduction and seizure control in temporal lobe gangliogliomas associated with a longstanding medically in-tractable seizure disorder may involve a resection, defined by spatially registered electrocorticography, which is broader than simple le-sionectomy (Fig. 20). The three-dimensional orientation afforded by

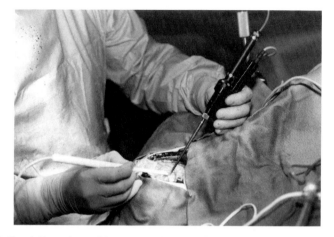

FIG. 19 Spatially registered intraoperative stimulation mapping of angular gyrus region prior to resection of ganglion cell tumor.

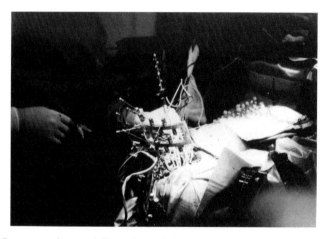

FIG. 20 Intraoperative spatially registered electrocorticography. Reproduced with permission from Maciunas RJ. Surgical aspects and general management of ganglion cell tumors. *In* Apuzzo MLJ (ed). *Benign Cerebral Gliomas: Neurosurgical Topics* Book 22, vol II. American Association of Neurological Surgeons, Park Ridge, IL, 1995, pp 427–444.

superimposing a narrow-angle endoscopic field of view onto preoperative triplanar tomographic images often helps to speed the initial positioning of the endoscope within the surgical work space to better predict what lies just ahead of the field and to maintain the endoscope's close relation to a known bleeding point when the neurosurgeon has to deal with abrupt intraventricular hemorrhage. An intriguing possibility presently under investigation is the real-time control of intracranially focused ultrasonic deep tissue ablation, using feedback from sequentially changing Mrimaging relaxation times of the ultrasonically annealed tissue.

Confirming the extent of resection by sweeping the probe along the resection cavity can prevent the neurosurgeon from leaving residual pockets of unresected solid tumor tissue buried under infolded edematous brain parenchyma, especially in ergonomically inconvenient corners (Fig. 21). While this is exceedingly helpful when operating on malignant gliomas, medulloblastomas, and ependymomas, it is also

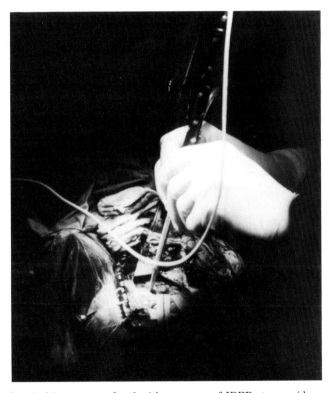

FIG. 21 Surgical instrument fitted with an array of IREDs to provide navigational guidance. Confirming the extent of resection of glioma, guided by MR-defined margins. Reproduced with permission from Maciunas RJ. Surgical aspects and general management of ganglion cell tumors. *In* Apuzzo MLJ (ed). *Benign Cerebral Gliomas: Neurosurgical Topics* Book 22, vol II. American Association of Neurological Surgeons, Park Ridge, IL, 1995, pp 427–444.

surprisingly useful on occasion when resecting benign extra-axial tumors. Painstaking efforts to resect the entire T2-weighted MR imaging abnormality caused by low-grade glial tumors, although unlikely to be curative, might appear to be associated with an improved long term survival and time to progression.

FUTURE BENEFITS

Although many neurosurgeons are subjectively impressed by the utility of these advanced systems of intraoperative cranial navigation, the cost-effectiveness of such systems remains to be convincingly and rigorously demonstrated. Measurements of incision length, degree of resection, operating time, or length of hospitalization are poor measures for comparison in studies, with analysis being confounded by the impact of individual practice preferences, case selection bias, and changing patterns of hospital practice under the influence of managed care contracts. Perhaps ultimately, the most significant effect of these navigational systems will be to standardize clinical outcome after neurosurgical intervention for a variety of disorders by allowing maximal flexibility to appropriately individualize surgical approaches, by optimizing and quantitatively defining the degree of resection, and by minimizing the collateral injury associated with surgery (Table 10). Standardization of neurosurgical results may become valued at least as highly as any other parameter, including cost-effectiveness, under a universal schema of rationalized, capitated health care delivery.

In addition to improving the performance of established neurosurgical operations, accurate intraoperative cranial navigation enables us to conceive of a new generation of surgical procedures for the implantation of neural prostheses (Table 11). Advanced surgical navigation systems will provide the vehicle for targeted delivery, whether the implanted elements are structural supports, electrode, or chemode arrays, mechanical effectors; or cellular and subcellular transplants.

We are all part of a fundamental transition in surgical navigation: from an era sustained by art to one that is informed by science and technology (Table 12). This comes at a time when quantitative clinical

---

TABLE 10
Long-Term Effects of Intraoperative Navigation upon Cranial Resective Surgery

- Individualize approach
- Optimize resection
- Minimize collateral injury
- Standardize outcome

TABLE 11
Neural Prosthetics

- Structural therapies and supports
- Chemodes
- Electrodes
- Mechanical effectors
- Cell transplantation
- Gene therapy and cellular function

TABLE 12
The Art and Science/Technology of Surgical Navigation

The Art of Surgical Navigation	*The Science/Technology of Surgical Navigation*

• Maps as illustrative pictures
• Reliance upon landmarks
 	
• "Hugging the shore"
 	
• A premium upon:
  skill, judgment, experience
• The need for:
  apprenticeship and lore
	I. Rigid body maps
	  • Linkage interactive localization devices
	  • 2-D tomogram slices and renderings as video display
	II. Dynamic, nonrigid body maps
	  • Nonlinkage interactive localization devices
	  • Integration of real-time data and video display
	
	III. Visualization
	  • Digital video
	  • Holography
	  • Augmented/virtual reality
	  • Intraoperative MR tomography
	
	IV. Mechanical effectors for holding, aiming, motion scaling
	  • Tactile feedback
	  • Control mechanisms
	  • Telesurgery
	  • Robotics

practice tracking methods are being brought to bear upon the task of creating a technology of decision-making and practice standards that are intended to produce cost-effective, optimized clinical outcomes in populations of covered lives. In the context of our times, these trends promise to radically alter the pattern of neurosurgical practice in the coming decades. Our abilities will be tested as we navigate between the past and the future of cranial surgery.

REFERENCES

1. Brown, RA: A computerized tomography-computer graphics approach to stereotaxic localization. **J Neurosurg** 50:715–720, 1979.
2. Maciunas RJ, Galloway RL, Jr, Latimer J: The application accuracy of stereotactic frame systems. **Neurosurgery** 35:682–695, 1994.
3. Evans AC, Peters TM, Collins DL, *et al.* Image registration based on discrete anatomic structures. *In* Maciunas RJ (ed): *Interactive Image-Guided Neurosurgery.* Park Ridge, IL, American Association of Neurological Surgeons, 1993, pp 63–80.
4. Maciunas RJ, Fitzpatrick JM, Galloway RL, Allen GS. Beyond stereotaxy: Extreme levels of application accuracy are provided by implantable fiducial markers for interactive image-guided neurosurgery. *In* Maciunas RJ (ed): *Interactive Image-Guided Neurosurgery.* Park Ridge, IL, American Association of Neurological Surgeons, 1993, pp 259–270.
5. Barnett GH, Kormos DW, Steiner CP, *et al.* Use of a frameless, armless stereotactic wand for brain tumor localization with 2-D and 3-D neuroimaging. **Neurosurgery** 33(4):674–678, 1993.
6. Benabid AL, Lavalee S, Hoffmann D, *et al.* Potential use of robots in endoscopic neurosurgery. **Acta Neurochir Suppl** (Wien) 54:93–97, 1992.
7. Bucholz RD, Smith KR. A comparison of sonic digitizers versus light emitting diode-based localization. *In* Maciunas RJ (ed), *Interactive Image-Guided Neurosurgery.* Park Ridge, IL, American Association of Neurological Surgeons, 1993, pp 179–200.
8. Drake JM, Prudencio J, Holowka S. A comparison of a PUMA robotic system and the ISG viewing wand for neurosurgery. *In* Maciunas RJ (ed): *Interactive Image-Guided Neurosurgery.* Park Ridge, IL, American Association of Neurological Surgeons, 1993, pp 121–133.
9. Heilbrun MP, McDonald P, Wiker C, *et al.* Stereotactic localization and guidance using a machine vision technique. **Stereotact Funct Neurosurg** 58:94–98, 1992.
10. Maciunas RJ, Galloway RL, Fitzpatrick JM, *et al.* A universal system for interactive image-directed neurosurgery. **Stereotact Funct Neurosurg** 58:108–113, 1992.
11. Mosges R, Schlondorff G. A new imaging method for intraoperative therapy control in skull-base surgery. **Neurosurg Rev** 11:245–247, 1988.
12. Oikarinen J, Alakuijala J, Louhisalmi Y, *et al.* The Oulu neuronavigator system: Intraoperative ultrasonography in the verification of neurosurgical localization and visualization. *In* Maciunas RJ (ed). *Interactive Image-Guided Neurosurgery.* Park Ridge, IL, American Association of Neurological Surgeons, 1993, pp 233–247.
13. Roberts DW, Strohbehn JW, Hatch JF, *et al.* A frameless stereotaxic integration of computerized tomographic imaging and the operating microscope. **J Neurosurg** 65:545–549, 1986.
14. Watanabe E, Watanabe T, Manaka S, *et al.* Three-dimensional digitizer (Neuronavigator): New equipment for computed tomography-guided stereotaxic surgery. **Surg Neurol** 27:543–547, 1987.
15. Adler JR, Jr. Image-based frameless stereotactic radiosurgery. *In* Maciunas RJ (ed): *Interactive Image-Guided Neurosurgery.* Park Ridge, IL, American Association of Neurological Surgeons, 1993, pp 81–89.
16. Pelizzari CA, Chen GTY, Spelbring DR, *et al.* Accurate three-dimensional registration of CT, PET, and/or MR images of the brain. **J Comput Assist Tomogr** 13:20–26, 1989.
17. Kwoh YS, Hou J, Jonckheere EA, *et al.* A robot with improved absolute positioning

accuracy for CT-guided stereotactic brain surgery. **IEEE Trans Biomed Eng** 35:153–160, 1988.

18. Galloway RL, Jr, Berger MS, Bass WA, Maciunas RJ. Registered intraoperative information: Electrophysiology, ultrasound, and endoscopy. *In* Maciunas RJ (ed): *Interactive Image-Guided Neurosurgery.* Park Ridge, IL, American Association of Neurological Surgeons, 1993, pp 247–258.

19. Zamorano L, Nolte LP, Jiang Z, *et al.* Image-guided computer-assisted spine surgery—A pilot study on spinal pedicule fixation. Presented at the Quadrennial Meeting of the American Society for Stereotactic and Functional Neurosurgery, Marina del Rey, CA, March 11, 1995.

20. Thomas DGT, Doshi P, Colchester A, *et al.* Craniotomy guidance using a stereo video-based tracking system (Vislan). Presented at the Quadrennial Meeting of the American Society for Stereotactic and Functional Neurosurgery, Marina del Rey, CA, March 11, 1995.

21. Kato A, Yoshimine T, Hayakawa T, *et al.* A frameless, armless navigational system for computer-assisted tomography. **J Neurosurg** 74:845–849, 1991.

CHAPTER

26

Magnetic Neurosurgery: Image-Guided, Remote-Controlled Movement of Neurosurgical Implants

M. A. HOWARD III, M.D., M. M. HENEGAR, M.D., R. G. DACEY, JR., M.D.,
M. S. GRADY, M.D., R. C. RITTER, AND G. T. GILLIES

A novel means of carrying out stereotactic procedures is under development and preparation for human clinical testing. The technique uses externally controlled magnetic fields to control the movement of an implanted object through the parenchymal tissues, opening the possibilities of nonlinear stereotactic procedures for spatially optimized drug delivery, brachytherapy, biopsy, etc. The system uses six superconducting magnets to create the fields needed to obtain movement of the implant. The surgeon-controlled computer interface, the superconducting "helmet" containing the cryogenic components and the overall status of the development effort will be described.

A magnetic surgery system (MSS) capable of nonlinear stereotaxis is being developed to advance the field of minimally invasive surgery. Neurosurgical applications will make use of the ability of the MSS to move intracerebral devices through the brain tissues by means of externally generated magnetic field gradients.

The remote, noncontact manipulation a brain implant will make it possible to: 1) navigate tetherless implants, 2) follow complex, non-linear trajectories, and 3) move an implant serially without "reoperation." With these fundamental implant control capabilities a wide range of new functional neurosurgical clinical applications may become possible.

Over the last 12 years, a multi-institutional, interdisciplinary research and development team has sought to reduce the principles of magnetic surgery to practice. We describe here the fifth-generation MSS apparatus, which is now being used in a series of animal trials in preparation for clinical testing. Test results of MSS component performance are presented as well as data from related in-vivo measurements of the force needed to move an implant through human brain. Plans for future development of the MSS will also be outlined.

MATERIALS AND METHODS

The principle subsystems of the MSS are the 1) external drive magnets (which are contained in the MSS helmet), 2) the implant and fiducial marker imaging system, and 3) the command computer and surgeon interface system. Each of these subsystems is described below.

MSS Helmet

All of the different MSS implants will have a small Nd-B-Fe permanent magnet positioned at their leading tips. A given implant might consist of an untethered probe or a single or multiple lumen catheter which is to be guided through the parenchymal tissues. Implant movement occurs when the permanent dipole in the tip is acted on by a magnetic field gradient produced by six superconducting electromagnets positioned in orthogonal pairs about the patient's head as suggested in Fig. 1. By varying the strengths of the persistent electrical currents running through these coils, it is possible to control the structure and orientation of the resulting magnetic field gradient within the region of the helmet corresponding to the location of the patient's brain. The product of the helmet's gradient and the implant's dipole moment yields the force that acts to move the implant. By selecting appropriate

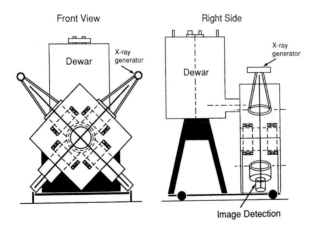

FIG. 1 Schematic diagrams of front and side views of the Magnetic Surgery System (MSS). Liquid helium is stored within the dewar and bathes the six superconducting drive magnets positioned within the MSS helmet. The patient's head passes through the central circular opening so that the brain is positioned within the center of the operating space of the MSS. Real time magnetic implant imaging is carried out using the two fluoroscopic x-ray systems shown.

combinations of currents it is possible to produce a movement-inducing magnetic gradient that can, in turn, navigate the implant in any direction desired.

The superconducting drive magnets must be operated at a temperature of 4 K (*i.e.*, 4 above absolute zero). Therefore, the helmet containing them must serve as a cryostat that continuously bathes the magnets in liquid helium, while allowing the patient's head to be positioned in the room-temperature center-region of the structure, and the conjunction of the three magnetic axes. The cryostat and coils have open axial bores, thus enabling the beams from the bi-planar fluoroscopy system to pass through the patient's head along the axes of the "x-" and "y- direction" coil pairs. The current human- compatible prototype MSS helmet is shown in Fig. 2.

Imaging System

Accurate imaging is essential in order to localize the implant's position within the brain, and hence to enable successful operation of the MSS. The method currently in use relies on an atlas of preoperative MR images onto which are superimposed the implant position data obtained from bi-planar fluorograms obtained intra-operatively. Before the MR study, fiducial markers are placed about the skull to serve as

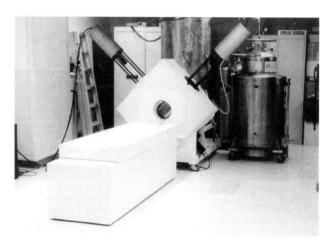

FIG. 2 Photograph of the first human MSS prototype located at the Neurosurgical Service, Barnes Hospital, Washington University, St. Louis. Magnetic surgery patients will lie on the gantry shown in the foreground. The patient's head and neck will be positioned within the central opening of the MSS helmet. The MSS superstructure is considerably smaller than a clinical MRI unit.

common volume-registration points for both imaging modalities. The MR views provide accurate spatial locations of structures in the patient's brain relative to the fiducial markers. During a magnetic surgery procedure, biplanar fluoroscopic images are obtained at rates up to a few times per second, and from them, three-dimensional information on the location of the radio-opaque implant (relative to the fiducial skull markers) can be derived. The MSS imaging computer transforms the fluoroscopic imaging data to the MR based imaging volume and presents the surgeon with a view depicting the current location of the implant on each appropriate slice of the MR atlas. Many of the general principles involved in this localization strategy are similar to those employed in the typical approach to frameless stereotaxis.

The MSS fluoroscopic imaging system must perform in the presence of strong magnetic fields; an environment that is unsuitable for standard electrostatic image intensifiers. To address this constraint, a magnetically impervious fluoroscopic system was developed based on microchannel plate technology [2]. With this adaptation it is possible to obtain useful x-ray images even in the presence of strong magnetic fields, and at very low x-ray doses. It is estimated that a 2 hour MSS procedure would expose a patient to a radiation dose of < 1.5 R [3].

Command Computer

The MSS is controlled by the neurosurgeon via a command computer. The neurosurgeon selects the desired target pathway for the implant based on the preoperative imaging data. Once the magnetic surgery procedure has begun the computer will direct currents into the drive magnet to generate a series of step-wise movements. By constantly updating the display to show the particular MR images that correspond to the implant's progressive locations, the user interface of the command computer allows the neurosurgeon to monitor the progress of the operation. Should any intended or actual movement vector be clinically unacceptable, the neurosurgeon can discontinue the movement protocol and generate the implant displacement vectors manually using a mouse or other convenient input device.

In vivo Force Measurement Experiments

Successful navigation of an intracerebral implant is critically dependent on the ability of the external drive magnets to generate adequate magnetic gradients to insure reliable implant movement through the full range of tissue rheologies encountered in both normal and diseased (e.g., tumor infiltrated) brain. Implant movement is impeded by frictional resistance of the surrounding brain tissue. In the past, measurements of the resistance of brain tissue to penetrative forces have been carried out in freshly harvested experimental animal brains as well as phantom gels [4]. To obtain resistance measurements that most closely simulate conditions during a clinical magnetic surgery procedure, *in vivo* force measurements have been carried out in human subjects scheduled for craniotomy.

The human experimental protocols have been approved by the University of Iowa human subjects institutional review board. All patients are scheduled for brain tissue resection as part of their standard neurosurgical treatment plan. Just prior to tissue resection, probes are passed slowly through the planned region of resection using a strain-gauge- based force meter (Chatilon Model No. DGGS-R-250g) that is advanced using an electrically controlled microdrive. The forces necessary to advance the probes are recorded continuously via an intra-operative computer, with the data stored on disk for off-line analysis. The overall experimental arrangement is shown in Fig. 3.

RESULTS

A human-compatible prototype of the MSS was constructed in Livermore, California (Stereotaxis, Inc.) and then transported for further testing to the Neurosurgical Service at Barnes Hospital, Washington

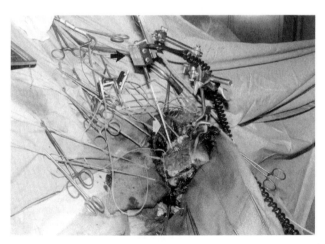

FIG. 3 Intraoperative photograph of a force measurement experiment. A standard silastic ventricular catheter (white arrow) is being slowly advanced through a portion of anterior temporal lobe scheduled to be subsequently resected.* The forces exerted on the catheter as it advances through brain tissue are constantly measured using a force measurement device (black arrow). Measurement results are collected using a lap top computer outside the operating field.

University School of Medicine, St. Louis, Missouri. The design and performance characteristics of the MSS subsystems are summarized below.

Cryostatic Helmet

The cryostatic helmet housing the superconducting drive magnets weighs approximately 1,800 lb. and holds 150 liters of liquid helium. The six suspended magnets are constructed of 6,600 and 3,900 turns of superconducting wire for the x and y, and z coil systems, respectively. With maximum current of 90 A, a pair of the coils generates roughly 11 tons of force on the helmet superstructure. Following several dozen test cycles, the magneto-mechanical properties of the magnets have been quite carefully characterized, and the system's performance found to be highly reliable with only rare quenches.

The patient passes his head through a 27-cm diameter clear bore of the z-axis coil positioned at the front of the helmet. Two x-ray ports are diagonally oriented such that the beams intersect at a location approximating the position of the patient's brain. The amount of space occupied by the entire helmet assembly is considerably smaller than that of a standard MRI.

X-ray imaging

The biplanar fluoroscopic imaging system functions reliably, operating at low beam currents but high energy, producing pulses at 0.25-s intervals. The x-ray detectors and image processing computer are able to detect and track an implant of 2-mm cross-sectional diameter passing through a brain phantom placed within the MSS treatment volume. When the implant is moving along a straight-line path, the tracking error has a standard deviation of approximately 0.25 mm. The image capture systems shows no detectable distortion in the presence of the magnetic fields and gradients associated with the operation of the helmet, which are typically on the order of 0.8 T and 5 T/m respectively.

Command Computer

The primary imaging interface with the surgeon is based on the frameless stereotactic imaging software developed by Surgical Navigation, Inc. (Denver, Colorado). Instead of using positional references based on a wand pointer, implant position is calculated based on the x-ray imaging data. Representative coronal axial and cut-away MR images are presented to the neurosurgeon who then uses a mouse to identify the entrance point, a terminal target point, and any number of intermediate points along the intended path of motion. The computer generates a "best fit" curve that indicates the resulting planned pathway. During simulated biopsy procedures using human MR data, the mouse pointing technique proved to be a convenient method for navigating around sulci to deliver a vehicle to a deep-seated target site.

The evolving magnetic control algorithms are extremely complex because of the large number of possible combinations of coil current that can in principle be used to effect each movement sequence. Highly accurate (< 1 mm SD) movement of an untethered implant is routinely achieved while activating 2 coil pairs simultaneously. Movements of this accuracy have not yet been achieved in situations that might require all three pairs of drive magnet simultaneously. However, an improved algorithm designed to address this eventuality is currently being tested.

Force measurements

In vivo measurements of the forces needed to move an implant in human brain have been carried out in six patients. During these experiments ventricular catheters, metal spheres (3-mm cross-sectional diameter) on the end of a thin (1-mm diameter) rigid shaft, and a multi-linked titanium catheter have been used to make a total of 12 passes through anterior temporal lobe tissue to a distance of 0.8 - 2.0 cm from the pial surface. A wide range of resistance characteristics were noted. All catheters displayed a steady linear increase in resistive force as more of the implant entered the brain (Fig. 4), but resistance was significantly greater for the titanium catheter than the silastic catheter. Abrupt rises in resistance were noted periodically which seemed to correlate with the tip of the implant abutting a subsurface sulcus. The metal-sphere implant showed nearly flat resistance characteristics as it traversed brain tissue. These results indicate that a free-floating magnetic implant as well as a silastic catheter could be reliably manipulated through human brain tissue with the current MSS apparatus. The greater resistance encountered with the titanium catheter suggests that modifications may be necessary for this particular application.

DISCUSSION

To date, stereotactic neurosurgical procedures have been carried out using linear probes. This is a treatment delivery configuration that is not optimally suited to access the complex curvilinear shapes of anatomical structures in the human brain. This technical limitation becomes clinically relevent in the modern brain imaging era when high resolution MRI scans are capable of precisely defining the optimal tar-

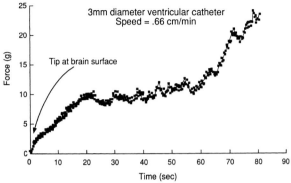

FIG. 4 Representative force measurement data. In this experiment a 3 mm diameter silastic catheter was advanced through brain tissue at a speed of 6.6 mm/minute. Resistive forces are depicted along the vertical axis. As more of the catheter enters brain tissue, cumulative resistance increases in a near linear fashion. Approaching the end of the run, the slope of the curve changes, indicating a rather abrupt increase in resistance. Based on previous force measurement studies, it is likely that this increase results from the catheter tip encountering a sulcus below the brain surface.

get-treatment volumes for a wide range of neurological diseases. To take full therapeutic advantage of this elegant anatomical information, it is desirable to have a treatment delivery system with complete freedom of movement, thus enabling intracranial navigation along even highly curvilinear paths.

Although a number of different probe movement systems have been investigated over the years for the purpose of remotely manipulating objects within the brain, magnetic stereotaxis is the only technique that has actually been able to move a probe in a noncontact manner through brain tissue. In this report, we have described a magnetic surgery system that is capable of performing image-guided, magnetic manipulation of an intracerebral implant. Even though most of this system's components are individually quite complex, most of the major subsystems have proven to be highly reliable and relatively inexpensive compared to other advanced medical technologies. This is predominantly a reflection of the remarkable pace of recent technological advances in the fields of computer science, superconducting technology, and brain imaging.

Large superconducting magnets have been commercially available for several years now. Even so, the design of the six-coil drive-magnet system within the MSS is quite novel in many of its particulars. Its performance is excellent, though, with unexpected quenches being rare events. When the magnets are purposely quenched, however, as is done in performance verification studies, the result is that the implant remains stationary and is not subject to large transient movements. Magnetically immune image intensifiers track the position of the implant during intracranial navigation and the surgeon is presented with a highly refined set of representative brain images based on a commercially-available frameless-stereotaxis imaging system. The computational and image processing requirements of the MSS are easily handled by commercially available workstations, and much of the present work has been accomplished with processors made, *e.g.,* by the SUN and Datacube Corporations.

From the physicist and engineer's perspective, the principle technical challenges that remain are to optimize the drive magnet-control algorithms and to develop methods of moving smaller and smaller implants through the brain with roughly the same level of magnetic field gradient as is produced by the existing helmet. Controlling six simultaneously activated superconducting magnets is a highly complex process. In particular, rapid ramping of the coils is something that has not been done previously in any related industrial or medical application. While algorithms have been developed which meet all theoretical control requirements, exhaustive trials must be carried out to confirm the reliability of the resulting software.

Smaller implants (*i.e.,* those with a maximum dimension of <3 mm) have a mechanical advantage over larger ones in that they face less rheological resistance when traveling through the brain tissue. The disadvantage of going to a smaller-sized magnetic tip, of course, is that the corresponding magnitude of the permanent magnet's dipole moment decreases as well. It is unlikely that long implants with very small cross-sectional diameters, such as flexible microelectrodes, will be implantable using magnetic forces alone. Such an implant would have a large cumulative drag, but only a small magnetic moment at the tip to couple to the external gradient. In this situation, a combination of magnetic control of the implant's tip and mechanical "boost" to aid in translational advance of the body (perhaps by use of an actuator located at the skull's surface) may prove to be effective. The feasibility of this approach is currently under investigation.

The eventual clinical success of magnetic surgery is critically dependent on demonstrating the safety and efficacy of hardware and software components of the overall system. As the MSS matures, issues such as ease of use and cost-effectiveness are likely to be equally important. In the final analysis, however, superior treatment efficacy will only be achieved if volume-contoured therapy treatment hypotheses prove to be correct [1].

ACKNOWLEDGMENTS

The authors thank Stereotaxis, Inc. for supporting this research. They also thank the Margaret W. and Herbert Hoover, Jr. Foundation, the Huston Foundation, the Beirne Carter Foundation, and the Kopf Foundation for financial assistance with the project.

REFERENCES

1. Howard MA, Gross A, Grady MS, Langer RS, Mathiowitz E, Winn HR, Mayberg MR. Intracerebral drug delivery in rats reverses lesion-induced memory deficits. **J Neurosurg** 71:105–112, 1989.
2. Ramos PA, Allison SW, Molloy JA, Lawson MA, Quate EG, Ritter RC, Gillies GT, Grady MS, Howard III MA. "Electro-Optic Imaging Chain for a Biplanar Fluoroscope for Neurosurgery," Optical Engineering 32, 1644–1656 (1993).
3. Ritter RC, Werp PR, Lawson MA, Egan JM, Howard III MA, Dacey Jr, RG, Grady MS, Broaddus WC, Gillies GT. "Magnetic Stereotaxis: An Application of Magnetic Control Technology to the Needs of Clinical Medicine," in Proceedings of the MAG'95 Conference, ed. P. Allaire (Technomic Publishing, Lancaster, Pennsylvania, 1995), pp. 186–193.
4. Molloy JA, Ritter RC, Grady MS, Howard III MA, Quate EG, Gillies GT. "Experimental Determination of the Force Required for Insertion of a Thermoseed into Deep Brain Tissues," **Ann Biomed Engin** 18, 299–313, 1990.

27

Thoracoscopic Spinal Surgery

CURTIS A. DICKMAN, M.D. AND DEAN G. KARAHALIOS, M.D.

Endoscopic techniques have substantially affected almost every sphere of medicine and surgery. The impetus for this movement is multifaceted. Patients find minimally incisional techniques attractive from an aesthetic standpoint. The clinical benefits include less dissection of superficial tissues, which can result in less postoperative pain, less blood loss, shorter intensive care unit (ICU) and hospital stays, and faster recovery times. In turn, these techniques have a potential to lower the costs of health care and to facilitate the speed of recovery and the patient's return to normal activities.

Technological advances in endoscopic imaging devices have played a critical role in the development of minimally invasive surgery. The resolution of endoscopic images now far surpasses those previously obtained because of improved technology such as computer interfacing, optical chips, fiber-optic cables, video endoscopy, and three-dimensional (3-D) imaging. Endoscopes provide illumination, visualization, magnification, and a conduit to access almost every region of the human body through very small skin incisions. We prefer the term minimally incisional surgery rather than minimally invasive surgery because "conventional" operations with extensive anatomical dissections can be performed through very small incisions. Endoscopes have become increasingly employed as diagnostic and therapeutic tools in almost every surgical specialty. A large proportion of surgical procedures that were previously performed solely with open techniques are now performed almost exclusively using endoscopic techniques as the primary procedures of choice. Endoscopes have been used extensively as arthroscopes in orthopedics; as laparoscopes in general surgery and gynecology; as cystoscopes and ureteroscopes in urology; and as thoracoscopes in cardiothoracic surgery. Only recently has endoscopy found its respective niche in neurosurgery.

Minimally invasive techniques in neurosurgery, including stereotactic surgery, endovascular techniques, radiosurgery, specialized microsurgical approaches, and intracranial endoscopy, have changed the way neurosurgeons approach some of the most challenging clinical problems. Intracranial endoscopy has been successfully applied to the treatment of a variety of intracranial and intraventricular processes. Only during the past few years has endoscopy been applied in the treatment of spinal pathology.

Endoscopic approaches to the spine include posterolateral percutaneous approaches to the lumbar disc spaces and neural foramina, anterior laparoscopic and anterolateral retroperitoneal endoscopic approaches to the lumbar spine, and thoracoscopic approaches to the thoracic spine/(1-14). All of these techniques have primarily used rigid rod-lens endoscopes for visualization of the anatomy and pathology. Flexible fiberoptic endoscopes have also been used as an adjunct to open spinal surgical procedures to inspect the cauda equina, spinal cord, and neural foramina and to assess the internal anatomy of syringomyelic cavities (7-10, 13, 15). Flexible fiberoptic endoscopes have poorer resolution and image quality compared to rigid endoscopes. The wide range of potential spinal uses for endoscopy is beyond the breadth of this monograph, which focuses on the application of thoracoscopy for the treatment of thoracic spinal pathology.

Thoracoscopy has been widely employed by cardiothoracic surgeons during the past few years; the techniques for thoracoscopic spinal surgery are adapted from their methodologies (16-19). Thoracoscopic access is achieved by temporarily deflating the lung on the ipsilateral side of the spinal exposure using a double-lumen endotracheal tube. The chest cavity becomes a wide empty corridor or working space to access the thoracic spine. Narrow portals are strategically positioned in small incisions in the intercostal spaces. One portal is used for the endoscope, which is usually a 1-cm diameter, rigid, high-resolution endoscope. Two or three other portals are used to insert working tools. The endoscopes have video cameras mounted on them, which then relay the images to video monitors. The operative procedure can be observed by the entire surgical team on the video monitors.

HISTORICAL OVERVIEW

Thoracoscopy was introduced in the early 1900s and was used initially as a diagnostic tool for the evaluation of pleural diseases (20-23). During the late 1980s, techniques and instrumentation for laparoscopic surgical procedures improved dramatically, facilitating new applications for thoracoscopy. During the early 1990s, thoracoscopic techniques evolved rapidly and were applied to a broad spectrum of pathology involving the thorax (16-19). Today, many thoracic procedures previously performed via thoracotomy are routinely performed preferentially using thoracoscopy. These procedures include biopsy or resection of pleural or lung lesions, lymph node biopsy, dissection for tumor staging, biopsy and resection of mediastinal masses, lobectomy, pneumonectomy, pleural sclerotherapy, treatment of blebs, esophageal procedures, sympathectomy, and other procedures (16-19, 24). Several clinical studies have found significant advantages to thoracoscopy compared with thoracotomy for the treatment of thoracic pathology (24-26). Studies examining the results of resection of pulmonary lesions have demonstrated significant clinical advantages to thoracoscopy (24-26); small incisions with minimal dissection and retraction of the chest wall resulted in decreased blood loss, reduced postoperative pain, better postoperative pulmonary and shoulder function, shortened intensive care unit and overall hospital stays, fewer complications, and faster recovery times (16-19, 24-26). The morbidity, pain, and time of recovery were significantly lower with thoracoscopy compared to thoracotomy.

Thoracoscopic spinal surgery is still in its infancy and its history is relatively brief. In the early 1990s the spinal techniques were independently developed by John Regan and co-workers (27) in the United States and by Daniel Rosenthal and his colleagues (5) in Germany. The first published report of thoracoscopy for spinal diseases appeared in 1993 by Mack et al. (27) who described 10 patients with diverse spinal pathology who were effectively treated thoracoscopically without major complications. Their only complication consisted of postoperative pneumonia in one patient. In 1994, Rosenthal et al. (5) and Horowitz et al. (4) published separate reports that described the techniques for thoracic microdiscectomy using thoracoscopy. During 1994 and 1995 clinical interest in this topic increased dramatically and a few clinical series were published (Table 1) (1-3, 6, 28). These reports documented the ability to achieve operative dissections comparable to thoracotomy, with less morbidity than similar spinal procedures performed using thoracotomy.

TABLE 1
Thoracoscopic Spinal Surgery: Clinical Series to Date

Author	Year	No. of pts.	Procedures		
			Discectomy	Vertebrectomy	Anterior release
Rosenthal and Lorenz (28)	1994	20	8	12	0
Regan, et al. (6)	1995	12	6	1	5
McAfee, et al. (2)	1995	78	41	13	24
Dickman et al (1)	1996	17	0	17	0

INDICATIONS FOR THORACOSCOPIC SPINAL SURGERY

Thoracic spinal pathology commonly involves either the vertebral bodies or the disc spaces. Thoracoscopy can be used to access the discs, vertebral bodies, and ipsilateral pedicle; however, it cannot access the posterior surfaces of the spine. A wide variety of thoracic spinal pathology is amenable to treatment using thoracoscopy. Thoracoscopic approaches have been used to treat herniated thoracic discs (2-6, 27); to drain vertebral epidural abscesses; to debride vertebral osteomyelitis and discitis; to decompress fractures; to biopsy and resect neoplasms (1-3, 27); and to perform vertebrectomies and interbody fusions, vertebral body reconstructions and instrumentation (1-3, 27, 29), sympathectomies (30-32), and anterior releases for the treatment of kyphosis and scoliosis (2, 3, 6, 27, 29).

COMPARISONS OF THORACOSCOPY WITH OTHER SURGICAL APPROACHES

The relative merits and disadvantages of the three primary surgical approaches to the thoracic spine are compared in Table 2. Spinal surgeons have often been reluctant to use thoracotomy for access to the ventral thoracic spine, primarily because of the morbidity and pain associated with thoracotomy and the need for a cardiothoracic surgeon for exposure and closure (33-43). However, a transthoracic approach vastly improves visualization of the ventral surfaces of the thoracic spine and spinal cord to facilitate decompression, reconstruction, and internal fixation. Thoracoscopy has some advantageous characteristic (*i.e.*, minimal muscular incisions or rib resection) that both thoracotomy and costotransversectomy lack. Thoracoscopy reduces the morbidity and pain associated with the transthoracic approach yet fully provides a broad direct view and access to the ventral surfaces of the spine and spinal cord. Decompression, reconstruction, and instrumentation can be performed using thoracoscopy. Thoracoscopy also provides a more direct, complete view of the entire ventral surface of the spinal cord than costotransversectomy.

Educational Issues

Clinical application of thoracoscopic techniques should only follow an educational program that includes comprehensive lectures and extensive practice of surgical skills in a surgical laboratory. Surgeons must recognize that their previous surgical experience and training inadequately prepares them for competency with these new techniques. We performed extensive dissections in animal models and in human cadavers before attempting clinical surgeries and emphatically recommend this practice.

TABLE 2
Comparisons of Operative Approaches to the Thoracic Spine

	Costotransversectomy	Thoracotomy	Thoracoscopy
Direction of approach	Posterolateral	Anterolateral	Anterolateral
View of ventral surface of spinal cord	Oblique, indirect	Full, direct	Full, direct
Size of incisions	4 to 12 in	6 to 15 in	1/2 to 1 in (x 3-4)
Muscle transection	Moderate or extensive	Extensive	Minimal
Relationship to pleura	Extrapleural	Intrapleural	Intrapleural
Postoperative chest tube	No	Yes	Yes
Access to posterior spinal elements for decompression or fixation	Yes	No	No
Access to vertebral bodies for screw-plate fixation	No	Yes	Yes
Extent of rib resection or rib retraction	3 to 7 in of rib removed/ moderate retraction	6 to 12 in of rib removed/ extensive retraction	1 in of rib head and proximal rib removed/no retraction
Incidence of postoperative intercostal neuralgia	Uncommon/often transient	Common/often prolonged	Uncommon/usually transient

Thoracoscopic surgery requires acquiring new psychomotor skills, adapting and modifying how tools are manipulated, developing new ways of perceiving the operative anatomy, developing strategies to maintain a patent image, and navigating in a "different" environment, through restricted portals of entry.

These techniques have a very steep "learning curve" that must be mastered prior to clinical application. Many experienced spine surgeons have commented that they "felt disoriented, inexperienced, and poorly prepared to pursue these techniques," during their first few laboratory training sessions. However, skill acquisition and facility with these techniques can develop fairly rapidly and each surgeon has a different aptitude for developing these techniques.

Once sufficient laboratory skills have been developed, a transition to clinical work is recommended. It is extremely helpful to observe other surgeons performing clinical cases and to have some type of supervisory preceptorship to minimize potential morbidity during these initial procedures. Additionally, thoracoscopy should be performed in conjunction with a cardiothoracic surgeon so that an immediate thoracotomy can be performed if needed.

These caveats and prerequisites to thoracoscopy are important; surgeons should not attempt these techniques in a clinical setting without comprehensive training. Failure to recognize the high degree of difficulty during the initial acquisition of knowledge of skills will result in unnecessary serious complications. These ethical and educational issues also confronted general and cardiothoracic surgeons during initiation of their experiences with endoscopic techniques, and training and practice guidelines were established (15, 44). Spinal surgeons can benefit by adopting similar recommendations and guidelines so that clinical complications are minimized.

THORACOSCOPIC TECHNIQUE

General Considerations

Thoracoscopic spinal surgery requires a thorough familiarity with the anatomy of the thoracic spine, spinal cord, thorax, and mediastinum. The decision to approach the spine from the left or right side depends upon several factors including location, lateralization, and extent of the pathology. The position of the great vessels is also important to consider and may be evaluated on preoperative computed tomography (CT) or magnetic resonance (MR) imaging studies. A right-sided approach is more commonly used for midline lesions because more spinal surface area is usually available behind the azygous vein than behind the aorta. If a lesion is lateralized to the left, a left-sided approach is more appropriate. Also, if a lesion is located below T9, a left-sided approach is preferred because at this level the diaphragm rides high on the right side. In general, an exposure from T1-T2 to the T11-T12 interspace is possible via the thoracoscopic approach.

Thoracoscopic Imaging

In thoracoscopy, the endoscope is used for illumination, visualization, and magnification. Unlike other endoscopic techniques, working channels within the scope are usually not used. Several separate portals are inserted in the chest wall for the endoscope and for the passage of instruments. A standard 1-cm diameter rigid-rod lens endoscope with a 0 to 30° angle of view is connected to a 2- or 3-dimensional camera, which transmits the image to a video monitor (Fig. 1). High-resolution 3-dimensional endoscopes can vividly represent the complex anatomical relationships between structures and markedly enhance the surgeon's ability to manipulate instruments in this region. Xenon or halogen light sources are primarily used, and the light is delivered to the end of endoscope via fiber-optic cables. The endoscope may be affixed to a table-mounted endoscopic holder to free the surgeon's and assistant's hands.

A clear endoscopic image is provided by using several strategies. The endoscopic lens must remain free from debris. Debris and blood may be

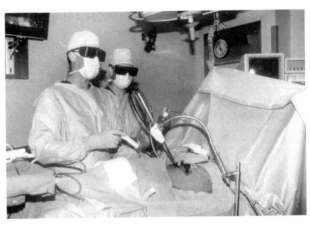

FIG. 1 A rigid-rod lens endoscope is mounted on an endoscope holder. The 1-cm diameter endoscope is inserted into a portal into the chest. A video-camera on the end of the endoscope transmits the images to video monitors in the surgical suite. Three dimensional endoscopy requires that the surgeons wear glasses while observing the images on the video monitor. The depth perception permits precise appreciation of the extent of dissection to facilitate working safely around the spinal cord.

cleared manually. Alternatively, there are irrigating and automated wiper mechanisms on the tips of some endoscopes. Fogging can be a problem and is avoided by prewarming the endoscope, by using warmed irrigation solution, and by wiping the lens with an antifogging agent. Finally, blood pooling in the thoracic cavity will absorb a significant amount of light and will darken the operative field. Frequent irrigation and suctioning will avoid this problem.

Instruments for Thoracoscopic Spinal Surgery

Instruments used in performing the thoracoscopic spinal dissection are longer versions of conventional instruments to accommodate for the working distance from the chest wall to the spine. This distance ranges from 14 to 30 cm depending upon the size of the patient and the position of the portals in relationship to the spinal pathology. Tools often require two hands for precise control during manipulation and during dissection. Long tools amplify motions differently than short surgical tools; however, precise control of the tips of instruments is easily obtained with two-handed techniques.

Laparoscopic and thoracoscopic soft tissue dissection tools, which are commercially available, may be used in thoracoscopic spinal surgery. These tools include microscissors, fine tissue forceps, Babcock clamps, Allis clamps, right-angled tissue forceps, suction-irrigation tools, monopolar and bipolar cautery, peanut dissectors, and other tools. Long bone and disc dissection tools consist of curved and straight curettes, Kerrison rongeurs, Leksell rongeurs, Penfield instruments, nerve hooks, Cobb periosteal elevators, rib dissectors, disc space rongeurs, osteotomes, and bone graft impactors (Fig. 2). For many applications, a high-speed drill is necessary. A pistol grip is used on the drill to help stabilize the shaft during drilling. Long drill bits and attachments, which are commercially available, can be used for thoracoscopic spinal surgery.

Hemostatic Agents

One of the most common questions from surgeons is "can hemostasis be adequately achieved using thoracoscopic techniques?" The techniques to obtain hemostasis are identical to methods used in open surgery and pose no limitations. A number of tools and methods may be used for hemostasis in thoracoscopic spinal surgery, including vascular clips, monopolar cautery, and bipolar cautery. As in "open" procedures, monopolar cautery should be used with caution in the region of the spine and avoided near the dura to avoid injury to the nerve roots and spinal cord. Cotton-tipped peanut dissectors may be used to apply

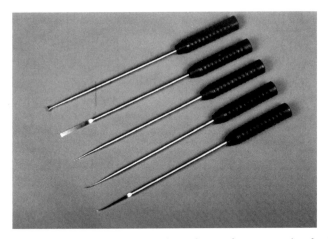

FIG. 2 Thoracoscopic spinal dissection tools are longer than conventional spinal tools to accommodate the distance from the chest wall to the spine, which ranges from 14 to 30 cm.

bone wax. Gelfoam®, Endoavitene®, and Nuknit® also may be used as in "open" procedures to gently tamponade epidural venous bleeding. Cottonoid paddies with long strings can be used, but the end of the string must be anchored outside the chest wall to prevent loss of the paddie within the thoracic cavity. Finally, in the event of massive hemorrhage resulting from injury to the great vessels, a tightly-rolled 4 × 4 sponge on a long clamp (sponge stick) may be used to provide gentle tamponade until the chest is opened. A thoracotomy tray should always be readily available for rapid conversion of the procedure. Fortunately, we have never had an injury to a major vascular or visceral structure and have never had to convert any of our thoracoscopic cases to a thoracotomy.

Operating Room Setup and Patient Positioning

Video-monitoring screens are placed at several locations throughout the operating room so that all members of the operating team can monitor the procedure as it is being performed. A complete set of instruments for both thoracoscopic spinal surgery and open thoracotomy are available on the back table.

The patient is intubated with a double-lumen endotracheal tube and is placed in the lateral decubitus position on a radiolucent operating room table in an identical position that would be used for thoracotomy. The dependent axilla is padded and the upper arm is abducted, elevated anteriorly, supported, and padded. The arms and legs are padded to prevent compressive neuropathies. The patient is secured to the table to allow safe rotation during the procedure.

The scapula, portal sites, and the site for a potential thoracotomy incision are marked on the chest wall (Fig. 3). The location of the portal incisions are adjusted based on the level of the spinal pathology. the iliac crest also can be marked if a bone graft will be required.

After the patient is prepared and draped, the surgeon stands anterior to the patient's chest facing the spine. Initially, the patient is placed in a true lateral position to maintain the surgeon's orientation. Intraoperatively, the table may be rotated 30 to 40° anteriorly to allow the deflated lung to fall away from the spine, obviating the need for lung retraction.

Portal Insertion

Three to four portals are inserted for access into the thoracic cavity (Fig. 4). They are usually placed into the intercostal spaces centered over the middle or anterior axillary lines and are spaced apart to triangulate over the level of pathology. The portals should be spaced widely enough to provide room for the surgeon's hands to work with tools over the surface of the chest, without interfering with the ma-

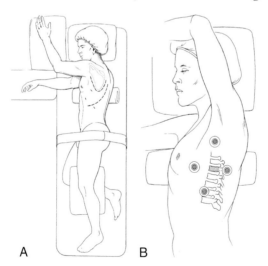

A   B

FIG. 3 (**A**) Patients are positioned in a lateral decubitus position on the operating table. The scapula, portal sites, and a potential thoracotomy incision are marked on the chest wall. (**B**) The portals are placed in the anterior, middle and posterior axillary lines, spread over the surface of the chest and centered around the level of the pathology (shaded). [Reprinted with permission of Barrow Neurological Institute.®]

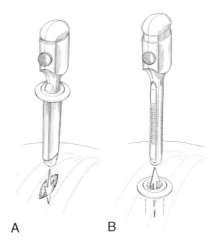

A   B

FIG. 4 (**A**) Flexible portals are inserted through the intercostal spaces to access the pleural space using a trochar. The portals are inserted like chest tubes over the upper surfaces of the ribs to avoid injuring the neurovascular bundles. (**B**) The trochar is removed leaving the portal in place in the chest wall. (Reprinted with permission of Barrow Neurological Institute.®)

nipulation. This problem has been referred to as "fencing" or "sword fighting." Flexible portals are used because they are less likely to cause intercostal neuralgia from nerve compression.

Portal incisions (15-20 mm in length) are made over the intercostal spaces near the superior surface of the rib to avoid injury to the neurovascular bundles. The portals are inserted into the chest in a manner almost identical to a chest tube. A trochar is used to pass the flexible portals through the intercostal space into the chest cavity. After the first portal is inserted, all subsequent portals are inserted under endoscopic visualization to avoid visceral injury. Caution must be exerted to avoid injury to the diaphragm when portals are passed below the T7 level.

Initial Spinal Exposure

The first portal is usually placed in the sixth or seventh intercostal space. As the lung is deflated, the thoracoscope is inserted to visualize the thoracic cavity. If necessary, the operating room table may be rotated 30 to 40° anteriorly to allow the lung to fall away from the spine to minimize the need for retraction. An endoscopic fan retractor may be used through another portal for gentle lung retraction; however, this instrument must be opened and closed under visualization to avoid lacerating the lung. Pleural adhesions, when present, may be detached with cautery and scissors to mobilize the lung.

Spinal Localization

Identification of the appropriate spinal level can be challenging. Counting the ribs endoscopically from within the thoracic cavity is an excellent way of initially localizing the proper level. The first visible rib at the apex of the thoracic cavity is usually the second rib. Each subsequent rib is directly visualized, palpated, and counted. A long, blunt-tipped needle may then be inserted into the disc space and a radiograph obtained (Fig. 5). Anteroposterior images are preferred over lateral images to enable reliable rib counting.

Pleural and Paraspinal Tissue Dissection

Endoscopic scissors and endoscopic forceps are used to dissect the pleura and soft tissue from the rib heads and vertebral bodies. In the midbody region, care is taken to avoid injuring the segmental vessels. These vessels do not always need to be divided for anterior release or discectomy, but they must be mobilized and ligated to perform a vertebrectomy. To divide these vessels, scissors and right-angle forceps are used to dissect the vessels from the surrounding soft tissue. The vessels are ligated individually with endoscopic hemoclips and divided

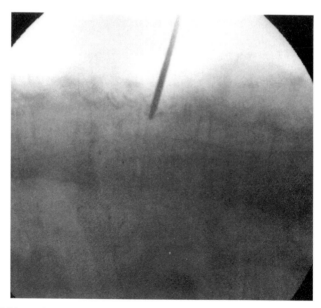

FIG. 5 A blunt-tipped, long needle is inserted into the disc space under direct vision with the thoracoscope. An anteroposterior radiograph is obtained to accurately identify the correct level of operative exposure.

with endoscopic scissors. Coagulation alone is insufficient because the blood vessels communicate directly with the great vessels. If a left-sided exposure is required in a region where the aorta is covering the surface of the spine, the aorta can be mobilized and gently retracted anteriorly to allow access to the thoracic spine.

Thoracic Spinal Dissection:

TECHNIQUES FOR DISCECTOMY, VERTEBRECTOMY, AND FUSION

We have extensively described the details of the operative techniques for thoracoscopic discectomy, anterior release, vertebrectomy, reconstruction and fixation in other publications (1, 29, 45) and only summarize the most salient points here. The sequences of operative steps used for thoracoscopic spinal surgery are virtually identical to those used for open procedures.

Several key aspects of the thoracic spinal anatomy should be emphasized to facilitate the safety of the operative dissection. The rib articulates with the transverse process, the pedicle, and the vertebral body just caudal to or at the level of the disc space (Fig. 6). The safest approach for exposing the dura involves removing a portion of the pedicle and proximal rib rather than dissecting through the neural foramen. To expose the pedicle adequately, 2 to 3 cm of the rib head and

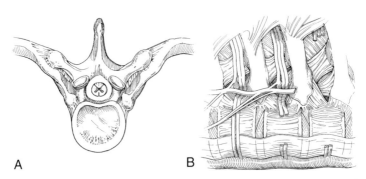

A   B

FIG. 6 (**A**) Illustrations of the relationship of the rib head, pedicle, and spinal canal. The proximal rib, which overlays the dorsal disc space and pedicle, must be removed to access the pedicle. The pedicle is then removed to clearly visualize the dura during the surgical maneuvers. (**B**) The segmental vessels course over the concave surface of the vertebral bodies, halfway between each of the disc spaces. The vessels join the thoracic nerves on the undersurfaces of the ribs. [Reprinted with permission of Barrow Neurological Institute.®]

proximal rib must be removed first. The pedicle is then removed with a Kerrison rongeur to expose the dura. Early identification of the dura allows the surgeon to visualize the anterolateral border of the spinal canal and enables constant visual orientation to the position of the spinal cord during any subsequent dissection.

A consistent anatomical relationship exists between the intercostal vessels and nerve. The segmental artery and vein course over the concave surface of the middle of the vertebral body and are joined by the intercostal nerve at the neural foramen (Fig. 6B). As the neurovascular bundle courses laterally from cephalad to caudad, the vein, artery, and nerve run in the groove on the undersurface of each rib. Care should be exercised throughout the procedure to insure that the neurovascular structures are not injured.

Thoracoscopic Discectomy

The intercostal nerve and segmental vessels and muscles are carefully detached from the proximal rib using subperiosteal dissection with curettes and periosteal elevators. The costotransverse and costovertebral ligaments are sharply detached from the rib and then the proximal rib and pedicle are removed. Once the pedicle is removed, the dura is identified to allow protection of the spinal cord. Next the annulus of the disc is incised. Drills and curettes are used to create a 1- to 1 1/2-cm wide cavity within the dorsal edge of the disc space and the adjacent vertebral bodies to serve as a working space. The herniated disc material and any osteophytes are precisely curetted away from the spinal cord into the cavity in the spine (Fig. 7).

Thoracoscopic Anterior Release of Spinal Deformity

Anterior release refers to the transection of anterior spinal soft tissue attachments (i.e., annulus, anterior longitudinal ligament, and scar tissue) required for correction of chronic progressive kyphotic or scoliotic curvatures. This technique consists of modified multilevel discectomies and has been used extensively in orthopedic spinal deformity surgery (2, 29, 46). The pleura is incised over the disc spaces of interest; however, the dura need not be exposed and the rib heads are not removed (unless a thoracoplasty is being performed with the correction of the curvature). At each disc space, the annulus is incised, disc material is removed with curettes and rongeurs, and the end plates are decorticated with curettes or drills. After the anterior release is performed, the curvature is reduced and fixated, typically with a posteriorly applied universal hook-rod system. After the spine is reduced and

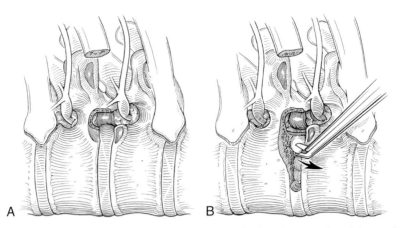

FIG. 7 A discectomy is performed. (**A**) The proximal rib and upper edge of the caudal pedicle are removed to expose the dura. (**B**) A 1- to 1.5-cm wide cavity is made in the dorsal edge of the disc space. Disc material is removed using microdissection with fine microsurgical tools. The disc material is pulled away from the spinal cord into the cavity created in the spine. (Reprinted with permission of Barrow Neurological Institute.®)

fixated, bone grafts can be impacted into the disc spaces to facilitate interbody fusion.

Thoracoscopic Corpectomy and Reconstruction

The initial techniques for vertebral body resection and decompression of the spinal cord resemble the basic steps initially used for discectomy. The pleura is dissected off the vertebrae and the proximal ribs at the region of the pathology. The segmental vessels are ligated and divided, and the proximal 2 to 3 cm of the ribs and the pedicles are removed to expose the lateral aspect of the dura. Discectomies are performed to define the cephalad and caudal limits of the bone dissection. A large cavity is created in the center of the involved vertebral bodies using high-speed drills, osteotomes, rongeurs, and curettes. Posteriorly, the remaining thin shell of cortical bone, the posterior longitudinal ligament, and any pathology compressing the spinal cord are removed by curetting the material into the cavity in the bodies, thus safely decompressing the spinal cord under direct visualization (Fig. 8).

Reconstruction of the osseous defect is readily performed using bone grafts. The length, width, and depth of the vertebral defect are measured precisely with a ruler. Reconstructive grafts are placed into the chest end on through a 20-mm portal. The grafts are wedged into po-

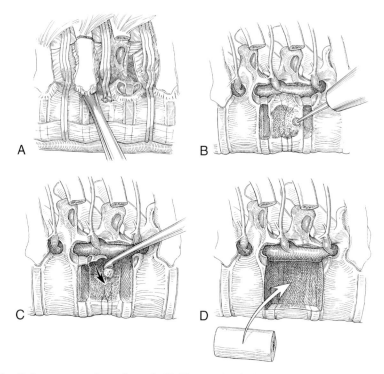

FIG. 8 A corpectomy is performed. (**A**) The proximal ribs and pedicles are removed to expose the dura. (**B**) A large cavity is made in the involved vertebral body. (**C**) The compressive pathology and the posterior aspect of the vertebral bodies are removed with curettes and rongeurs. The spinal cord is decompressed by removing the pathology away from the spinal canal into the cavity in the vertebral body. (**D**) Reconstruction is performed with precisely sized bone grafts that are inserted through the endoscopic portals end on and carefully compressed into the corpectomy defect. (Reprinted with permission of Barrow Neurological Institute.®)

sition in the corpectomy bed using a bone graft impactor. By sizing the grafts precisely and slightly beveling one edge of the graft, the grafts can be compressed into the surrounding bone. The dura is visualized constantly during graft insertion to prevent injury.

Methylmethacrylate can be used for vertebral body reconstruction after resection of tumors with thoracoscopy (1, 45), using a technique described by Errico and Cooper (47). A silastic tube is used as a mold or template within the corpectomy defect. Liquefied methacrylate is injected into the tube and is allowed to harden. Thoracoscopic internal fixation can be performed with screw plate instrumentation using similar procedures as in open surgery (1, 45, 48). The portals are strategically positioned on the chest wall using fluoroscopy so that the portals are coaxial with the trajectories needed to insert the screws and bolts into the bone. The plate can be inserted into the chest, end on, through a 20-mm diameter thoracoscopic portal. The plate is anchored to the spine using bolts and nuts and screws.

Wound Closure and Postoperative Management

At the termination of the procedure, the thoracic cavity is thoroughly irrigated to remove pooled blood and tissue debris. The thoracoscope is used to inspect the lung and the thoracic cavity. Before lung reinflation, chest tubes are placed through the preexisting portal incisions. The insertion of the chest tubes is visualized with the thoracoscope to ensure optimal positioning of the tubes. An apical chest tube is used to help reinflate the lung, and a posteroinferior tube is used to facilitate fluid drainage.

The wounds are closed in a layered fashion with absorbable suture material. The skin is closed using subcuticular sutures. The chest tubes are placed to 20 cm H_2O suction, and the entry sites are covered with an occlusive dressing. Patients are usually extubated at the end of the procedure. Chest and spine radiographs are obtained in the recovery room to assess the spine and to exclude a pneumothorax. Postoperatively, patients are placed on aggressive pulmonary physiotherapy routines. The chest tubes are removed when drainage diminishes to less than 100 ml/day.

CASE EXAMPLES

Thoracoscopic Discectomy

A 49-year-old woman presented with a 3-year history of progressively worsening incapacitating dysesthetic and crushing pain that began between her shoulders and radiated anteriorly into the middle and lower chest region bilaterally. Her workup revealed no cardiac pathology. She had no signs or symptoms of myelopathy. Radiographic studies demonstrated a large, central calcified disc herniation at the T6-T7 level (Figs. 9A and B) (20, 21). She underwent, without complications, a thoracoscopic discectomy that achieved complete resection of the disc (Fig. 9C). Postoperatively, she was intact neurologically and her preoperative radicular pain resolved completely.

Thoracoscopic Anterior Release

A 14-year-old girl was involved in a roll-over motor vehicle accident. She sustained multiple injuries including T8 and T9 burst fractures but was neurologically intact. She was initially managed at another

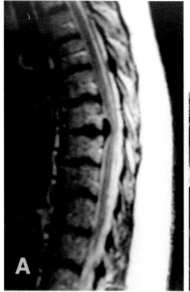

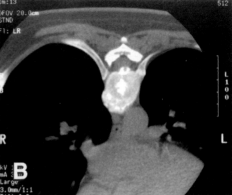

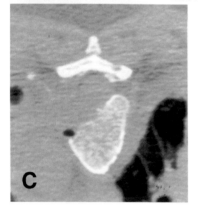

FIG. 9 (**A**) and (**B**) Preoperative magnetic resonance image and preoperative computed tomography (CT) scan of a 49-year-old woman who underwent thoracoscopic discectomy for excision of a T6-7 disc. (**C**) The postoperative CT demonstrates that all of the disc material was removed. The patient's radicular pain resolved completely.

hospital where she underwent a decompressive laminectomy at T8 and T9, followed by T4-T11 posterior segmental fixation with hook-rod instrumentation. Two months later she presented to our institution with wound dehiscence and a deep wound infection. The patient underwent removal of the instrumentation and debridement of the wound. Her infection resolved after debridement and intravenous antibiotics, but she developed a progressive kyphosis (from 15 to 70°) despite management in a thoracolumbosacral orthosis (Figs. 10**A** and **B**). After several months, she developed signs of myelopathy and became disfigured by

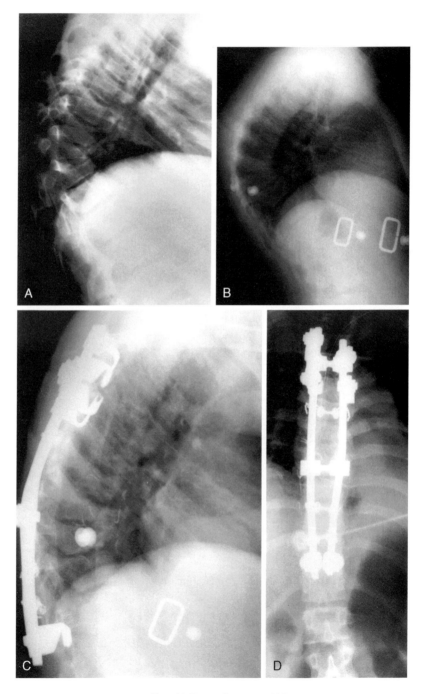

FIG. 10 Legend on page 411

a prominent hunchback. MR imaging revealed that the spinal cord was stretched over the severe kyphotic deformity.

An uncomplicated thoracoscopic anterior release and interbody fusion were performed in conjunction with posterior instrumentation and fusion. The kyphosis was reduced from 70° to 30° (Figs. 10C and **D**). Immediately after reduction of the kyphotic deformity, the amplitude and latency of patient's somatosensory evoked potentials (SSEPs) improved dramatically. Postoperatively, the patient's motor and sensory function progressively improved. She experienced no postoperative complications and was discharged home on the 5th postoperative day. At her 9-month follow-up visit, she was neurologically normal, had developed an osseous union, and her reduction was maintained at 32°.

Thoracoscopic Corpectomy, Fusion, and Fixation

A 72-year-old woman presented with a progressive myelopathy. At another hospital she had previously undergone a posterolateral approach to treat a large calcified midline T8-T9 disc. The disc was incompletely removed, and the procedure was terminated because the patient's SSEPs disappeared with attempted manipulation of the calcified disc fragment. Her postoperative course was complicated by the development of a *Staphylococcal* deep wound infection, which was treated with 3 months of intravenous antibiotics. She presented 6 months later with an acute myelopathy due to collapse of the T8 and T9 vertebral bodies, a kyphotic deformity, and compression of the spinal cord (Figs. 11A and **B**).

A thoracoscopic approach was performed with microsurgical removal of the ossified disc fragment. Corpectomies of T8 and T9 were required for exposure and excision of the disc. The vertebral bodies were reconstructed with a humerus allograft filled with the patient's rib. Anterior instrumentation was performed with a locking screw plate (Figs. 11C-**F**). A staged posterior spinal fixation was performed 2 days later because the patient had a prior laminectomy with posterior element instability and a moderately severe kyphosis (Fig. 11**G**). Postoperatively, her myelopathy slowly improved. Six months later she was ambulating independently and had recovered almost full motor function.

FIG. 10 This 14-year-old girl developed a progressive kyphotic deformity that caused a subsequent myelopathy. (**A** and **B**) The preoperative radiographs demonstrate progression of the kyphosis from 40° to 70° over a 6-month period. An anterior release was performed using thoracoscopy in conjunction with a posterior reduction and fixation. (**C**) Lateral and (**D**) anteroposterior postoperative radiographs demonstrate that the kyphus was reduced to 32° (29).

CLINICAL NEUROSURGERY

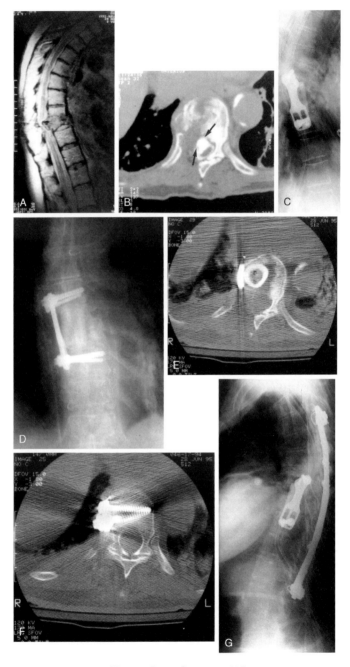

FIG. 11 Legend on page 413

CLINICAL RESULTS

Table 3 represents the clinical experience with 17 cases of thoraco-scopic spinal surgery performed at the Barrow Neurological Institute® from 1994 to 1995. Twelve patients underwent thoracic discectomies, one patient had a multilevel anterior release, and four patients were treated with corpectomy and reconstruction. Pathology included her-niated thoracic discs ($n = 12$), thoracic fractures ($n = 2$), spinal infec-tions ($n = 3$). Indications for surgery included treatment of myelopathy ($n = 11$), thoracic radiculopathy ($n = 6$), and associated spinal instabil-ity ($n = 5$).

All operative procedures were performed satisfactorily with thora-coscopy; no cases were converted to a thoracotomy. There were no in-traoperative vascular or visceral injuries. The extent of the anatomical dissection was evaluated postoperatively in every case with radi-ographs, and CT or MR imaging. A complete decompression was achieved in every instance and no patient had residual compressive pathology. In one case, the wrong spinal level was initially localized and a discectomy was performed; however, this was recognized and the correct level was decompressed without sequelae.

There were no intraoperative injuries to the nerve roots or spinal cord. Postoperatively, two patients developed mild intercostal neural-gia, which resolved completely (one within 1 week and one within 1 month). All six patients who presented with intractable thoracic radic-ular pain had complete resolution of the radicular pain. Among the 11 patients who presented with myelopathy, 5 patients recovered normal neurological function; three patients had improved neurological func-tion but had mild residual motor deficits; and three patients' symptoms stabilized. No patients' myelopathy worsened postoperatively or as a surgical complication.

FIG. 11 This 72-year-old woman developed progressive paraparesis after a calcified T8-9 disc was incompletely excised using a posterior surgical approach. A kyphosis and pathologic collapse of the vertebrae occurred and caused her myelopathy to worsen. (**A**) The preoperative magnetic resonance imaging study demonstrates the spinal cord com-pression and collapse of the T8 and T9 bodies. (**B**) Preoperative myelogram computed to-mography (CT) shows the residual calcified disc (*arrows*) compressing and distorting the spinal cord. (**C**) Lateral and (**D**) anteroposterior postoperative radiographs after the tho-racoscopic corpectomy, reconstruction, and fixation. Postoperative CT scans show that the spinal cord was completely decompressed and the (**E**) bone graft and (**F**) hardware were satisfactorily positioned. (**G**) A staged posterior fixation was performed for supple-mental stabilization of the spine.

TABLE 3
Clinical Summary of Thoracoscopic Spinal Surgery Performed at the BNI, 1994–1995.

| | | | | Surgical indications | | |
Case	Age/ sex	Thoracoscopic procedure	Spinal levels	Neurological symptoms	Spinal instability	Other spinal procedures
1	14/F	Anterior release inter- body fusion(b)	T7-T8 and T8-T9	Myelopathy	Yes	Posterior instrumentation
2	61/F	Microdiscectomy	T8-T9	Radiculopathy	No	
3	73/F	Microdiscectomy	T9-T10	Myelopathy	No	
4	64/F	Microdiscectomy	T9-T10	Radiculopathy	No	
5	42/F	Microdiscectomy	T7-T8	Myelopathy	No	
6	49/F	Microdiscectomy	T6-T7	Radiculopathy	No	
7	65/M	Microdiscectomy	T8-T9	Radiculopathy	No	
8	62/F	Microdiscectomy	T6-T7	Myelopathy	No	
9	37/F	Microdiscectomy	T7-T8	Radiculopathy	No	
10	54/M	Microdiscectomy	T6-T7	Radiculopathy	No	
11	78/F	Microdiscectomy	T3-T4	Myelopathy	No	
12	69/F	Microdiscectomy	T6-T7	Myelopathy	No	
13	50/M	Microdiscectomy	T8-T9	Myelopathy	No	
14	33/M	Corpectomy(a)	T8-T9	Myelopathy	Yes	Prior laminectomy and posterior hook-rod instrumenta- tion
15	68/F	Corpectomy(b)	T4-T5	Myelopathy	Yes	Luque rods
16	50/M	Corpectomy and screw plate(c)	T6-T7	Myelopathy	Yes	None
17	72/F	Corpectomy and screw plate(d)	T8-T9	Myelopathy	Yes	Prior laminectomy Luque rods

F=female; M=male; (a)=*Staphylococcus* osteomyelitis; (b)=fracture; (c)=tuberculosis osteomyelitis and epidural abscess, (d)=incompletely excised calcified disc, pathologic fracture, and kyphotic deformity.

There were no inadvertent intraoperative dural tears. However, two patients were treated who had large calcified disc herniations that extended intradurally. Under thoracoscopic visualization, the dura was opened and the intradural portions of the discs were removed using microsurgical techniques. After the discs were removed, the dura was covered with blood-soaked pieces of gelfoam, but the dura was not sutured closed. To prevent accumulation of postoperative CSF, one patient was treated with a lumbar drain and the other patient had a lumboperitoneal shunt inserted.

Five patients were treated with fixation and fusion procedures: four were performed in conjunction with corpectomies, one was performed with an anterior release. All have maintained stable spinal alignment. In one patient an anterior screw loosened one week after surgery and was removed with a second thoracoscopic procedure without sequelae. There were no other instances of hardware failure or hardware-related complications.

Pulmonary complications included one case of pleural effusion that required drainage, three cases of mild atelectasis, and one postoperative case of pneumonia. To minimize atelectasis and pulmonary complications, we began ventilating the collapsed lung 5 to 10 minutes after every hour of operating time. This strategy has reduced subsequent pulmonary complications. There were no intraoperative pulmonary lacerations or episodes of postoperative air leakage. The patients' chest tubes were usually removed 24 to 48 hours after surgery.

Comparison of Thoracoscopy and Costotransversectomy for Discectomy

Table 4 compares the 12 patients treated with thoracoscopic discectomy with a concurrent cohort of 10 patients treated for herniated thoracic discs with costotransversectomy at our institution from 1993 to 1995. There are no significant differences between the two groups in terms of demographic characteristics, levels of involvement, or severity of neurological deficits. There also were no significant differences in operative times, blood loss, the immediate amount of postoperative pain, or the length of the ICU or hospital stay between the two procedures.

TABLE 4
BNI Clinical Data for Thoracic Discectomy: 1993–1995

	Thoracoscopic Discectomy mean (range) $n=12$	Costotransversectomy for Discectomy mean (range) $n=10$
Operative time (min)	245 (129-390)	290 (155-440)
Estimated blood loss (ml)	600 (200-2100)	370 (200-900)
Duration of chest tubes (days)	2.2 (0.5-6)	N/A†
Amount of chest tube drainage (ml)	515 (65-1660)	N/A
Narcotic pain medications* (days)	2.1 (1-6)	2.0 (1-3)
ICU stay (days)	1.2 (0-3)	1.2 (1-2)
Hospital stay (days)	4.9 (2-8)	5.0 (4-6)

ICU=intensive care unit. *Duration of intravenous, intramuscular, or epidural narcotic analgesic administration.

†Two patients had chest tubes after costotransversectomy because of pleural tears. All patients had chest tubes after thoracoscopy.

TABLE 5
BNI Complications of Thoracic Discectomy

	Thoracoscopy	Costotransversectomy
	n	n
Inadequate decompression	0	2*
Wrong level	1	0
Intercostal neuralgia	2	1
Pleural effusion	1	1
Atelectasis	2	1
Neurological complications	0	1

*One calcified disc, one midline soft disc. Both required reoperation ventrally to remove the pathology.

Thoracoscopy was significantly better than costotransversectomy for achieving decompression of the spinal cord (Table 5). Two of the 10 patients treated with costotransversectomy had significant residual pathology compressing the spinal cord that caused progressive myelopathy in one and persistent myelopathy and radicular pain in the other. Both patients required reoperation using a ventral approach to treat their pathology. One of these patients had a calcified midline disc that narrowed the spinal canal by 50%. The other patient had a midline soft disc herniation.

Thoracoscopy provided better visualization and access to the ventral spinal cord than costotransversectomy. It provided a complete decompression of midline discs ($n = 6$) and calcified discs ($n = 5$) without any residual compressive pathology.

Our learning curve for thoracoscopy is demonstrated in Figure 12, which examines the operative times for our sequential thoracoscopic discectomies. The first four surgeries required 5 to 6 hours to complete. However, as we gained experience, increased skill, and confidence with our operative techniques, the surgical time was reduced to 2 to 3 hours, which is less than the average surgical time for costotransversectomy (4-5 hours).

Comparison of Thoracoscopy and Thoracotomy for Corpectomy

Table 6 compares thoracoscopy with thoracotomy for a concurrent cohort of patients undergoing anterior corpectomy and reconstruction. These thoracoscopy data were derived from our published report of a combined series of 17 thoracoscopic corpectomies performed at Johan Wolfgang Goethe University, Frankfurt, Germany and at the Barrow Neurological Institute® (1). The two groups of patients did not differ with regards to age, sex distribution, type of pathology, severity of neu-

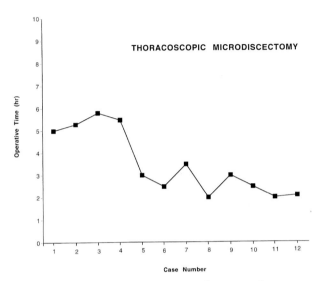

FIG. 12 The duration of surgery for thoracoscopic discectomy demonstrates our clinical "learning curve." The first few cases lasted 5 to 6 hours for a thoracic discectomy. Subsequently, the operative time has been reduced to between 2 and 3 hours for a one-level thoracic microdiscectomy.

TABLE 6
Comparative Clinical Data for Thoracic Vertebrectomies

	Thoracoscopic Vertebrectomy	Thoracotomy for Vertebrectomy
	mean (range) $n=17$	mean (range) $n=7$
Operative time (min)	347 (133-712)	393 (235-510)
Estimated blood loss (ml)	1117 (250-2000)	1557 (300-2500)
Duration of chest tube (days)	2.8 (1-8)	3.9 (1-10)
Chest tube drainage (ml)	1309 (120-3500)	1741 (128-4800)
Narcotic pain medications* (days)	4.1 (0.5-24)	8.9 (1-20)
ICU stay (days)	2.6 (1-17)	6.4 (1-22)
Hospital stay (days)	8.7 (4-31)	15.8 (5-60)

*Duration of intravenous, intramuscular, or epidural narcotic analgesic administration.
ICU-intensive care unit.

rological defects, or the extent of decompression and stabilization procedures performed.

There were no differences in the extent of decompression, reconstruction and fixation achieved between the two groups. No patients had residual compressive pathology. There were no significant differences between the lengths of the procedures. Thoracoscopic procedures were associated with less blood loss, less chest tube drainage, less pain medication usage, and shorter ICU and hospital stays compared to thoracotomy patients.

Complications in the thoracotomy group included pneumonia (n = 2), pleural effusion (n = 1), tension pneumothorax (n =1), deep venous thrombosis (n = 1), and intercostal neuralgia (n = 3). Complications in the thoracoscopy group included myocardial infarction leading to one postoperative death, transient intercostal neuralgia (n = 2), pleural effusion (n = 1), and pneumonia (n = 1). Intercostal neuralgia and postthoracotomy pain syndromes were more common and more severe after thoracotomy. Two of the patients with thoracotomy had prolonged, moderately severe pain syndromes. In both patients who experienced intercostal neuralgia after thoracoscopy, the symptoms were mild and transient (Table 7).

Contraindication and Limitations

Contraindications to a thoracoscopic approach include coagulopathy, inability to tolerate single lung ventilation, irrecoverable terminal illness, severe cardiac or pulmonary disease, or extensive pleural adhesions from prior chest trauma or prior thoracotomy. Evaluation by a pulmonologist or internist should be pursued for a patient with a potential contraindication. When thoracoscopy is infeasible, other opera-

TABLE 7
Comparative Clinical Complications of Thoracic Corpectomy and Reconstruction

	Thoracoscopy (n=17)	Thoracotomy (n=7)
MI and Death	1	0
Pneumonia	1	2
Pleural effusion	1	1
Tension pneumothorax	0	1
Incomplete decompression	0	0
Spinal cord injury	0	0
Intercostal neuralgia	3	3
(transient)	3	1
(prolonged)	0	2

MI = myocardial infarction

tive alternatives include thoracotomy, sternotomy, or costotransversectomy, depending upon the level and extent of the pathology.

The thoracoscopic approach is only able to access the anterior and anterolateral aspects of the vertebrae and spinal canal (*i.e.,* the vertebral bodies, ipsilateral pedicles, and transverse processes). This approach cannot adequately expose the posterior elements, nor the contralateral pedicle or transverse process. Thoracoscopy has not yet been widely applied for intradural procedures; however techniques currently being developed are anticipated to facilitate intradural applications and dural closure.

Biomechanically, the anterior thoracoscopic approach for reconstruction and instrumentation significantly increases the axial load-bearing capabilities of the spine. More than 80% of the compressive loads of the spine are borne by the anterior and middle columns. However, in the case of multilevel pathology, prior laminectomy, severe osteoporosis, or a large kyphotic deformity, the anterior approach alone may be insufficient to achieve reduction and fixation. A posterior approach to the spine may be needed for adequate fixation in these instances.

There are several additional limitations of thoracoscopic spinal surgery. Currently available data are limited to the experience of a few clinical centers. Objective comparative clinical outcome data and prospective clinical trials would be a more ideal method to obtain a satisfactory comparison of the different surgical techniques.

Application of these new surgical techniques requires tremendous patience and dedicated laboratory practice to acquire the proper surgical skills. The operations initially take longer than open surgeries and are technically difficult for surgeons to perform. However, with experience, the time and ease of the surgical procedures are reduced significantly.

The costs of endoscopic equipment can be relatively high. However, most operating rooms have existing tools and endoscopes that can be used for thoracoscopy without requiring major capital expenditures.

CONCLUSIONS

1. Thoracoscopic spinal surgery is technically feasible, and it can be performed safely with acceptable rates of morbidity and excellent clinical and neurological results.

2. Thoracoscopic techniques can be performed for biopsy, discectomy, vertebrectomy, vertebral reconstruction, and application of internal fixation devices to treat a wide variety of pathological processes affecting the spine.

420 CLINICAL NEUROSURGERY

3. This minimally incisional access technique can achieve the identical extent of spinal exposure, dissection, decompression, and reconstruction as those obtained with open techniques.

4. Thoracoscopy provides much more complete visualization and access of the ventral aspect of the spine and spinal cord compared to costotransversectomy. Compared to thoracotomy, it achieves identical visualization and access to the spine yet has substantially less postoperative morbidity and pain and faster recovery times.

5. The techniques for this surgical procedure are initially very difficult and require the surgeon to learn new psychomotor skills, to adapt existing techniques, and to develop new perceptions of operative anatomy. This steep learning curve must be mastered prior to clinical applications. To practice these techniques safely, surgeons must devote attention to instructional seminars, surgical skills laboratories, and clinical preceptorship programs.

REFERENCES

1. Dickman CA, Rosenthal D, Karahalios DG, Paramore CG, Mican CA, Apostolides PJ, Lorenz R, Sonntag VKH. Thoracic vertebrectomy and reconstruction using a microsurgical thoracoscopic approach. *Neurosurgery* 1996. (In Press)
2. McAfee PC, Regan JR, Zdeblick T, Zuckerman J, Picetti GD, III, Heim S, Geis WP, Fedder IL. The incidence of complications in endoscopic anterior thoracolumbar spinal reconstructive surgery. A prospective multicenter study comprising the first 100 consecutive cases. **Spine** 20:1624–1632, 1995.
3. Regan JJ, Mack MJ, Picetti GD, III, Guyer RD, Hochschuler SH, Rashbaum RF. A comparison of video-assisted thoracoscopic surgery (VATS) with open thoracotomy in thoracic spinal surgery. **Today's Theur Trends** 11:203–218, 1994.
4. Horowitz MB, Moossy JJ, Julian T, Ferson PF, Huneke K. Thoracic discectomy using video assisted thoracoscopy. **Spine** 19:1082–1086, 1994.
5. Rosenthal D, Rosenthal R, de Simone A. Removal of a protruded thoracic disc using microsurgical endoscopy. A new technique. **Spine** 19:1087–1091, 1994.
6. Regan JJ, Mack MJ, Picetti GD, III. A technical report on video-assisted thoracoscopy in thoracic spinal surgery. **Spine** 20:831–837, 1995.
7. Burman MS. Myeloscopy or the direct visualization of the spinal canal and its contents. **J Bone Joint Surg** 13:695–696, 1931.
8. Pool JL. Direct visualization of dorsal nerve roots of the cauda equina by means of the myeloscope. **Arch Neurol Psychol** 39:1308–1312, 1938.
9. Pool JL. Myeloscopy: Diagnostic inspection of the cauda equina by means of the endoscope. **Bull Neurol Inst NY** 7:178–189, 1938.
10. Pool JL. Myeloscopy: Intrathecal endoscopy. **Surgery** 11:169–182, 1942.
11. Onik G, Helms CA, Ginsberg L, Hoaglund FT, Morris J. Percutaneous lumbar discectomy using new aspiration probe. **AJR** 144:1137–1140, 1985.
12. Kambin P, Schaffer JL. Percutaneous lumbar discectomy. Review of 100 patients and current practice. **Clin Orthop** 238:24–34, 1989.
13. Ooi Y, Satoh Y, Morisaki N: Myeloscopy. The possibility of observing the lumbar intrathecal space by use of an endoscope. **Endoscopy** 5:901–906, 1973.
14. Mathews H. First International Symposium on Lasers in Orthopaedics. (Abstract). San Francisco, September, 1991.

15. McKneally MF. Video-assisted thoracic surgery: Standards and guidelines. **Chest Surg Clin North Am** 3:345–351, 1993.
16. Kaiser LR. Video-assisted thoracic surgery. Current state of the art. **Ann Surg** 220:720–734, 1994.
17. Landreneau RJ, Mack MJ, Hazelrigg SR, Dowling RD, Acuff TE, Magee MJ, Ferson PF. Video-assisted thoracic surgery: Basic technical concepts and intercostal approach strategies. **Ann Thorac Surg** 54:800–807, 1992.
18. Coltharp WH, Arnold JH, Alford WC, Jr., Burrus GR, Glassford DM, Jr., Lea JW, IV, Petracek MR, Starkey TD, Stoney WS, Thomas CS, Jr., Sadler RN. Videothoracoscopy: Improved technique and expanded indications. **Ann Thorac Surg** 53: 776–779, 1992.
19. Mack MJ, Aronoff RJ, Acuff TE, Douthit MB, Bowman RT, Ryan WH. Present role of thoracoscopy in the diagnosis and treatment of diseases of the chest. **Ann Thorac Surg** 54:403–409, 1992.
20. Jacobaeus HC. Possibility of the use of the cystoscope for investigation of serious cavities. **Munch Med Wochenscr** 57:2090–2092, 1910.
21. Jacobaeus HC. The practical importance of thoracoscopy in surgery of the chest. **Surg Gynecol Obstet** 34:289–296, 1922.
22. Jacobaeus HC. The cauterization of adhesions in pneumothorax treatment of tuberculosis. **Surg Gynecol Obstet** 32:493–500, 1921.
23. Jacobaeus HC. Endopleural operations by means of a thoracoscope. **Beitr Klin Tuberk** 35:1, 1915.
24. Landreneau RJ, Hazelrigg SR, Mack MJ, Dowling RD, Burke D, Gavlick J, Perrino MK, Ritter PS, Bowers CM, Defino J, Nunchuch SK, Freeman J, Keenan RJ, Ferson PF. Postoperative pain-related morbidity: Video-assisted thoracic surgery versus thoracotomy. **Ann Thorac Surg** 56:1285–1289, 1993.
25. Hazelrigg SR, Landreneau RJ, Boley TM, Priesmeyer M, Schmaltz RA, Nawarawong W, Johnson JA, Walls JT, Curtis JJ. The effect of muscle-sparing versus standard posterolateral thoracotomy on pulmonary function, muscle strength, and postoperative pain. **J Thorac Cardiovasc Surg** 101:394–401, 1991.
26. Ferson PF, Landreneau RJ, Dowling RD, Hazelrigg SR, Ritter P, Nunchuch S, Perrino MK, Bowers CM, Mack MJ, Magee MJ. Comparison of open *versus* thoracoscopic lung biopsy for diffuse infiltrative pulmonary disease. **J Thorac Cardiovasc Surg** 106:194–199, 1993.
27. Mack MJ, Regan JJ, Bobechko WP, Acuff TE. Application of thoracoscopy for diseases of the spine. **Ann Thorac Surg** 56:736–738, 1993.
28. Rosenthal D, Lorenz R. The use of the microsurgical endoscopic technique for treating affections of the dorsal spine: Indications and early results (abstract). **J Neurosurg** 82:342A, 1995.
29. Dickman CA, Mican CA. Multilevel anterior thoracic discectomies and anterior interbody fusion using a microsurgical thoracoscopic approach. **J Neurosurg** 1995. (In Press)
30. Krasna, MJ and Mack MJ. Sympathectomy. In: Krasna, MJ and Mack, MJ. (eds). **Atlas of Thoracoscopic Surgery.** St. Louis, Quality, 1994, p 139.
31. Robertson DP, Simpson RK, Rose JE, Garza JS. Video-assisted endoscopic thoracic ganglionectomy. **J Neurosurg** 79:238–304, 1993.
32. Kao M-C, Tsai J-C, Lai D-M, Hsiao Y-Y, Lee Y-S, Chiu M-J. Autonomic activities in hyperhidrosis patients before, during, and after endoscopic laser sympathectomy. **Neurosurgery** 34:262–268, 1994.
33. Bohlman HH, Zdeblick TA. Anterior excision of herniated thoracic discs. **J Bone Joint Surg (Am)** 70:1038–1047, 1988.

34. Benjamin V. Diagnosis and management of thoracic disc disease. **Clin Neurosurg** 30:577–606, 1983.
35. Crafoord C, Hiertonn T, Lindblom K, Olsson S-E. Spinal cord compression caused by a protruded thoracic disc. Report of a case treated with antero-lateral fenestration of the disc. **Acta Orthop Scand** 28:103–107, 1958.
36. Fidler MW, Goedhart ZD. Excision of prolapse of thoracic intervertebral disc. A transthoracic technique. **J Bone Joint Surg (Br)** 66:518–522, 1984.
37. Kaneda K, Abumi K, Fujiya M. Burst fractures with neurologic deficits of the thoraco-lumbar spine. Results of anterior decompression and stabilization with anterior instrumentation. **Spine** 9:788–795, 1984.
38. Kostuik JP. Anterior spinal cord decompression for lesions of the thoracic and lumbar spine, techniques, new methods of internal fixation results. **Spine** 8:512–531, 1983.
39. Kostuik JP. Anterior fixation for fractures of the thoracic and lumbar spine with or without neurologic involvement. **Clin Orthop** 189:103–115, 1984.
40. Yuan HA, Mann KA, Found EM. Early clinical experience with the Syracuse I-plate: An anterior spinal fixation device. **Spine** 2764:13056–13248, 1988.
41. Perot PL, Jr., Munro DD. Transthoracic removal of midline thoracic disc protrusions causing spinal cord compression. **J Neurosurg** 31:452–458, 1969.
42. Ransahoff J, Spencer F, Siew F, Gage L, Jr. Transthoracic removal of thoracic disc. Report of three cases. **J Neurosurg** 31:459–461, 1969.
43. Otani K, Nakai S, Fujimura Y, Manzoku S, Shibasaki K. Surgical treatment of thoracic disc herniation using the anterior approach. **J Bone Joint Surg (Br)** 64:340–343, 1982.
44. Statement of the AATS/STS Joint Committee on Thoracoscopy and Video Assisted Thoracic Surgery. **Ann Thorac Surg** 54:1, 1992.
45. Dickman CA, Mican C. Thoracoscopic approaches for the treatment of anterior thoracic spinal pathology. **BNI Quarterly** 1995. (In Press)
46. Dwyer AF, Schafer MF. Anterior approach to scoliosis. Results of treatment in fifty-one cases. **J Bone Joint Surg (Br)** 56:218–224, 1974.
47. Errico TJ, Cooper PR. A new method of thoracic and lumbar body replacement for spinal tumors: Technical note. **Neurosurgery** 32:678–681, 1993.
48. Zdeblick, TA. Z-plate anterior thoracolumbar instrumentation. In Hitchon, PW, Traynelis, VC and Rengachary, SS. (eds) **Techniques in Spinal Fusion and Stabilization.** New York, Thieme, 1995, p 279.

28

Percutaneous Lumbosacral Fixation and Fusion: Anatomical Study and Two-Year Experience with a New Method

MICHAEL MAC MILLAN, M.D., RICHARD G. FESSLER, M.D., PH.D,
MARK GILLESPY, M.D. AND WILLIAM J. MONTGOMERY, M.D.

Fusion of the adult lumbosacral spine is indicated for some cases of spondylolisthesis, degenerative disease, trauma, and postsurgical instability. One proposed reason for the highly variable success rates of this procedure is that extensive soft tissue disruption is required during the procedure. To address this problem we are developing a new technique for fixation and fusion of the L5-S1 vertebral segment. Phase one of this study determined an anatomic pathway through the sacrum that allowed access to the L5-S1 disc and L5 vertebral body. In phase two, 13 patients underwent fixation of the lumbosacral segment with accompanying bone grafting. Twelve of the 13 patients successfully fused. No complications were experienced. We feel that this minimally invasive lumbosacral fusion technique shows promise for application to the lumbosacral spine, which may allow improved clinical outcomes.

Despite the large number of lumbar spinal fusions routinely performed, the indications and techniques for these procedures are not well established. Relatively well-accepted indications include trauma, spondylolisthesis, and iatrogenic instability; however, more controversial indications are degenerative disc disease, lumbar stenosis, and low back pain. In addition to this controversy, diagnostic accuracy is made more difficult because patients with similar symptoms may have different underlying pathologic etiologies and a defined structural cause of low back pain has not been universally accepted (1). These dilemmas in surgical indications and diagnoses have contributed to wide variations in reported clinical outcomes of spinal fusions. Published results also vary widely depending on the methodology used (2) and even the geographic locations of the surgery (3). Yet despite these controversies, there are certain conditions for which lumbar fusion has been proven successful through prospective, randomized studies (4).

The lumbosacral joint or L5-S1 segment requires special considerations when fusion is attempted. Specifically three questions must be answered. First, what anatomic structures influence the surgical approach and success rate? Second, what is the optimal fusion technique for this region? Finally, is instrumentation of L5/S1 necessary, or is fusion alone adequate? From an anatomic standpoint this area is difficult to access. It is positioned deep within the iliac crests and is farthest from the skin surface. The thick muscular cover and over-hanging iliac crests make exposure of the transverse processes and access to the pedicles difficult. Mechanically, the lumbosacral joint is the transition between the flexible lumbar spine and the relatively rigid pelvis. In addition this joint receives significant translational stress between the relatively vertical lumbar spine and a more oblique pelvis. Several fusion techniques have been utilized in this region.

The standard posterolateral fusion of the lumbar spine was developed because of dissatisfaction with earlier posteromedial techniques (5). For single-level lumbosacral disease, fusion rates over 90% have been reported. However, these patients were kept at bed rest for long periods of time or were placed into body casts. Also, reported fusion rates with this technique were based on radiographic evaluations alone. Biomechanical evaluation has revealed that posterolateral fusions of the lumbosacral spine allows residual motion across the disc at this level (6). These authors have suggested that this motion could be clinically significant. Finally the wide exposure necessary for posterolateral fusions has recently been implicated in denervation of the lumbar paraspinal muscles (7), which could be an etiology of chronic low back pain (8).

Fusion techniques that place the graft in the disc space may have advantages over the posterolateral method. Posterior lumbar interbody fusion (PLIF) is performed via a laminectomy and discectomy after which structural bone graft is placed into the disc space through the spinal canal. Although early reports of this technique were favorable (9, 10), later studies suggested that acceptable fusion rates could only be obtained by the addition of rigid internal fixation (11). Other authors have not had favorable results (12).

Fusion of the L5-S1 disc space through the anterior approach has also been reported. This technique places graft in the biomechanical center of the segment and avoids posterior tissue trauma. Despite some studies showing excellent fusion rates, other reports suggest nonunion rates as high as 40% without rigid internal fixation (13, 14). In addition, independent review of anterior lumbar fusions has shown vascular complication rates of 18% (15). Thus, simple anterior lumbar fusion alone may be ineffective in achieving fusion of the lumbosacral spine.

The final question in lumbosacral arthrodesis is whether rigid internal fixation is a necessary adjunct to achieve acceptable fusion rates in posterolateral fusion. At the lumbosacral level, this issue is most pertinent when addressing isthmic spondylolisthesis. Certainly in children and adolescents successful lumbosacral fusion is readily accomplished without spinal instrumentation (16, 17). However in adults it appears that fusion may not be as predictable. Kim *et al* reported that simple bracing resulted in almost 30% pseudoarthrosis as opposed to a 10% non-union rate when a rigid body cast was used postoperatively (18).

Although Peek *et al* suggested that simple onlay fusion is successful in adults, of the eight patients in his study, four were 21 years old and all were under 30 years (19).

These results suggest, therefore, that regardless of the surgical approach, rigid stabilization postoperatively is required to achieve acceptable rates of fusion in adults. To avoid postoperative body casts internal fixation may be used; however, the extensive tissue disruption necessary to apply standard spinal hardware systems may contribute to persistent painful complaints after surgery (8). In an effort to achieve rigid fixation of the lumbosacral spine with the least amount of damage to the posterior soft tissues, we have developed a new technique for discectomy, bone grafting and fixation of the lumbosacral spine. The following sections describe the anatomic pathway through which this can be achieved, the surgical techniques, and the preliminary clinical results.

Phase One: Determination of Anatomic Pathway

Clinical observations of the continuity of S1 pedicle with the sacral alae were made by studying inlet views of the sacrum. In this projection, the dorsal and ventral sacral foramina are superimposed and a continuous bony corridor from the S1 pedicle outward to the iliac crest is revealed. A review of the literature pertaining to the anatomy of the sacrum describes the sacral pedicle as the narrowest isthmus of a pathway from the outer cortex of the ilium to the S1 endplate (20, 21). The width of this pedicle has been shown to average over 18 millimeters (22). To verify that this pathway to the L5-S1 disc was reliably accessible, we placed 30 implants through this pathway in 15 cadaver specimens.

MATERIALS AND METHODS

Because the narrowest portion of this pathway lies within the confines of the S1 pedicle, a technique was developed to control the passage of a guide wire through the pedicle as it approached the sacral endplate. In this technique, one limb of a triangulation guide was placed into the pedicle of S1 through a standard posterior approach, while the other limb could rotate and arc to align with the transsacral pathway (Fig. 1). With the use of the prototype guide, 10 cadavers were used for 20 approaches through the described bony pathway. Each was screened for evidence of spinal abnormalities. The cadaver was placed in the prone position and secured on a radiolucent table. With the use of either fluoroscopic (14 specimens) or computed tomographic (6 specimens) control, one arm of the triangulation guide was fixated into the S1 pedicle. All 10 specimens then had the triangulation guide attached to the fixed arm allowing the free arm to rotate and arc into the appropriate trajectory. Once the guide was aimed, a 5-millimeter Steinmann pin was drilled across the iliac crest into the sacral ala and finally across the S1 endplate into the L5 vertebral body (Fig. 2). Twenty pins were placed after which the sacrum and lower lumbar spines were harvested and 3 mm contiguous axial computed tomographic images were obtained along the length of the pathway. These images were analyzed and the distance from the pin to the L5, S1, S2, and S3 nerve roots was recorded (Fig. 3). Also, the accuracy of the guide was evaluated by observing the position of the Steinmann pin in relation to the guide arm in the S1 pedicle. These results demonstrated that the bony pathway between the iliac wing and L5 via the S1 pedicle could be safely and reliably accessed (see below).

To determine whether fixation screws could safely be placed into the pathway, each of five cadavers was placed in the prone position in

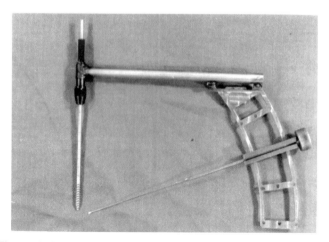

FIG. 1 The vertical member of this triangulation guide is placed into the S1 pedicle. The thin guide pin can then be drilled carefully through the sacrum to the pedicle.

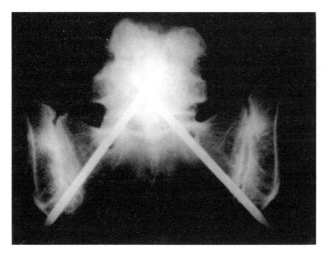

FIG. 2 A cadaveric specimen with Steinman pins placed along the described pathway.

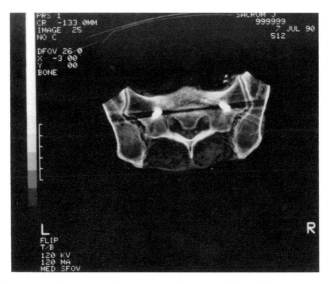

FIG. 3 A cross-sectional computer tomographic view of the Steinman pin within the bony confines of the sacrum.

the CT scanner. The gantry was tilted until it paralleled the L5 inferior endplate, and positioned over the S1 pedicle. The narrowest portion of the pathway in the S1 pedicle was then identified. With the use of radiopaque markers on the surface of the cadaver, a 2-mm guide pin was introduced at the proper angle into the S1 pedicle and positioned in the middle of the pathway (Fig. 4). A second guide pin was placed in a similar fashion on the contralateral side. The cadaver was then taken to a radiolucent table and under fluoroscopic control, a 4.5-mm cannulated, threaded post was placed over the guide pin and inserted to the precise depth of the pin. The triangulation guide was then attached to the post. The movable arm of the triangulation guide could then be aimed directly toward the center of the pathway. A .062-inch guide wire was then directed down the length of the pathway, through the base of the S1 pedicle and across the L5-S1 disc. For this portion of the study, a 7-mm cannulated drill was used to ream over the length of pin. Finally, a threaded, headless screw, 9 mm in diameter, was placed through the pathway across the L5-S1 disc and into the body of L5. This was repeated on the contralateral side. The specimen with the screws in place was returned to the CT scanner and scanned over the length of screws in 3mm contiguous slices.

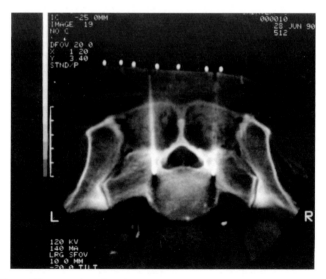

FIG. 4 Two-millimeter pins placed under computer tomographic guidance into the S1 pedicles. These guide pins will be used to permit exact location of the triangulation guide into the S1 pedicle.

RESULTS

Analysis of the position of each Steinman pin in the first 10 cadavers demonstrated the bony pathway to be consistently present. The angles formed by the Steinmann pins revealed that the pathway is angled 43° toward midline (ranging 40–60°) and is angled dorsally 76° the endplate of L5 (ranging 68–85°). In 20 passes of the Steinmann pin through this region there were 40 possible sites of neural contact (20 with L5 and 20 with S1). Three transgressions out of vertebral confines were noted, two at S1 and one at L5. In the second portion of the anatomical study, five specimens were studied. These specimens had 9 mm diameter, headless, cannulated screws placed with the aid of triangulation guide, which was installed under CT guidance. The average minimum distance from the screw edge to the L5 nerve root was 5.0mm (range 2.5–8.9mm). The average minimum distance from the screw edge to the S1 nerve root was 7.5mm (range 4.7–13.0mm). The total width of the pathway at its narrowest portion was 21.5mm (range 18.4–25.5mm).

We concluded that, with strict radiographic control this transilio-sacral pathway can reliably be used to fixate L5-S1.

Phase Two: Clinical Evaluation

The results of phase one suggested that the transilio-sacral pathway was consistent, of adequate dimension, and that guided screw placement through it could be performed safely. Clinical application of the technique required development of instrumentation and surgical technique to safely perform this technique in patients with L5-S1 segmental instability. The procedure consists of four separate parts.

The first component is, of course, fixation across the L5-S1. The implant we designed is a 9-mm diameter, fully threaded, headless screw. This screw is made of titanium and has a minor diameter of 7mm. It is headless so that it can cross the sacroiliac joint without transfixing it. The biomechanical characteristics of this device have been studied but not yet published (23).

The second aspect of the procedure was a paraspinal muscle splitting approach to the sacral alae similar to the technique described by Wiltsie (24). This technique was minimized by fluoroscopically localizing the L5 transverse process and exposing it with a speculum-type retractor used for microdiscectomies. Each incision was approximately 1-in long and permitted decortication of the transverse process and the adjacent sacral ala with a high-speed drill and placement of bone graft. This standard transverse process fusion was included to guarantee the patients "standard of care" fusion, in the event the investigational technique of interbody fusion failed. It is not intended to be a permanent part of this technique.

In addition to the laterally applied bone graft, graft was also packed into the disc space. With the use of bilateral 7 mm diameter drilled tunnels as portals (accessed as described in phase one), specialized curettes were introduced into the L5-S1 disc space and both endplates were abraded (Fig. 5). The endplate and disc fragments were removed with pituitary rongeurs. Morcelized bone graft was then packed into the disc space via cannulas. The graft was further compressed as the screws were placed down the drill tunnels and across the disc.

The final portion of the procedure is the iliac crest bone graft. This was taken in a standard fashion.

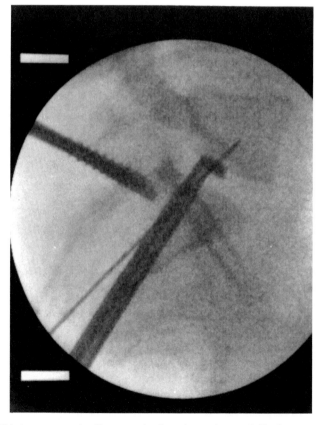

FIG. 5 This intra-operative fluoroscopic view shows the specialized curette within the L5-S1 disc. The disc fragments are then removed with pituitary rongeurs.

Fourteen patients were selected who had disease limited to the L5-S1 disc level. Five patients had debilitating low back pain following L5-S1 discectomy. These patients were found to have nonunion of a previously attempted fusion. Five patients had an L5-S1 spondylolisthesis. One patient suffered instability from primary degenerative disc disease. In this group of 14 patients, the first procedure was performed in January of 1992 and the last in June of 1995.

The first seven patients underwent CT guided localization of the S1 pedicle and intra-operative use of the triangulation guide to access the trans-ilia-sacral pathway. This technique was described in the Phase I study. After the seventh patient, we had developed sufficient familiarity with the procedure to use biplanar fluoroscopy and eliminate the need to transfer the patient from the CT scanner to the operating room. All patients had intraoperative electromyographic monitoring of L5 and S1 nerve roots.

All patients had a preoperative CT scan to assess the dimensions of the pathway to the L5-S1 disc. Each patient also had postoperative radiographs at approximately 3-month intervals after surgery. All patients underwent CT scan reconstructions between 9 to 12 months postoperatively to assess fusion status. All CT scans were independently read by a staff radiologist. No preoperative or postoperative data were collected to assess pain relief. Fourteen patients were disabled from workers' compensation injuries and were referred from a pain management program. The remaining patients were receiving disability payments from Social Security. The objective of this study was to assess the reliability of attaining fusion through this technique. Therefore, the clinical parameters measured were intraoperative complications, hardware problems, posterolateral fusion status, and intradiscal fusion status.

RESULTS

At the time of follow-up, there were 14 patients who ranged from 7 to 30 months postsurgery. (Table 1).

Intra-operative complications were evaluated in relation to discectomy, bone graft placement or fixation. No intraoperative neurologic complications were noted in any of these patients. Based on radiographic evaluation, neurologic evaluation, intraoperative EMG evaluation, and the patient's report, there was no effect of this procedure on the L5 or S1 nerve roots. Likewise, no nonneurologic intra-operative complications were recorded during discectomy or bone graft placement. There was one intra-operative complication specific to screw placement. In one patient, the left and right screws were inadvertently

TABLE 1
Percutaneous Lumbosacral Fixation and Fusion: Anatomical Study and Two Year Experience with a New Method

Number	Age	Sex	Diagnosis	D.O.S.	Months Follow Up	Neurologic Complication	Implant Complication	CT or Flouro	Lateral Fusion	Disc Fusion	Additional Surgery
1	27	M	Spondylolisthesis	01/31/92	30	None	None	CT	Yes	Yes	Right L5 Foraminotomy
2	33	M	Degenerative Disc	03/27/92	28	None	None	CT	No	Yes	Repeat Facet Fusion
3	32	M	Post-Laminectomy	05/8/92	26	None	None	CT	Yes	Yes	L4-L5 Post-Fusion
4	38	F	Post-Laminectomy	07/17/92	24	None	None	CT	Yes	Yes	None
5	41	M	L5-S1 Non-union	09/14/92	22	None	Intersecting Pathways: One Screw	CT	Yes	No	None
6	32	M	Recurrent L5-S1 Discectomy	10/12/92	21	None	None	CT	Facet Fusion	Yes	Concomitant L5-S1 Discectomy
7	25	M	Spondylolisthesis	05/17/92	14	None	None	CT	No	Yes	Subsequent Posterolateral Fusion
8	35	F	Spondylolisthesis	09/8/93	10	None	None	CT	Yes	Yes	None
9	49	F	Non-union	12/15/93	7	None	None	CT	Yes	Yes	None
10	49	F	Pseudoarthrosis	12/15/93	13	None	None	Fluoro	No	Yes	Revision pseudo-arthrosis
11	37	M	Post-laminectomy	5/13/94	8	None	None	Fluoro	No	Yes	L5/S1 facet fusion
12	54	F	Spondylolisthesis	5/27/94	8	None	None	Fluoro	No	Yes	Infected bone graft site
13	24	F	Spondylolisthesis	6/10/94	7	None	None	Fluoro	No	Yes	No
14	41	F	Instability	6/20/94	7	None	None	Fluoro	No	Yes	Posterolateral fusion

angled so that their paths intersected in the L5-S1 disc. Given the nine millimeter diameter of the screw, we did not feel that it was prudent to try to create an entirely new pathway, yet it was impossible for both screws to cross the L5-S1 disc and enter the L5 vertebral body. We elected to just place one screw. The drill hole for the unplaced screw was used for discectomy access and bone graft placement.

Because the posterolateral fusion procedure is mechanically, anatomically and biologically distinct from the intradiscal fusion, the two potential sites of fusion were evaluated separately. Both fusion sites were examined by CT evaluation between 9 and 12 months. Bony fusion within the L5-S1 disc was present in 13 out of 14 patients (Fig. 6). The posterolateral graft was determined to be fused in 13 of the 14 patients (Fig. 7). In one of the questionable posterolateral fusions, a patient with spondylolysis was returned to the operating room at 6 months after surgery for prophylactic posterolateral bone grafting. A second suspected posterolateral fusion failure had an initial diagnosis of degenerative disc disease. His fusion was augmented by percutaneously decorticating and bone grafting the L5-S1 facet joints bilaterally. Of note, these two patients were heavy smokers who resumed tobacco use postoperatively despite constant admonishments from their physician.

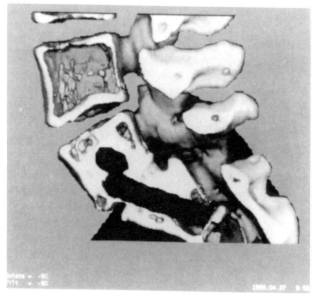

FIG. 6 This three-dimensional computed tomography image shows the intra-discal fusion between L5 and S1. The screw position is well demonstrated with this technique.

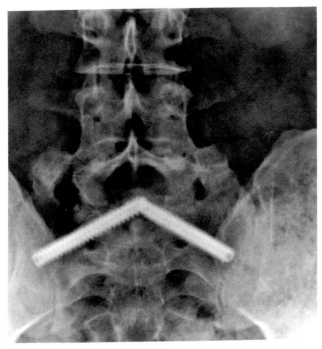

FIG. 7 This anteroposterior view shows the consolidated posterolateral fusion mass.

Finally, the one solitary screw was the only implant that showed any radiographic signs of loosening.

DISCUSSION

This chapter reports a posterior approach to the L5-S1 disc that travels obliquely and anteriorly across the sacral ala through the S1 pedicle and exits the sacrum at the S1 endplate. Our anatomic study found this pathway to be approximately 2 cm in width. It was consistently present in the 15 cadavers we studied and could reliably accept a threaded screw that was 9 mm in diameter. We proceeded to develop a surgical procedure that used this approach for the fixation and fusion of the L5-S1 level. Using this method, we were able to successfully fuse 14 patients treated during our study period.

The importance of this study lies not only in the operative technique but also because of the level that is addressed.

The operative technique is designed to avoid extensive dissection of paraspinal muscles. The harmful effects of this have been described previously (8). In addition to muscle denervation, L5-S1 paraspinal stripping also effects the insertion of the paraspinals on the sacrum. This decreases their ability to generate force to support the upper body.

The potential clinical applications of this technique are related to the prevalence of disease at this level. Ninety-five percent of disc surgery is performed at the L4-L5 and L5-S1 level, and half of these surgeries are performed at the L5-S1 level (25). Twelve percent of patients with discectomies develop debilitating low back pain (26). If the frequency of low back pain can be decreased by reducing paraspinal muscle dissection, then a large number of patients could benefit from a minimally invasive fusion procedure at L5-S1.

This technique may also have advantages over other evolving techniques of minimally invasive fusion. Specifically, a number of techniques have used a posterolateral approach to L4-L5 to perform a discectomy and bone grafting (27). These posterolateral percutaneous techniques are difficult to apply at the L5-S1 levels because of the adjacent iliac crests, the position of the nerve roots and the significantly narrower disc heights.

Recently laparoscopic techniques have been used to perform fusions at L5-S1 (28). Apparently this technology allows good visualization of the anterior disc and permits adequate disc removal. Whether laparoscopic methods will allow fixation and fusion is unknown and we await further reports.

In summary, therefore, this procedure enables discectomy, fusion and fixation, of L5 to S1 via a minimally invasive technique. It is based on consistent and adequately sized anatomy. When applied to 14 patients, fusion was reliably achieved and no complications directly attributed to individual screw placement occurred.

REFERENCES

1. Zimmerman J. The diagnosis and misdiagnosis of back pain. Brunswick Maine: Biddie Publishing Co. 7–9, 1991.
2. Wennberg JE, McPherson K, Caper P. Will payment based on diagnosis-related groups control hospital costs? **N Engl J Med** 311:295–300, 1984.
3. Deyo RA. Practice variations, treatment fads, rising disability: do we need a new clinical research paradigm? **Spine** 18:2153–2162, 1993.
4. Zdeblick TA. A prospective, randomized study of lumbar fusion: preliminary results. **Spine** 18(8):983–999, 1993.
5. Thompson WAL, Gristing AG, Healy WA. A method of bilateral posterolateral fusion combined with a Hibbs fusion. **JBJS** 56(A):1643–1647, 1974.
6. White AA III, Panjabi MM. Clinical Biomechanics of the Spine Second Edition, Lippincott, Philadelphia PA, 1990.
7. Hayashi N, Tamaki T, Yamada H. Experimental study of denervated muscle atrophy following severance of posterior rami of the lumbar spinal nerves. **Spine** 17:1361–1367, 1992.

8. Sihvonen T, Herno A, Paljarvi L, Airaksinen O, Partanen J, Tapaninaho A. Local denervation atrophy of paraspinal muscles in post-operative failed back syndrome. **Spine** 18:575–581, 1993.

9. Cloward RB. The treatment of ruptured lumbar intervertebral discs by vertebral body fusion. **J Neurosurg** 10:154–158, 1953.

10. Lin PM, Cautilli RA, Joyce MF. Posterior lumbar interbody fusion. **Clin Orthop** 180:154–168, 1983.

11. Brantigan JW, Steffee AD, Keppler L, Bisap RS, Enker P. Posterior lumbar interbody fusion using the variable screw placement spinal fixation system. **Spine** 16:175–200, 1992.

12. Verlooy J, DeSmedt K, Selosse P. Failure of a modified posterior lumbar interbody fusion technique to produce adequate pain relief in isthmic spondylolytic Grade 1 spondylolisthesis patients. A prospective study of 20 patients. **Spine** 18(11): 1491–1495, 1993.

13. Flynn JC and Hogue MA.: Anterior fusion of the lumbar spine. JBJS 6(A): 1143–1150, 1979.

14. Kumar A, Kuzak JA, Doherty J, Dickson JH. Interspace distraction and graft subsidence after anterior lumbar fusion with femoral sntn allograft. **Spine** 18: 2393–2400, 1993.

15. Baker JK, Reardon PR, Reardon MJ, Heggeness MH. Vascular injury in anterior lumbar surgery. **Spine** 18:2227–2230, 1993.

16. Boxall D, Bradford D, Winter R, Moe J. Management of severe spondylolisthesis in children and adolescents. **JBJS** 52(A):529–535, 1970.

17. Wiltsie L, Jackson D. Treatment of spondylolisthesis and spondylolysis in children. **Clin Orthop** 117:92–100, 1976.

18. Kim SS, Denis F, Lonstein JE, Winter RB. Factors affecting fusion rate in adult spondylolisthesis. **Spine** 15:979–984, 1990.

19. Peek RD, Wiltsie LL, Reynolds JB, Thomas JC, Guyer DW, Widell EH. In Situ arthrodesis without decompression for grade III or grade IV isthmic spondylolisthesis in adults who have severe sciatica. **JBSJ** 71(A):62–69, 1989.

20. Asher MA, Strippgen WE. Anthropometric studies of the human sacrum relating to dorsal transsacral implant designs. **Clinical Ortho Rel Res** 203:58–62, 1986.

21. Whelan MA, Gold RP. Computed tomography of the sacrum: 1. normal anatomy. **AJR** 139:1183–1190, 1982.

22. Bernard TN and Seibert CE. Pedicle diameter determined by computed tomography. **Spine** 17(65):S160–S163, 1992.

23. Mac Millan M, Cunningham B. Biomechanical comparison of trans-sacral-vertebral fixation versus variable screw position plating for L5-S1 stabilization. Unpublished Results.

24. Wiltsie LL, Bateman JG, Hutchinson RH, Nelson WE. The paraspinal sacrospinalis-splitting approach to the lumbar spine. **JBJS** 50(A):919–926, 1968.

25. Deyo, RA, Leser JD, Bigos SJ. Herniated lumbar inter-vertebral disk. **Ann Int Med** 112(8):598–603, 1990.

26. Hanley EW, Shapiro DE. The development of low back pain after excision of a lumbar disc. **JBJS** 72(A):719–721, 1989.

27. Lev JF, Schreiber A. Percutaneous fusion of the lumbar spine: a promising technique. **Spine** 6(3):593–604, 1992.

28. Stein SC, Slotman GJ. Laparoscopic lumbar discectomy. Presented at the Joint Section on Disorders of the Spine and Peripheral Nerves, AANS/CNS. 10th Annual, Ft. Lauderdale, Florida, 1994.

CHAPTER

29

Clinical Neurosurgery Interactive Audience Participation 1995

MARK N. HADLEY, M.D.

An interactive audience participation system was used during the general scientific sessions of the 1995 Congress of Neurological Surgeons annual meeting, held in San Francisco, California. Speakers were encouraged to create questions that could be presented to the audience for immediate electronic response, using one of 500 IRIS electronic response terminals placed throughout the general scientific session auditorium. Unfortunately, the system was not well used, either by presenters or by respondents, and therefore its maximum potential remains unrealized. Ideally these types of interactive audience response systems allow "real-time" audience participation and interaction with topic presenters. They allow presenters, via well-constructed propositions, to assay the contemporary thought processes and the knowledge base of active neurological surgeons. Perhaps more importantly, this type of interactive dialogue can be used to poll neurosurgeons about current neurosurgical practices, health care reform, medical-legal issues, and concerns of mainstream neurosurgery. It appears that this format of interactive audience participation at our national meetings is not a viable means of obtaining this information. Despite having large audiences for most of the general scientific sessions in which the IRIS system was used, rarely more than 200 of the 500 electronic response terminals were used at any time during the meeting. Few of the many speakers who provided general scientific session presentations offered questions to the audience via the IRIS system. Without well-conceived, carefully designed questions, meaningful responses cannot be collected from even the small number of individuals who might choose to participate.

The following represents the majority of questions for which responses were generated during this year's annual meeting. Several questions had to do with general information about practice type and experience. Several questions addressed issues related to stroke, carotid endarterectomy, and the management of patients with asymptomatic but significant carotid artery stenosis. A large number of questions focused on the management of patients following head injury, controversial areas of treatment, and the need for guidelines and suggestions to help direct contemporary care. The Joint AANS/CNS Section of Neurotrauma and Critical Care has completed a 2-year project addressing 15 major aspects of the management of severe head injury. Their work, "the Guidelines for the Management of Severe Head Injury, 1995," represents a landmark contribution to neurological surgery and is a comprehensive compendium of the available data on the most essential aspects of the management of patients with severe head injury. For each major issue, standards, guidelines, and options are discussed, and a thorough overview of the existing clinical and scientific literature is presented in a concise format. This year, and in years past, the need for evidence-based guidelines for the management of head injured patients has been strongly voiced, including responses via the IRIS audience participation system during this year's meeting (Questions 22–24). The leaders of the Joint Section of Neurotrauma and Critical Care have responded to these needs, and in an impressive fashion.

Vascular Neurosurgery

1. Who manages the stroke patient in your community?
   (215 respondents)

Neurologist	51.5%
Primary Physician	18.1%
Neurosurgeon	3.7%
Team Approach	17.2%

2. How soon after initial symptoms are stroke patients evaluated in your Emergency Room? (195 respondents)

1–3 hours	14.4%
3–6 hours	45.6%
24 hours	37.4%

3. What do you advise the patient who calls with first-time TIA symptoms? (198 respondents)

Go directly to Emergency Room	76.8%
Call Neurologist in AM	8.1%
Arrange for radiological evaluation in AM	9.6%
Take an Aspirin	5.1%

4. Which x-ray do you start with first? (197 respondents)

CT Scan	73.1%
Carotid ultrasound	7.6%
MRI/MRA	14.2%
Angiogram	4.1%

5. Do you have a stroke team? (200 respondents)

Yes	21.0%
No	51.5%
Incomplete team	26.5%

6. Do you perform carotid endarterectomies?
(199 respondents)

Yes	61.8%
No	20.1%
Did in training, would like to resume	16.1%

7. Would you operate on an asymptomatic patient with 75%, nonulcerative stenosis? (293 respondents)

Yes	64.8%
No	12.6%

8. Would you perform angiography on this patient?
(217 respondents)

Yes	77.4%
No	18.4%

9. How many carotid endarterectomies do you perform a year?
(164 respondents)

1–15	53.7%
16–30	12.8%
30–50	6.1%
>50	10.4%

10. Do you operate on the basis of carotid ultrasound only?
(73 respondents)

US + MRA	15.1%
MRA + TCD	4.1%
Angiography	75.3%
US only	0.0%

11. On diagnostic imaging basis do you operate?
(120 respondents)

US + MRA	16.7%
MRA + TCD	6.7%
Angiography	75.0%
US only	1.7%

12. When the cranial CT shows evidence of ischemic stroke, do you consider: (122 respondents)

Anticoagulation	36.1%
Volume expansion	38.3%
Carotid endarterectomy	20.5%

Head Trauma

1. Are you a: (244 respondents)

Neurosurgeon in private practice	43.0%
Neurosurgeon in an academic practice	22.5%
Resident	17.2%
Medical student	1.2%
Other	9.4%

2. If you are a neurosurgeon, how long have you been in practice? (184 respondents)

0–5 years	29.3%
6–10 years	16.8%
11–15 years	1.4%
16–20 years	14.1%
21+ years	27.2%

3. What is the most active trauma hospital in which you work? (205 respondents)

Level 1	51.2%
Level 2	33.7%
Level 3	12.2%
Not sure	2.9%

4. What proportion of your practice consists of head injury? (199 respondents)

51–100%	4.0%
25–50%	15.1%
11–24%	34.2%
1–10%	43.7%
None	2.5%

5. In your institution how are head injured patients managed? (207 respondents)

By Neurosurgeons with other consultants needed	69.1%
By Trauma surgeons with NS consulting	28.0%
By Intensivits with NS consulting	2.4%
Other	0.5%

6. In what proportion of GCS 3–8 patients do you monitor ICP? (208 respondents)

100%	25.0%
75–99%	39.5%
50–74%	13.2%
25–49%	7.9%
0–24%	13.2%

7. What ICP monitoring device do you use most often?

Ventricular catheter	41.4%
Parenchymal device (Codman, Camino, etc.)	45.2%
Subdural bolt	5.2%
Subdural catheter	3.8%
Epidural catheter	3.8%

8. Which of the following do you use as your primary measure?
(207 respondents)

ICP	47.3%
CPP	35.7%
Neither—clinical exam only	15.5%

9. In what ICP level do you initiate treatment?
(209 respondents)

30	2.4%
25	17.7%
20	57.4%
15	15.3%
Do not use	6.2%

10. What CPP level do you aim for? (206 respondents)

90	3.9%
80	12.1%
70	45.1%
60	16.0%
Do not use	21.8%

11. Do you use hyperventilation? (control, 214 respondents)

Continuously for days without ICP monitoring	9.3%
Continuously for days only if ICP is elevated	49.1%
For acute deterioration only (*e.g.* blown pupil)	38.3%
Never	2.3%

12. What pCo2 level do you aim for? (211 respondents)

As low as necessary to get ICP down	5.2%
20	4.3%
25	45.0%
30	37.9%
35+	6.6%

13. Do you use Mannitol? (217 respondents)

Always	11.1%
Sometimes	87.6%
Never	1.4%

14. Do you use Lasix to control ICP? (222 respondents)
    Always 5.0%
    Sometimes 53.6%
    Rarely or never 40.5%
15. How do you like to keep the patient's hydration?
    (control, 214 respondents)
    Normovolemia 71.0%
    Dehydrated ("dry") 22.4%
    Hypervolemic 6.5%
16. When do you use pentobarbital (217 respondents)
    Prophylactically to prevent elevated ICP 0.9%
    When ICP goes up as first-line treatment ... 4.1%
    Late—when all other therapies have failed .. 74.7%
    Never 15.2%
    I use agents other than pentobarbital 4.6%
17. Do you use dexamethasone? (233 respondents)
    Always 8.5%
    Often 7.2%
    Occasionally 22.0%
    Never 61.0%
18. When do you usually initiate feeding? (217 respondents)
    Day 1 postinjury 22.6%
    Day 3 .... 41.0%
    Day 7 .... 9.7%
    Uncertain/variable 25.8%
19. What type of nutritional support do you usually order?
    (219 respondents)
    Tube feeds 84.9%
    TPN 11.9%
    Uncertain 0.5%
20. What do you use for seizure prevention?
    (211 respondents)
    Phenobarbital 1.8%
    Phenytoin 77.4%
    Other 3.2%
    None 17.6%
21. How long do you keep patients on seizure meds?
    (218 respondents)
    Do not use 7.0%
    1–2 weeks 22.9%
    1–2 months 19.3%

Several months	32.6%
Year or more	7.3%

22. Do you believe that EVIDENCE-BASED guidelines for severe head injuries are: (79 respondents)

A good idea	78.5%
A bad idea	11.4%
Uncertain	10.1%

23. What is your MAIN concern relating to guidelines? (71 respondents)

Increased malpractice exposure	38.0%
Loss of independence	12.7%
Other	9.9%
I have no major concerns	38.0%

24. From a medicolegal viewpoint, do you believe the guidelines will? (79 respondents)

Help the neurosurgeon	50.6%
Hurt the neurosurgeon	26.6%
Have no significant effect	19.0%

Index

Page numbers in *italics* denote figures; those followed by "t" denote tables.